Chiropractic spinal manipulation and nutritional therapy are missing links to health — largely ignored by mainstream medicine. In this book you will learn how Martin Gallagher, D.C., has used these and other natural healing techniques for more than 20 years to help thousands of patients. Dr. Gallagher draws on his vast clinical experience to offer new hope for many common conditions and practical information for escaping the grip of hopelessless, pharmaceutical side effects, and potentially-harmful medical treatments. Read this book for insights and inspiration, both from Dr. Gallagher and from dozens of his patients who have regained lost health through natural healing.

"I was facing two total knee replacements. Today, I walk with no cane and my knees have been rehabilitated to most of their original motion. I am now actually playing tennis."
– Father Vernon Holtz, O.S.B., Ph.D., arthritis patient

"My son is tall, strong and healthy. He is rarely ill, has no coughing spells or allergy attacks. He needs no antihistamines, antibiotics or breathers. His learning difficulties gradually disappeared and today he is once again back on the honor role. When I compare him now to the pale, fat 12-year-old who could not function in school, read, or hang out with friends because he was too weak and tired, it brings tears to my eyes."
– Linda Benninger, mother of allergic son

"I believe I am in better health now than any time in my life. I work full time, do yard work, swim, walk, play ball with my son, paint the house, walk up steps, no limit."
– Charles Hodges, heart disease patient

"The change in Brandon's personality is so dramatic he appears to be a different child. He started taking naps...he is happy and busy. He loves to run, jump and climb. He has been exposed to numerous children with colds and has yet to come down with a cold or ear infection since treatment started."
– Maureen Juliano, mother of child
with multiple pediatric health problems

DR. GALLAGHER'S
GUIDE TO 21ST CENTURY MEDICINE

*How To Get Off The Illness Treadmill
and Onto Optimum Health*

MARTIN P. GALLAGHER, M.S., D.C.

Atlas Publishing Company
P.O. Box 455
Greensburg, PA 15601
(724) 523-5505

ISBN 0-965-7433
Library of Congress Catalog Card Number 97-061522
Printed in the United States of America
Second Printing
How to order:
Copies may be ordered from Atlas Publishing Company, P.O. Box 455, Greensburg, PA 15601, (724) 523-5505

NOTE TO THE READER

This book is not intended to replace medical care. It is meant exclusively for informational and educational purposes only.

If you have symptoms or a disease, please consult a physician, preferably a wholistic practitioner such as a chiropractic doctor (D.C.), medical doctor (M.D.), naturopath (N.D.), or osteopath (D.O.).

If you are under the care of a physician, you may like to show this book to your doctor.

If you are currently taking prescription drugs, do not discontinue or substitute natural remedies without consulting your doctor.

Any individual natural health care therapy should be used in conjunction with a total health care plan and lifestyle modification.

DEDICATION

I
t is rare in one's life that you meet a true mentor. God placed such a person in my life 25 years ago. Although technically speaking a mentor is a teacher or counselor, I must take literary license to transcend this definition to include enduring friend.

And like all great teachers, he saw something in his student that the student, to date, had not materialized.

Such was the vision of my mentor (and father-in-law) John Ciotti, who planted the seed of this book in my consciousness decades ago, who nurtured each aspect by encouragement, compassion and love, and who never asked for anything in return.

I return you this — my dedicated manuscript.

ACKNOWLEDGMENTS

I want to thank my wife, Charlotte, who is my best friend and associate, whose unwavering love and support inspires and sustains me;

To our son Todd, whose ideas have helped guide this book;

To my parents, Jeff and Marie, who taught me self-reliance;

To my mother-and-father-in-law, John and Laura, whose unconditional love is the greatest natural prescription.

To my friends, associates and staff who keep the principles of natural healing alive and well;

To the many patients who allowed their stories to be told so that they might help others;

And finally to God who has given me the opportunity to see and feel his presence in the composite experience we call life.

Martin P. Gallagher, M.S., D.C.
Jeannette, Pennsylvania
July 3, 1997

DR. GALLAGHER
ON TV AND RADIO

Learn about the latest breakthroughs in alternative medicine and how chiropractic, homeopathic, herbal medicine, acupuncture, chelation therapy, exercise, prayer, relaxation and lifestyle management can restore vital health in your life.

In simple language that everyone can understand, Dr. Gallagher explains the latest developments in health research and how he success- fully applies natural healing methods in his clinic to help patients prevent and overcome many common conditions.

See Dr. Gallagher, and his wife, Dr. Charlotte Ciotti, as they host a nationally-syndicated half-hour weekly health show seen on many cable stations across the country. The program features interviews with leading physicians and researchers in the alternative medicine field as well as dramatic first-person stories by patients who have recovered from serious illnesses that conventional medical treatments were unable to help. In addition, Dr. Gallagher offers practical health tips and home remedies to help viewers, and their families, overcome health problems safely and effectively.

In the Pittsburgh area, the program is seen every Tuesday on Cornerstone Television, WPCB — Channel 40, at 7 p.m., and every Saturday at 1:30 p.m.

Cable subscribers: check with your local cable system.

Satellite subscribers: the program can be picked up worldwide on C Band, Satellite GE1, Channel 7, and on Echostar Dish Network Sky Angel Channel 273.

On radio, you can hear Dr. Gallagher's popular call-in program, "Alternatives 2 Medicine," live on Pittsburgh's WEDO (810 on the AM dial) every Saturday morning from 9-11 a.m., and during the week daily on WEDO from 1-2 p.m. The program is heard in many areas of Pennsyl- vania, Ohio, West Virginia and Maryland. To call in with questions con- cerning natural health care, dial WEDO at (412) 664-4444 during the Saturday show.

WHJB (620 AM) in Greensburg, Pennsylvania, carries the second hour of the radio broadcast — at 11 a.m. — each Saturday, plus each Thursday at 11 a.m.

"And God said, Behold I have given you every herb bearing seed, which is upon the face of all the earth and every tree in which is the fruit of a tree yielding seed, to you it shall be for meat."

Genesis 1:29

TABLE OF CONTENTS

PART ONE THE ILLNESS TREADMILL

PART TWO THE GALLAGHER WELLNESS PROGRAM: YOUR PERSONAL "HEALTH BLUEPRINT"

PART THREE NATURAL REMEDIES FOR SPECIFIC HEALTH CONDITIONS

The Illness Treadmill

CHAPTER ONE

What's the treadmill?

A treadmill is something that you run or walk on and get nowhere.

An illness treadmill is something that snares you in an endless web of diagnoses, tests, prescriptions, and procedures and gets you nowhere, or even makes you sicker.

Unfortunately, the illness treadmill snares many people.

Once you are on the treadmill, you may get some temporary relief from symptoms. But all too often the cause of your problem is ignored, so things just gets worse. Meanwhile, the treatments used to suppress the symptoms often cause side effects and new symptoms.

The illness treadmill can kill.

Over the years I have helped thousands of individuals desperate to get off the treadmill, patients such as Dianne Burkhart, a medical researcher from Pittsburgh, and Bill Heinz, a pharmaceutical representative from Pittsburgh.

Dianne Burkhart's case

Dianne had suffered from Crohn's Disease, an intestinal disorder, since the age of 16. She was not improving, despite all the powerful medication her doctors could unleash on her. Far from improving, she was feeling worse because of side effects.

"I became moody and depressed," she told me. "I developed an insatiable appetite and gained 50 pounds. My vision became blurry. I developed hair growth on my face. A blood clot formed in my leg. My skin started to peel and split apart. I fractured a rib from coughing. A steroid medication had leached the minerals out of my bones. I became bloated and my face swelled up like a big balloon. I was literally falling apart from the side effects of the medications."

Dianne was now facing an operation to remove her colon, but as you will see if you turn to page 269, she was able to avoid surgery, stop the drugs, keep her colon intact, get off the treadmill, and make a full recovery.

Bill Heinz's case

From the age of 6, Bill's life revolved around baseball. He rose up through the ranks of Little League, played in high school, later at the University of Iowa, and continued playing after graduation. "A life of running, twisting, throwing, jumping, diving, sliding, bending and long bus rides," as he put it, finally caught up with him in 1984, when he developed low back pain as a college freshman.

Over the next dozen years, he underwent two back surgeries, multiple spinal injections, electrical spinal probes to neutralize irritated nerves, and countless prescriptions for painkillers, tranquilizers, anti-inflammatories and antibiotics. He developed post-surgical infections and side effects of constipation, rectal bleeding and drowsiness from his medications.

Bill was stuck on a nightmarish treadmill with little hope for resolution. After all the years and treatments, he still had back pain. But, as Bill's story continues on page 200, you will learn how he, too, beat the pain and got off the illness treadmill.

The treadmill scenario

Dianne and Bill were fortunate. They were able to escape the treadmill.

Clinics like mine, where alternative medicine is practiced, have become asylums for "medical refugees" like Dianne and Bill. We see such patients every day, with all sorts of conditions for which they unnecessarily receive painkillers, tranquilizers, anti-depressants and surgery.

A typical example in my clinic is the patient who initially goes to the family doctor with pain in the back, neck, shoulder or knee. The doctor does a physical examination, X-rays, and other tests, and diagnoses arthritis, tendonitis, bursitis, headaches, migraines or some degenerative disease. A routine prescription follows — often a non-steroidal anti-inflammatory drug such as Motrin, Feldene, Advil, Nuprin or Aleve.

The patient begins taking medication, thinking the condition is being cured. But two to four weeks later, digestive problems develop, such as abdominal pain, bloating, gas, or diarrhea.

The patient returns to the doctor.

"The pain is not so bad in my back," the patient says, "but I'm having these things going wrong with my digestion."

The doctor says there may be a gallbladder problem or an irritable bowel syndrome or suggests that "you may be under a lot of stress and tension."

With that, the physician refers the patient to a gastrointestinal specialist. The specialist does a gastroscopic examination and a gallbladder study, looks into the stomach, and checks out the upper and lower intestine. A diagnosis follows, such as gastritis, or irritable bowel syndrome, or gallbladder problem, or ulcers. A new round of pharmaceuticals is prescribed, medications like Tagamet, Zantac, or Prilosac. Not only do these drugs not cure the cause of the condition, but in many cases they cause depression, anxiety or impotence.

The patient still has the tendonitis, bursitis, back problem or arthritic pain, plus the additional digestive upsets that have been blamed on gastritis, irritable bowel or gallbladder problems. Now there may be impotence, which affects relationships, or bouts of depression and anxiety.

The patient goes back to the doctor complaining of these problems and is sent to a urologist for an evaluation, or to a psychiatrist, who says the problem is depression. Maybe an anti-depressive drug such as Prozac is prescribed, leading to additional side effects.

There are countless cases like this — medical histories bulging with one ineffective and damaging treatment after another, testimonials to a system that at large is unable to heal and only able to manage symptoms.

A patient starts with one problem. But the real underlying cause, be it a structural misalignment, a nutritional deficiency, or a lifestyle error, is rarely corrected. The consequence is a series of medical stresses that compound the original problem. Now the patient is fatigued, stressed, depressed, with low sex drive, headaches, back pain, and a bag of prescription drugs to mask the symptoms.

This is the illness treadmill — a trap for millions. The lucky person manages to escape. Many, however, are wounded on the treadmill. They limp, crawl, or, unfortunately, are carried off, the quality of their lives diminished by a vicious cycle of varying diagnoses, "learn to live with it" advice, redundant and maiming drugs, and multiplying side effects.

I am deeply troubled by what I have seen during my more than 20 years in practice. I know many medical doctors and respect their professional skill, concern for patients, and sincerity. Yet the medical education system that has trained them is deeply flawed and the form of medicine they practice, as a result, is extremely limited. They deal primarily with symptoms and not causes. Their use of pharmaceutical drugs and surgery as primary treatment options is questionable, risky business, and all-too-often not in the best interest of the patient. A whole universe of safe, effective and direct natural treatments are ignored. I, and other alternative medical practitioners, see the fallout from this system on a daily basis in the form of patients who are actually sicker after conventional treatment than before.

This book is your wake up call

This book, and the true stories in it, offers a startling view of a global medical system gone haywire. At the same time the book offers hope for people who are not getting well under the conventional system, who have become fed up, and who are seeking alternatives.

This book is intended to make you aware of the medical treadmill. It is a wake up call. The knowledge it contains can serve as your ticket off the treadmill and a roadmap leading to powerful opportunities for safely and naturally improving your health. As you read on you will learn how many of my patients took control of their health and turned their lives around. You will learn how you can do the same.

The book is divided into three parts. In the next chapter I will share my own personal experience on the treadmill and how I escaped it. In chapter three I describe the extent and seriousness of the treadmill phenomenon and how it is sapping the health of the nation. Chapter four focuses on the dynamic changes taking place within the current medical scene, namely a grassroots movement of patients breaking out of the narrow confines of our present disease-care system in the search of natural alternatives, and how this development is influencing the whole system.

In part two I will introduce you to my wellness program that has evolved over 20 years of clinical practice. During that time I have personally treated or supervised more than a half-million patients. I have personally administered over 1.5 million chiropractic adjustments, on newborn infants, teenagers, adults, pregnant women, and senior citizens as old as 92 years. For me, this experience has been a "living laboratory."

The program I have developed is based on the principle of achieving better health through structural, nutritional, emotional and spiritual balance. I will lay out the eight steps that I use in my clinic to reach this goal.

The Gallagher Wellness Program, as I call it, features methods that you can follow on your own or do with the cooperation of your personal physician. In either case, these methods offer significant potential for both the prevention and improvement of many conditions.

The methods include:

- **a healthier diet**
- **nutritional and herbal supplements**
- **identifying and eliminating hidden food allergies and chemical sensitivities**
- **a simple detoxification program to rid the body of harmful toxins**
- **chiropractic manipulation**

As a chiropractic physician, I have seen first hand how the various techniques of chiropractic correct spinal and joint misalignments and achieve remarkable healing effects. I am not just speaking about people with back pain, but with conditions you would never think had anything to do with structural misalignments in your spine, such as allergies, asthma, mental confusion and anxiety, PMS, sexual dysfunction, ear and sinus infections, tinnitus, chronic fatigue, and many many more. When you refer to specific conditions in part three of the book, you will find some fresh and surprising solutions to problems that often defy standard treatments.

You might never think, for instance, that chiropractic alone could possibly help your body's defenses to resist disease. Yet it can — in a major way. And scientific studies are confirming this. Chiropractic physicians are routinely helping people overcome recurring ear, sinus and other infections and improve weak immune systems.

Throughout this book you will encounter a recurring theme — that a spinal misalignment could possibly be the cause of poor health. I believe spinal misalignments represent, in fact, a massively overlooked source of unwellness. Medical doctors are not trained to recognize or treat such problems, which may be more common than cavities. But unlike our teeth, do any of us get a spinal checkup? The answer is no, and the consequences of ignoring the spine may be the cause of an enormous amount of suffering that frequently begins as a result of spinal trauma at the time of birth and extends through a lifetime.

This book will reveal how many common conditions — from infancy to the later years of life — can be caused by misalignments...and how they can be effectively and safely corrected, naturally.

Manipulations and nutritional therapies are critical missing links in the treatment of disorders, largely ignored by mainstream medicine. Yet we use them with great effect and success everyday in my clinic to restore balance and wellness for suffering patients.

In part three I will cover many different conditions and offer recommendations for natural healing that have worked well, and without side effects, for my patients. In this section you will find true life stories written by patients themselves. You may find some of these accounts similar to your situation. If this is the case, I hope you will become inspired to overcome your difficulties and go on, as my patients do, to lead healthier lives.

The body is a miraculous system equipped with an innate ability to achieve balance and health. We have, within each of us, the ability to work with, and nourish, this God-given gift. It is my sincere hope that this book helps cultivate and enhance that process.

The book is an extention of a profound desire to be of service. It is the distillation of my years in practice. My mission remains the same today as it was when I started in practice — to do my part to help create a state of perfect health within each person, each nation and, ultimately the world.

CHAPTER TWO

My escape from the treadmill

When I was 14-years-old, I injured my lower back playing high school basketball. As I limped off the court, bent forward in severe pain, I could see my athletic dreams vanishing.

For the next 18 months, I lived through a nightmare of daily pain. Seven different medical specialists diagnosed at least seven different conditions, from "muscle spasms" to "growing pains." They prescribed a variety of muscle relaxants, pain pills, and cortisone shots.

I wasn't getting better on this revolving door. In fact, I had new problems from the side effects of the prescription drugs. Colitis was one of the problems. I didn't realize it at the time but I had joined the ranks of millions of other unaware Americans. I was on the medical treadmill.

One day my father suggested I try a chiropractor. When I mentioned this to my family doctor, who appeared not to be making progress with me, he admitted that he himself went to a chiropractor for his own back condition. When I asked him who I should go to, he said that he saw someone "out of town."

I chose someone locally. When I entered the waiting room, I was curious...and apprehensive. There were no other patients waiting. There was no receptionist. After waiting what seemed a lifetime, the chiropractor descended from his upstairs home office and asked me about my lower back.

The treatment that fixed my back also changed my life

He told me to lie down on his treatment table. He checked my leg length, then pressed on certain parts of my low back, and then checked my leg length again. Within five minutes, I got up off the table and walked without pain and without a limp for the first time since the injury. I no longer needed pain pills, braces, heating pads or any other device. I had just received a chiropractic adjustment that fixed my back and altered the course of my life.

I went on to play varsity sports in high school and college. I visited the chiropractor on a regular basis to reduce the risk of re-injury. All went well until my senior year in college when I experienced another serious back injury while playing rugby. Once again, chiropractic came through for me and got me back on my feet.

I had been contemplating a career in law or psychology. But chiropractic had so impressed me that I began to reconsider. Maybe I should become a chiropractic physician. My college girl friend, whom I later married, encouraged me to take that direction. As it turned out we both eventually became chiropractors.

I remember clearly the graduation banquet at Wheeling Jesuit University when all members of the senior class were introduced along with their acceptances to graduate and professional schools. In a large room filled to capacity, my turn came:

"Martin Gallagher. Student Body Vice President. National Honor Society for psychology majors. Planning to attend Logan College of Chiropractic."

There was a deadening silence. Then a mixture of applause and laughter. Somewhat confused by this ambivalent response, it wasn't until well into my chiropractic education that I understood the societal prejudice perpetrated by the medical- pharmaceutical complex against natural healing, especially chiropractic.

A widespread disinformation program was in effect — generated by the American Medical Association — to poison the minds of medical consumers. During my years in chiropractic school I often heard class-mates tell stories of parents being jailed for practicing chiropractic in the 1940's and 50's in the U.S.

Against this backdrop were the daily miracles I was observing. I remember a fellow student who was cured of crippling arthritis. Another, of severe migraines. And yet another of ulcers. Students whose fathers and grandfathers were chiropractors and who had never been to a medical doctor, taken a drug, or been immunized, were rarely sick.

"Dr. Monty" — A reminder of the dangers of medicine

Then there was the case of Dale Montgomery, D.C., our anatomy instructor. "Dr. Monty," as he was affectionately known, had been a rising college football star whose life experiences and compassion were indelibly etched into his 6-4, 240-pound frame. He had become paralyzed and bed ridden at twenty years of age following a rabies shot!

One day, he and his father heard a chiropractor on the radio speak of remarkable results in seemingly hopeless cases. The chiropractor was promptly summoned to the Montgomery home and began a series of daily manipulation treatments. Within weeks the young man was on his feet, and although he would never play football or walk normally again, he became an ever-present reminder of the dangers of medicine and the healing power of chiropractic.

As I learned more, I began to bring back these incredible stories and new health concepts to my friends and family. The conversation would usually be quite upbeat until I mentioned the "C" word (chiropractic). I noticed the word evoked an array of emotional responses that ran the gamut from "quack" to "cult" to "bone crusher" to "faith healer." I was told that chiropractors weren't really doctors, that they preyed on the sick, that they took all of your money, that they took mail order courses, and that they couldn't make it to medical school.

As I returned to school feeling somewhat isolated and despondent, I decided to look into the sources of this animosity and bigotry. What I ultimately learned was that the AMA had spent more than 25 years and millions of dollars in an effort to disgrace chiropractic. From 1963 until 1975, the AMA's Committee on Quackery (originally called the Committee on Chiropractic) had mobilized the organization's massive prestige, money, influence and communication resources into a campaign to "contain and eliminate" chiropractic as a health care alternative.

Although it seemed hard to believe, the AMA was sponsoring a direct, vicious crusade designed to "eliminate the chiropractic threat." The AMA influenced doctors, who in turn influenced their patients. The organization prejudiced the media, and even educational institutions and guidance counselors against this "unscientific cult."

> **It was now perfectly clear to me that the real agenda of organized medicine was not healing patients or saving lives but rather creating a drug and surgical monopoly for prestige and wealth.**

As I continued my studies at Logan College, I became exposed to the role of clinical nutrition. As I delved further into this area, I learned that many of the common health problems like headache, fatigue, insomnia, depression, and digestive disorders were intimately linked to the American diet, food allergies and nutritional deficiencies.

I decided to put this new information to the test. I proceeded to spend the next three months detoxifying my body through a program of raw organic fruits, vegetables and grains. I began taking vitamin supplements and herbs and using colon cleansing techniques. After a short period of time, I felt my mind becoming clearer and more focused in a way I had never before experienced. An additional side benefit was a drop in weight from 209 to 155 pounds in three months and I've been there ever since.

As I moved into my clinical rounds as an intern, I began using these natural health techniques with my patients. The results were astounding. Through chiropractic manipulation, nutritional therapy, detoxification, fasting, and herbal medicines I marveled at my ability to help patients overcome conditions such as chronic migraines, back pain, ulcers, depression and psoriasis.

Following graduation, I entered private practice in St. Louis and also served as a faculty member at Logan College. I married my college sweetheart, Charlotte Ciotti, who had inspired me toward chiropractic and who herself was in the process of completing her studies at Logan.

While integrating the many natural health care techniques with my patients in St. Louis, I began treating many pregnant women, who preferred home deliveries. I developed a close relationship with an obstetrician who recommended chiropractic and nutrition for his patients and encouraged this care during the pregnancy and delivery stages.

This experience provided the preliminary steps for the home birth of our own son, one year later. We began to see the importance and power of natural healing techniques from conception through delivery. The positive role of chiropractic became obvious in overcoming nausea of pregnancy, back pain and pelvic misalignment to facilitate an uncomplicated delivery and the importance of bringing a child into the world without anesthesia, surgery or head and neck injuries. What better gift, we thought, than to bring a child into the world with love, compassion and natural healing.

Armed with this new "low tech, high touch" approach to healing, we moved back to Pennsylvania and established Chiropractic Nutritional Associates in the home of my wife's parents.

As we began to help growing numbers of people, the word about the effectiveness of alternative medicine began to spread in the community. Converted skeptics and reluctant non-believers became our best ambassadors. As this new wave of health care began to grow, we were invited to appear on several television and radio programs in the Pittsburgh area. The public, we found, had an insatiable desire to find the causes of their health problems in spite of their doctors' admonitions that natural health care was worthless or unproven.

Victims of monopolistic medical practices

By 1990, following a 14-year bitter legal battle, the U.S. Supreme Court dealt the AMA a major setback and found it guilty of "lawless" behavior. The high court censured the AMA's nationwide boycott of doctors of chiropractic that had declared it unethical for medical doctors to associate professionally with chiropractic physicians. This illegal boycott had forced hospitals under the control of medical doctors to bar diagnostic assistance and facilities to chiropractic physicians and their patients. The AMA campaign had also involved interference with chiropractic educational institutions and health insurance programs designed to reimburse patients for chiropractic health care services. In addition, there had been a covert, nationwide propaganda effort to ruin the reputations of chiropractic physicians.

Long ago, Benjamin Rush, M.D., a signer of the Declaration of Independence and physician to President George Washington, warned of the danger of a medical establishment running amok. He said that "unless we put medical freedom into the Constitution, the time will come where medicine will organize into an undercover dictatorship...to restrict the art of healing to one class of men and deny equal privileges to others... All such laws are un-American and despotic and have no place in a republic....The Constitution of this republic should make special privilege for medical freedom as well as religious freedom."

For many decades, and even continuing to this day, the medical establishment has waged an evil, relentless and greed-motivated campaign against alternative health practitioners and methods outside the narrow confines of what has become known as conventional medicine. Many sincere, innovative and independent-minded professionals, who simply have found other methods to be more effective or who have chosen to explore new and promising ideas, have been harassed, branded "quacks," lost their licenses, raided by government agents and even jailed.

The big losers in all this have been the American people who, as you will read in the next chapter, have been truly victimized by monopolistic medical practices. For more information on this medical madness, you may like to read "The Assault on Medical Freedom," by P. Joseph Lisa (Hampton Roads Publishing, Norfolk, VA, 1994) and "The Serpent on the Staff: The Unhealthy Politics of the American Medical Association," by Howard Wolinsky and Tom Brune (Tarcher/Putnam, New York, 1994).

Chiropractic research, suppressed by the AMA for decades, has emerged strongly in recent years. Studies conducted worldwide have shown chiropractic to be significantly more effective than any other form of medical care for back pain. Many more studies are revealing the benefits of chiropractic for ear infections, attention deficit disorders, hypertension, migraines, ulcers, depression, anxiety and other numerous other conditions.

Promising research suggests chiropractic may play a positive role in the treatment of immune related diseases including chronic fatigue, cancer, and AIDS. Recent HIV studies have demonstrated that chiropractic cervical manipulation of the neck significantly elevates immune activity in the blood.

From our humble beginnings and with a keen desire to "help sick people get well," our chiropractic office has grown, added staff, and expanded the natural health care options. We have established a 20,000 sq. ft. state-of-the-art clinic with chiropractic physicians, 65 paraprofessionals and integration of the best of chiropractic, nutrition, homeopathic, herbal medicine, relaxation and exercise rehabilitation techniques.

In addition, we created an educational outreach program called "Alternatives 2 Medicine" a conduit of information through radio, newsletters, TV and direct patient care that enables people to transform the quality of their health and lives.

In 1996 we reached a new stage — the combination of chiropractic and medicine. Our new name became Medical Wellness Associates. To our staff of five chiropractic physicians we added two medical doctors. We envision this type of "multi disciplinary practice" as a model for the future. We see it as a truly complementary approach offering patients the best and safest treatments available from both conventional and alternative medicine.

The medical system desperately needs this type of integrated approach. The next chapter will explain why.

CHAPTER THREE

The treadmill – How bad is it?

Deanna Johns' medical history reads like an Edgar Allen Poe story — pure horror. Deanna, from Bridgeport, West Virginia, is a 19-year-old college student who barely survived her doctors' prescriptions.

"From the time I was six I suffered bouts of tonsillitis, strep throat, sinusitis and severe headaches," she told me during her first appointment. "Almost all of these were treated with antibiotics by various physicians."

When Deanna began menstruating, she experienced severe cramps and irregular, heavy bleeding. Her doctor treated this with pain killers.

"At age 16, a large grapefruit-sized cyst was diagnosed on my right ovary," she said. "My gynecologist told me it would be a 'simple procedure' to remove it. Instead it was the beginning of a nightmare which I have lived with ever since.

"I had serious blood loss which required transfusions. I had a reaction to the anesthetic and an undiagnosed infection which was treated for nine days with numerous intravenous antibiotics.

"Afterward, I experienced a resumption of severe menstrual cramps. I was placed on birth control pills. I then began to have bad mood swings and crying spells which I could not explain. I was fatigued. I had difficulty concentrating. I had terrible stomach pains which would cause me to pass out. There were alternating episodes of constipation and diarrhea and I woke up every morning with nausea.

"An internist prescribed Zantac and Donnatel for what he called irritable bowel syndrome. They made me drowsy to the point where I slept through many of my senior year classes in high school. I felt like a zombie.

"In my freshman year at college, I developed sinusitis. My doctor prescribed amoxicillin, an antibiotic. A few days later I began feeling in a daze. My speech slowed and slurred and my thoughts were unclear. My doctor said to stop the antibiotics. I couldn't get out of bed for three days. I could only sleep.

"From then on my life became a constant battle to stay alert and cope with everyday activities. I started to get headaches that lasted three to five days, severe shakiness, memory lapses, fits of laughter, and extreme fatigue. I had a hard time staying awake in class. Sometimes I would fall into a stupor or semi-conscious state where I could not speak or move my arms and legs. My friends had to literally drag me out of my room.

"My doctors put me on three different medicines for migraines. I had MRI scans, Cat scans, blood and urine tests, EEGs. Everything was negative.

"I did test positive for hypoglycemia and was advised to eat a high carbohydrate and low sugar diet. I got worse.

"One day I began convulsing uncontrollably. An ambulance was called. By the time I reached the hospital I had stabilized. I then went through a series of tests for seizures, pancreatic tumors, and everything else imaginable. All were negative.

"I began to seek out the opinion of specialists. Neurologists. Endocrinologists. Internists. Gynecologists. They said that I was not having seizures but one neurologist prescribed Dilantin, which is for seizures.

"Finally, three neurologists and two endocrinologists concluded that I was 'stressed out and anxious.' They said I should seek counsel from a psychiatrist.

"I decided I would just live with it for the rest of my life. I quit taking all my medicine and vowed never to see another doctor again. My parents had spent thousands of dollars to find out nothing. I had had enough."

Deanna left for her sophomore year of college. After three days, she experienced two serious seizure-like episodes and was sent home. A loving grandmother who listened to my regular radio broadcasts brought the young woman in to see me.

In our evaluation of Deanna we found spinal misalignments and nutritional deficiencies that medical doctors either ignore, are not trained to look for, or don't have the time to deal with. In her case, she was deficient in several important nutrients. She had allergies to foods she had been eating her entire life. She had disturbed pineal gland function, which affected her sleep. Her intestinal tract was highly toxic from years of medication. She had spinal misalignments as a result of past injuries.

After starting a wholistic treatment program that included nutritional supplementation, intestinal cleansing, and chiropractic adjustments, Deanna made a gradual recovery.

"I began to sleep better," she said. "I began to regain strength, clarity of thought and a sense of happiness."

After three months of treatment, Deanna told me that her headaches, her seizures, sleep disorder, extreme fatigue, and stomach aches were all gone. "I cannot begin to describe the difference in my life. I feel like a brand new person," she said.

"The System"

What if Deanna Johns' grandmother had not pointed her in a healing direction? How many people like Deanna are out there on a medical treadmill? I know that in my clinical practice I see many patients just like her. How, you ask, in this day and age of modern medicine, can these things happen?

> "It seems as if an entire country has swallowed a philosophy of 'health care' that is killing us by the thousands and disabling many more."

"Nobody should go through what I went through, "Deanna told me. "I feel that I was a puppet of the medical system. It seems that many legal drugs are just as harmful to the body as illegal drugs, and that we have allowed pharmaceutical companies to dictate our way of life and even our thinking process. What's going on? It seems as if an entire country has swallowed a philosophy of 'health care' that is killing us by the thousands and disabling many more."

We grow up with fondness and reverence for the doctors and healers in our midst. It is this way now and it probably has always been so, for it is to them that we innocently turn when our bodies malfunction. Most care deeply about their patients and are committed professional human beings.

In our times, a powerful medical establishment composed of professional associations, the pharmaceutical industry, insurance companies, and government agencies dictates how medical doctors can practice in this country. The result is an immeasurable disaster that creates many Deanna Johns.

The system views the treatment of disease primarily from the limited perspective of pharmaceutical drugs and surgical procedures. This is what is taught in medical schools; this is what medical doctors read about in their medical journals.

The system, through its vast public relations resources, has hypnotized Americans to believe that all symptoms are bad and that medical doctors, like the U.S. cavalrymen, will come rushing to the rescue with drugs, surgery, and high-tech wizardry. As a result of this, patients often demand an antibiotic, a drug, or a surgical procedure to cure their ills and will go elsewhere if their doctor doesn't give it to them. They are locked into a consumer mentality limited to "what drugs or surgery are you giving me?"

This modern system has racked up brilliant achievements in emergency medicine, acute care treatment, and sophisticated and heroic surgical procedures. We all applaud and honor such accomplishments. The system, however, fails miserably to prevent disease and supports treatments, procedures and drugs that often cause substantial — and even deadly — new symptoms and complaints.

We are told we have the best medical system in the world. For sure, it's the most expensive. Our runaway national medical bill is $1 trillion a year and gaining momentum daily. Based on current trends, the figure is expected to increase to $1.7 trillion by the year 2000. Despite the high costs, we have some of the worst health statistics of all industrialized countries. In a 1993 ranking of health among the developed nations, the World Health Organization (WHO) listed the U.S. as 18th!

Against major chronic diseases, we have made little progress.

For an overall picture of health (or lack of it, would be a better term) in America, look no farther than a 1996 University of San Francisco study which made nationwide headlines. About 99 million of us are afflicted with some form of chronic ailment, the report said.

Will healthy Americans soon become a new minority? It's starting to look that way.

Where is America the beautiful? It's more like America the sick.

Something for sure is wrong.

The truth is we don't really have a health care system in America. Not by any stretch of the imagination. We have a disease care system — a massive industry almost wholly oriented to managing symptoms of disease with drugs and surgery.

Deepak Chopra, M.D., a well-known advocate of alternative medicine, describes modern medicine thusly: "The fascination is with disease, and not with health and the two are completely different things. It's like the difference between being rich and poor. If you want to study health, you can't study it by studying disease, which is what medicine does."

Ninety-nine percent of our "health sector budget" is used to treat illness after it occurs. One percent is allocated for prevention, even though the vast majority of chronic illness is preventable.

Incredibly, the government consistently ignores prevention-oriented

America The Beautiful or America The Sick?

- *33 million Americans suffer from arthritis.*
- *21 million are afflicted with heart disease. Two out of five of us are expected to develop cardiovascular disease during our lifetime.*
- *Nearly 50 million have high blood pressure.*
- *Some 400,000 will die this year of smoking-related disease.*
- *23 million suffer from cognitive, emotional or behavioral disorders.*
- *Perhaps a fifth of all Americans suffer from severe head aches and more than 10 million of them are moderately or severely disabled as a result.*
- *More than 25 million are affected by osteoporosis, 80 percent of them women.*
- *An estimated 22 million individuals suffer from irritable bowel symptoms such as abdominal pain, bloating, diarrhea or constipation.*
- *8 million Americans have diabetes.*
- *And cancer? Many billions of dollars have been spent since President Nixon declared "war on cancer" in 1971 and launched a national crusade against this dreaded illness. Yet, the number of new cases of every form of cancer has increased over the last 60 years and today more than 1,500 people die from it daily in the U.S. Cancer is expected to overtake heart disease as the deadliest killer. Currently, one in three of us will develop cancer during our lifetime. By 2000, experts think the odds will be two out of five.*
  "The costs in terms of suffering and death and the inflationary impact of cancer, now estimated at $110 billion annually (nearly 2 percent of the gross national product), are massive," wrote cancer expert Samuel Epstein of the University of Chicago in 1992.

approaches. Health care reform bills debated in congress deal only with disease-care financing and delivery and the goal of saving money by streamlining the system. There's no talk of improving health. Medicare, believe it or not, doesn't cover preventive services. It ignores it, even at a time when the cost of caring for the chronically-ill elderly in nursing homes is rapidly approaching a critical breaking point that can wipe out family savings.

No wonder Medicare is going broke. The government debate has degenerated into an argument over "who should pay for whose disease."

Real prevention (and not just merely early detection of disease) and alternative approaches are the only solution.

One major reason for the better health status of other industrial nations is that they maintain a pluralistic approach to health-care delivery, according to the World Health Organization.

This means many different methods are allowed to thrive in other countries and openly compete in the medical marketplace. Here in the U.S., by comparison, the government essentially supports a medical monopoly — namely the limited conventional approach of drugs and surgery, commented Alternative Medicine Digest, under the headline "America's Vast Sick-Care Economy."

"What is shameful here, even inexcusable, is that in most cases conventional medicine is unsuccessful in resolving chronic illness, while this is alternative medicine's strongest suit," the outspoken magazine said in a 1997 commentary.

The overwhelming majority of government-funded research pursues the myth of finding a silver bullet while results of treatment continue to be unimpressive and in many cases downright destructive. Our medical system relies primarily on drugs and surgery, and many of these treatments have serious side effects, risks, and questionable validity. According to the Office of Technology of the U.S. Government, 80 percent of conventional medical therapies have no basis in science.

The negative impact of these therapies is beyond belief.

- **The cost of iatrogenic disease — that is disease or mortality occurring as the result of treatment by a doctor or hospitals — is staggering, both in terms of human suffering and money.**

- **Iatrogenic disorders are estimated to affect about a third of patients in hospitals.**

- **The number of people dying in the U.S. as a result of medical treatment is equivalent to three Boeing 747 crashes every two days! As many as 1 million people may be in some way injured in hospitals each year and as many as 180,000 are estimated to die as a result.**

"Therefore, the iatrogenic injury rate dwarfs the annual automobile accident mortality of 45,000 and accounts for more deaths than all other accidents combined," the Journal of the American Medical Association said in 1995.

When you contrast the number of medical treatment deaths to the 50,000 American GI deaths during the entire 10-year war in Vietnam, the statistics become even more chilling.

The Surgical Epidemic

Unnecessary surgeries, and their complications, represent a major assault on our bodies.

• **Hysterectomies:** By age 60, more than a third of all American women will have undergone a hysterectomy — the highest rate in the world. Some 60 percent of these operations are performed on women under 45. In half of these cases, ovaries as well as the uterus are removed in order to spare the woman the risk of developing ovarian cancer. The removal of ovaries, however, raises the risk of osteoporosis and/or cardio-vascular disease. It also triggers a sudden "surgical menopause," the relief of which, women are told, can be obtained through prescribed hormonal therapy.

• **Heart surgery:** Most experts now agree that of the current 800,000 bypass and angioplasty surgeries performed each year, to suppos-edly "save your life," you are five to ten times more likely to die from the procedure and its complications than by the disease itself. Although 10 percent of heart disease patients may benefit from the procedure, 90 percent of all bypass is unnecessary. According to a ten-year follow-up of survival among heart attack patients, individuals with one, two or all three of their major heart blood vessels blocked do quite well without surgery.

Yet, our sophisticated medical system is geared up to perform surgery — which isn't cheap. Bypass surgery goes for $40,000 a shot and more than 250,000 Americans get bypasses each year. The cost: $18 billion. It's the No. 1 medical tab in the nation. Angioplasty — the balloon technique — is performed on some 400,000 patients a year. That goes for $10,000 per procedure. Despite the great medical technology involved in these procedures, up to a half of bypass grafts reblock after only five years, and a third to a half of angioplastied arteries reblock again after four to six months. The original procedure is often repeated at additional cost.

• **Back surgeries:** Back pain, the leading cause of work loss in the U.S., has become another favorite of surgeons. Currently up to 700,000 Americans receive "disc surgery" to supposedly remove pain-producing herniated discs from the back. Research now indicates that perhaps only one percent of these operations are necessary and that discs, in most cases, are not pain provoking.

This surgical "hit list" goes on and on from tonsillectomies, to gallbladder surgeries, to appendectomies, to ear tube surgeries, to hyster-ectomies, to breast, uterine and prostate biopsies.

The failed war against cancer

Let's turn to cancer. A revealing article in the May 1995 issue of the Journal of the National Cancer Institute disclosed the findings of a survey from 14 cancer centers and 10,000 cases where chemotherapy was used for Hodgkin's disease. Results: people who take chemo are 14 times more likely to develop leukemia. In addition, chemo also increased the risk of bone, joint and soft tissue cancer by 6 times. Radiation therapy increased the risk of developing lung cancer by 2.7 times and female genital cancer by 2.4 times.

John D. Bailar III, M.D., Ph.D., of McGill University, and the former editor of the Journal of the National Cancer Institute, along with Elaine M. Smith of the University of Iowa, published a historic study of overall cancer survival data in a 1986 issue of the New England Journal of Medicine. They concluded that "some 35 years of intense and growing efforts to improve the treatment of cancer have not had much overall effect on the most fundamental measure of clinical outcome — death. Overall, the effort to control cancer has failed — so far — to attain its objectives."

The only bright side to an otherwise dismal picture, they said, is the decreased mortality in those under 30. But such deaths account "for only one to two percent of total mortality from cancer."

Their main conclusion was that "efforts focused largely on improving treatment must be judged a qualified failure."

In 1997, Bailar updated his findings in the New England Journal of Medicine and reported that "the war against cancer is far from over. The effect of new treatments for cancer on mortality has been largely disappointing. The most promising approach to the control of cancer is a national commitment to prevention" with a parallel rebalancing and refocusing of cancer research funding.

Medical Drugs — Helping or Harming?

Pharmaceutical drugs represent big, big business — $200 billion in annual worldwide sales. There is no doubt that their use has a positive role in medicine and helps millions of people. But there is also no doubt that they are overused, are often ineffective and inappropriate, and that their side effects are contributing to illness and death at a massive scale unrecognized by the public.

Consider these shocking facts:

• Americans are now spending $75 billion annually on prescription drugs. But more is being spent — $76 billion — on the direct medical costs from adverse drug side effects, according to a 1995 study. The largest component of this total is $47.4 billion for the drug-related hospitalization of some 8.7 million individuals each year.

• Forty percent of patients suffer at least one major drug side effect.

• A 1993 analysis of eight popular drugs published in the Journal of Applied Nutrition determined they had 97 pluses (positive indications) and 2,449 minuses (drawbacks or dangers)! Prozac, a frequently-prescribed anti-depressant, for instance, scored 22 pluses and 597 minuses. Among the adverse reactions to Prozac are convulsions, hallucinations, aggression, delirium, violent hostility, psychosis, and even death by suicide.

• In March of 1995, a flurry of publicity surrounded the revelation that a popular type of anti-hypertensive drug called calcium channel blockers actually raise the risk of a heart attack by 60 percent. A report later that year in the Journal of the American Medical Association noted that another major category of anti-hypertensives, known as beta blocking drugs, elevates cholesterol levels and also increases the risk of heart disease.

• One group of popular prescriptions called non-steroidal anti-inflammatory drugs (NSAIDs) were responsible for 15-20,000 deaths in 1995 while a quarter of all patients taking them developed stomach ulcers within 4 weeks! These same drugs have been touted by pharmaceutical companies and doctors as a "safe and effective" alternative for steroids (cortisone). Outcome studies are showing that these drugs, often prescribed for the pain of arthritis, actually may accelerate joint and cartilage damage — the very thing that patients think they are curing.

• According to a 1994 article in the New England Journal of Medicine, people who often take acetaminophen (popular brands of over-the-counter, non-aspirin pain killers) and NSAIDs have an increased risk of kidney damage.

• In 1994, almost 70,000 incidences of acetaminophen overdose were reported to the Toxic Exposure Surveillance System of the American Association of Poison Control Centers.

• Twenty-five percent of all prescription drugs cause impotence in males and low libido in women. Additionally, more than 100 prescription drugs should not be taken if you drive an automobile.

- The average American completing his stay at a hospital will leave with an average of seven prescription drugs!

Wanted! A cure for antiobiotics!

- Antibiotics are prescribed at an alarming rate. Obstetrician and gynecologists write 2,645,000 antibiotic prescriptions every week and internists some 1,416,000. Pediatricians and family physicians alone prescribe more than $500 million worth of antibiotics each year to treat just one problem — ear infections in children. Another $500 million is spent on antibiotics for other pediatric illnesses.

According to a 1989 issue of Health Letter, a publication of Ralph Nader and Sidney Wolfe's Health Research Group in Washington D.C., congressional hearings and numerous academic studies has led to the "consensus that 40 to 60 percent of antibiotics are misprescribed."

The problem is so flagrant that the Centers for Disease Control drafted guidelines for physicians in 1996 in an effort to help reduce over-use. Obviously there are many situations where antibiotics are necessary. However, some medical studies question whether they are any more effective than doing nothing.

A 1996 report in the Journal of Internal Medicine declared that bacteria resistance to virtually all our most marketed antibiotics has become apparent. The main cause of this is overuse. Despite a dramatic increase in use of these medications during the last decade there is no corresponding decreases in deaths or illness from bacterial infections. One major reason for overuse of antibiotics is patient pressure!

One of the most critical and yet massively under-recognized side effects of antibiotics is their destructive impact on the beneficial intestinal bacteria. These colonies of micro-organisms help you stay healthy by producing enzymes, vitamins, and natural antibiotics to counteract harmful microbes. In addition, they enhance healthy bowel function and help prevent cancerous substances from forming. They have anti-viral, anti-fungal, and even anti-cholesterol properties.

Candida albicans, the infamous yeast organism that causes infections and suffering, can spread rapidly when the influence of friendly bacteria is weakened.

Research clearly shows that virtually every antibiotic taken orally affects the balance of intestinal bacteria. Even one single course of antibiotics can have a negative effect. The degree of damage caused depends on the type and strength of medication.

• Non-prescription cough and cold preparations sold over-the-counter came in for sharp criticism during a 1994 congressional hearing. "The sad fact is that much of the billion-dollar cold medication industry may be based more on hype than on health care," one congressman said. "The high use rate of these medications may be a tremendous waste of money and may unnecessarily expose children to toxicity."

In a commentary on this, the Journal of the American Medical Association pointed out that more than half of mothers in a national survey said they had given their three-year-olds an OTC medication, primarily Tylenol or cough or cold medicine, in the past 30 days. Given the high incidence of fever and upper respiratory tract illnesses in children, such usage is not surprising, the journal said, "however, we have no assurances that these medications are used correctly. Moreover, the use of cough or cold medications are increasingly called into question due to the striking absence of efficacy data."

Pill-taking: a doctor-sanctioned ritual for the elderly

Drug abuse in this country is not just limited to junkies and illicit stuff grown in a South American jungle or manufactured in an inner-city garage. It also includes the overuse, abuse and eventual addiction of medical drugs, particularly among the elderly.

Nobody knows precise numbers of people affected, but according to a 1996 front-page Los Angeles Times article, "some senior citizens, unwilling to bother far-off — and busy — children or grandchildren, stumble into trouble self-medicating themselves and wind up hooked. The tablets they take for sleeplessness or pain diminish the dread of losing control, of being poor or ill, of seeing friends pass away. Pill-taking becomes part of a comforting, doctor-sanctioned ritual, part of a daily routine with dwindling options."

While some doctors and geriatric specialists contend that elderly addicts are rare and that physicians are responsibly prescribing, addiction experts believe that doctors often do not have the time or the knowledge to diagnose underlying emotional problems such as depression. "Pressed for time, they too often use pills as band-aids for the complaints of the elderly," wrote Times reporter Tracy Weber.

According to medical research and federal reports cited in her article, 37 percent of Americans over 65 use five or more prescription drugs at the same time, or roughly a third of all medical pills consumed.

Many pharmacists can tell that their customers, seeking refills, are affected. Often they try to warn their customers.

"You are supposed to give drugs like Valium for short-term relief of anxiety — four to six weeks at the outside — not four to six years," said one Southern California pharmacist. "The doctors keep giving it to them. We get prescriptions for 300 Valium at a time. Some of these older people, you can tell before they open their mouths that they've taken too much of whatever they're on. It's cheaper to medicate them than to deal with their problem."

Experts envision the prescription epidemic will increase as the baby boomer generation comes of medical age. As one addiction expert in the Times article said, the boomers are "into instant gratification. They're used to the fact that there's a pill you can take to cure anything."

At a price, for sure.

• A 1994 Harvard study found that almost one-quarter of U.S. senior citizens are overmedicated, resulting in more than 650,000 hospitalizations.

• Drug-induced illness is the leading cause of preventable disease in older men and women, according to "Worst Pills, Best Pills II" by Sidney Wolfe, M.D. Pharmaceutical drugs each year cause some 61,000 cases of Parkinsonsim (tremors), 32,000 hip fractures from falls, and 163,000 cases of documented memory loss.

The Medical Vietnam

Conventional medical care has created a drug and surgical nightmare. How can you not but doubt the motivations of a system that persists in promoting questionable methods while at the same time conspiring to stifle alternatives and promising non-toxic treatments. This is scary stuff. This is nothing less than criminal. Whose welfare is being protected?

Despite the evidence, where is the public uproar? Why does the public continue to take it? Are we hypnotized lambs going to the slaughter?

The situation is nothing less than a "medical Vietnam," in the words of Peter Barry Chowka, a respected medical journalist.

Can we afford our present medical system and the poor lifestyle habits that feed it?

This predicament has saddled American businesses with crippling medical burdens. Employee health costs have skyrocketed from single digits to 25 percent and even up to 50 percent of profits in recent years.

Medical benefits have become the third largest expense after raw materials and straight-time pay for most manufacturers. Automakers pay more for the medical insurance of their employees than for the raw steel that goes into their cars. For most service businesses, this is the second largest expense. In the U.S. on any given workday, there are approximately one million absent employees, costing about $22 billion annually in lost productivity.

What is all this doing to the economic viability of America, and the cost of producing goods and services? In many cases, the cost of corporate health benefits precludes real salary increases for employees, and many otherwise profitable businesses are driven into bankruptcy by spiraling medical costs.

And look what's ahead: the baby boomers are coming of medical age. This is the largest generation in American history. Emergency rooms are already seeing the first wave of heart attacks. If we do nothing now, nothing will be left of government medical care funding when the first of the 76 million boomers become eligible for Medicare in 2015.

Our medical system needs to shift its priorities and vast resources to prevention and open itself to ideas and treatments that work. Just as we crave political and personal freedom, we — the public — need to demand health care freedom. Although many would argue that we live in an enlightened, high-tech medical era, future generations may look back at our society as a "dark age" in which people abdicated their health responsibilities to doctors, their fundamental health rights to a medical dictatorship, and went en mass from red-blooded to anemic Americans in the process.

Unless we act now we may be facing a catastrophic rise in medical costs that might drastically reduce our standard of living. According to aging experts L. Stephen Coles, M.D., of the California Institute of Technology, and Steven B. Harris, M.D., of UCLA, "the only rational economic answer to the specter of catastrophic health care costs is the development of anti-aging therapies to enable individuals to live healthier and more youthful lives while at advanced ages."

In many cases, these experts wrote in a new textbook on anti-aging medicine, "funding to support research on the cures of specific age-related diseases such as cancer, atherosclerosis, arthritis and immune failure, is a little like rearranging the deck chairs on the Titanic. In the future therapies will be developed to keep people healthy and youthful throughout their lives. Anti-aging and preventive medicine is growing and experts in the field are actively researching and finding practical solutions. They need the funding support that will result in lengthening our lives dramatically while postponing the ravages of old age. We must think ahead. We have to."

We already have the knowledge to do these things. The research on the efficacy of many "alternative" treatments is powerful, yet these methods are specifically excluded from the U.S. medical care system. This cannot continue. For everybody's sake.

CHAPTER FOUR

The shifting system: from disease-care to health-care

"Wisdom is the ability to find an alternative when something isn't working," said Bernard Jensen, D.C., a famous pioneer of chiropractic and nutrition, in a Let's Live Magazine interview back in the 1980s. "We find today that many of the drugs and methods in use are turning out to be detrimental to our bodies. We are living in side-effects, time bomb effects and genetic effects as a result of this. The age of alternative is coming in. It cannot be stopped because, as my mother used to say, if you give a man enough light he is bound to find his way."

Jensen was right. It's happening — now. When articles on alternative medicine and vitamins make the cover of Time and Life Magazines you know there's a big change going on.

There is, in fact, an enormous shift in public acceptance and use of alternative treatments. For sure this is not change driven by the medical establishment, but by patients like you who have become aware that the system isn't working. You have become a powerful force for change.

Some of the most noteworthy signs of this development include the following:

• In 1990, one-third of Americans visited an alternative doctor, spending about $11 billion out of their own pockets for 425 million office visits not covered by conventional insurance medical plans. The New England Journal of Medicine first published the Harvard study reporting this development. It sent shock waves through the medical establishment.

• A 1993 poll indicating that 70 percent of people are beginning to lose faith in doctors — an all-time low.

• A 1993 American Cancer Society survey estimated that 9 percent of cancer patients use complementary therapies, and among higher-educated and more influential groups the percentage is 14 percent. But other reports put the number much higher — as high as 50 or 60 percent.

• In 1991, one out of 15 Americans saw a chiropractor and 90 percent said the treatment was effective.

• The Internal Revenue Service now recognizes expenses for acupuncture and chiropractic.

• In 1995, the mass market sales of medicinal herbs grew by 35 percent, along with similarly impressive growth in sales of nutritional supplements and homeopathy.

• In response to public pressure, states are beginning to pass laws to protect licensed alternative practitioners and even authorize insurance coverage. In 1996, Washington became the first state to mandate reimbursement for treatment performed by any licensed or certified health practitioner. The treatment includes massage therapy, acupuncture, and more than two dozen other methods.

• Major medical schools, the bastions of orthodoxy, have started to offer courses in alternative medicine. Among them are Harvard, Columbia, Yale, Johns Hopkins and the University of Arizona. About 60 medical schools now teach complementary medicine.

• In November of 1996, the first publicly-funded natural medicine clinic opened in Washington State's King County.

• On the federal government level, an Office of Alternative Medicine was established at the National Institutes of Health (NIH) in 1992. In the words of Life Magazine's September 1996 cover article on "The Healing Revolution," it was given "modest" but "groundbreaking" funding for research on natural, non-toxic medical treatments.

• In 1996, a special NIH panel recommended that medical and nursing students be instructed in the use of nutritional supplements, acupuncture, and stress-reduction techniques. The recommendation was prompted by a University of Maryland poll of 800 U.S. physicians. In that poll, 70 percent of the doctors expressed interest in knowing more about alternative medicine. Moreover, some 40 percent of their patients desired alternative treatments.

• Even that arch-enemy of alternative medicine, the American Medical Association, is being forced by events to change its tune. In 1995, according to Life Magazine, it grudgingly advised its 300,000 members to "become better informed regarding the practices and techniques of alternative or unconventional medicine."

These developments indeed reflect a paradigm shift in progress — regular people, government, educators and professionals adopting prevention and natural, alternative medical ideas.

I see in my very own practice a prime example of how medicine is changing, of how medical doctors, chiropractors and other health professionals can work together in a spirit of cooperation to inspire patients to stay healthy and deliver to them the best and safest methods of treatment.

The best treatment may be:
- A spinal manipulation.
- A homeopathic remedy.
- A detoxification program.
- Certain vitamins and minerals.
- Chelation therapy.
- Colonic hydrotherapy.
- Or, when indicated, prescription drugs.
- Surgery.
- Or a combination of these.

Andrew Weil, M.D., who has developed a post-doctoral program in alternative medicine at the University of Arizona, calls this "integrative medicine."

I believe this is where the system is headed. I am extremely proud to be already involved in this. From my own experience, in my clinic, I see on a daily basis a real health care model where natural and medical techniques merge into an integrative practice that truly serves patients well in a cost-effective manner.

Alternative medicine saves money

Alternative medicine inspires individuals to become intimately involved in their own health. Studies show this has a powerful effect in elevating personal health...and saving money.

Insurance companies and managed care organizations, you would think, would pick up on this in a big way and broaden their coverage. Indeed there appears to be a dynamic trend in this direction.

A comprehensive article on the "Health Insurance Revolution" in the March/April 1997 issue of New Age Magazine said that "more and more health insurers are covering therapies that were once considered alternatives but are now accepted as mainstream." The article quoted a 1995 survey of the nation's largest HMOs which found that 86 percent of them cover chiropractic, 31 percent cover acupuncture, and 28 percent cover relaxation therapies.

According to a 1996 editorial in USA Today, alternative medicine is "slowly, but surely gaining credibility. Latest example: Oxford Health Plans, a Connecticut-based HMO, is preparing to offer its 1.4 million enrollees access to a panel of 1,000 non-traditional health-care providers, including chiropractors, homeopaths, naturopaths, yoga instructors and massage therapists."

A promising example of interest in alternative medicine by the insurance industry is Dean Ornish's Program for Reversing Heart Disease where patients are able to eliminate symptoms and become functionally normal through intensive lifestyle modification alone. No costly operations or a lifetime of cholesterol-lowering drugs are necessary.

Ornish is director of the Preventive Medicine Research Institute in Sausalito, Ca., and an assistant clinical professor of medicine at the University of California, San Francisco. Since the late 1970s, he has conducted clinical trials based on a program featuring a low-fat vegetarian diet, moderate regular exercise, smoke cessation, meditation, and professionally-supervised support group sessions.

When his first published study claimed improved heart function, Ornish's conservative peers called the program a radical idea with questionable elements.

By 1993 Ornish's studies had produced hard data showing the disease is reversible. As a result, it started to be offered at medical centers around the country. In addition, several large insurance companies have agreed to cover it, making it the first non-surgical, non-pharmaceutical therapy for heart disease to qualify for insurance reimbursement.

There are two reasons for such mainstream acceptance. One is the great cost savings, compared to expensive conventional treatments, which often have to be repeated.

The second reason is effectiveness. Followers of the program consistently report rapid and significant reductions of cholesterol and chest pain. They feel better, have more energy, with less anxiety and depression.

Writing in leading medical journals, Ornish has compared the results of his patients with others receiving usual and customary care. In regard to chest pain, his patients as a group attained <u>reductions</u> of 91 percent in frequency, 42 percent in duration, and 38 percent in severity. Patients in the comparison group averaged <u>increases</u> of 165 percent in frequency, 95 percent in duration, and 39 percent in severity.

"The major clinical reason for performing bypass surgery and angioplasty in most patients is to help reduce frequency of chest pain from heart disease," says Ornish. "We can generally achieve this through lifestyle changes alone, often within a few days or weeks."

Acceptance of Ornish's program serves perhaps as another signal of growing openness toward alternative medicine concepts in today's managed health care climate where cost and effectiveness are becoming absolutely critical. We still have a long way to go, but we appear at last to be moving in a positive direction.

There are many striking examples of how alternative practices can have a massive effect in lowering medical costs. Here is but a small sampling of them:

- At a 1996 conference on alternative medicine, Michael Janson, M.D., president of the American Preventive Medical Association, commented on a number of patients with diseased limbs that he treated with chelation therapy and who would otherwise have undergone amputation. In one case, a patient had "spent one third of his life ill, and now, three years after chelation treatment, he is golfing, bowling, and has had no difficulties. He spent $600,000 on his early treatments and about $6,000 on the chelation treatment. The $600,000 was reimbursed; the $6,000 was not." Chelation therapy is a series of safe intravenous procedures administered by many alternative doctors that dramatically improves circulation. It is an extremely effective option for people with cardiovascular conditions.

- At the same conference, Wayne Jonas, M.D., director of the NIH Office of Alternative Medicine, said there is "little doubt" that some alternative treatments can reduce costs. He pointed to a 56 percent reduction in C-sections in parts of the country where midwives were involved in deliveries. This alone represents vast savings, he said. A C-section costs several thousand dollars, while a midwife is paid far less.

- Powerful research has accumulated in recent years showing how antioxidant supplements, such as vitamins C and E, and CoQ10, a fat-soluble vitamin, can cut the incidence of heart disease.

- The late Linus Pauling chronicled in articles and books how large doses of vitamin C, along with other nutritional supplements, could dramatically extend survival rates and well-being among cancer patients.

- In a 1996 column in the Townsend Letter for Doctors and Patients, Seattle physician Alan Gaby, M.D., offered the following dramatic comparison of cost and effectiveness between conventional and alternative approaches: "I am reminded of a patient with a 7-year history of daily migraines, rheumatoid arthritis, and severe abdominal pain. He had spent $27,000 on numerous doctors and treatments, without obtaining relief. A simple elimination-and-rechallenge diet determined that corn allergy was the cause of all of these problems..."

No amount of "care managing" can alter the fact that "modern medicine is too expensive and in many instances ineffective," he added.

• Numerous studies with large numbers of patients have shown chiropractic to be enormously cost-effective when compared to medical management in the treatment of back-related pain and injuries, one of the most costly causes of illness, debility and lost work time. Medical treatments are four times more expensive, and the number of work days lost ten times higher! I'll be talking much more about the research on chiropractic benefits for not just back pain, but many other conditions, in Chapter 13.

• A decade-long study by the University of Michigan at Steelcase Corporation, a major manufacturer of office equipment, concluded that systematic programs of diet, exercise, and stress reduction, when targeted for subjects in high health risk categories, reduce total medical costs by 46 percent. (Medical Tribune, Feb 10 1994).

• According to a 1994 assessment by the Centers for Disease Control and Prevention, nearly 47 percent of premature deaths among Americans could be avoided by changes in individual behaviors and another 17 percent by reducing environmental risks. In contrast, the analysis suggested that only 11 percent of such deaths could have been prevented by improved access to medical treatments.

Taking personal responsibility for health

Research indicates that 50 percent of deaths and 70 percent of disease in America are self-inflicted. The vast majority of disease is thus preventable.

Most of our medical woes are, in fact, influenced by factors over which our disease-based system has little control — such as poor nutrition, stress, lack of exercise, structural misalignments, alcohol and substance abuse, societal problems, and exposure to environmental toxins. Consequently, in the absence of effective prevention and natural methods that activate the body's own healing mechanisms, our medical system, as it now exists, can never create a truly healthy society

We cannot really blame the healthcare crisis or our own health problems on the system. Nor can we blame viruses and bacteria. Blame lies clearly with each one of us for not taking responsibility for our own bodies.

We cannot really expect doctors or governments or technology to save us as we continue to pursue poor lifestyle habits and abuse ourselves.

In "The Kellogg Report: The Impact of Nutrition, Environment & Lifestyle on the Health of Americans," Joseph Beasley, M.D., former dean of the School of Public Health at Tulane University, laments that most people persist in believing that physicians, clinics, and the government are the primary protectors of health.

Wrong, he says: "While there is a crying need for reforms of the health-care system, the most needed reform of all is in our own attitudes — we patients must become activists for our own health. Health care, properly speaking, is what we should be doing ourselves, all our lives, to avoid the examining rooms and stunning bills of illness care."

Most people simply don't realize that they can take better care of their health. Some people know what to do but find it difficult to give up unhealthy ways of eating and living.

"These obstacles to self-care are enormous in practice," says Beasley, "particularly the complacent attitude that health care is not our individual duty but that of designated professionals. This has become a nearly impregnable attitude on the part of most patients AND doctors at a great cost in money and suffering to this nation."

Beasley is right.

We have a health crisis in America because there is an epidemic of poor health. Nobody can create health for us. Only we can do that for ourselves.

We need to be involved in making ourselves healthier.

We must develop a philosophy of self-reliance, empowerment, and natural health care first, drugs second, and surgery last.

We don't necessarily need more drugs, hospitals and doctors. We do need more personal responsibility.

We need to develop preventive strategies — personal, corporate and national — to minimize institutionalizing people and their illnesses.

Millions of Americans appear to be moving in this direction. They are crawling, walking, running or stumbling off the treadmill. They are seeking what the conventional disease-care system, despite its lucrative financial ties to the pharmaceutical industry, abusive political clout, and insurance industry connection, is incapable of providing: wellness.

Thus, a healthier America necessitates reform on two fronts:

1) the system shifting resources from its virtually total disease care emphasis to prevention, health education, and natural, effective treatment options;

2) a self-health reform where people take more responsibility for their own well-being.

The Great American Medical Myth: ═══════════
Symptoms Are Bad... We'll Remove Them

Through advertising, public education and media manipulation, the medical establishment long ago created the Great American Medical Myth that has hypnotized most of us in believing that symptoms are bad and that drugs, surgery or radiation are the means of eliminating them.

Whether you are aware of it or not, it's a big sales pitch for your business. You've been besieged from all sides to think of medicine...or surgery...for your every ache or illness.

How thoroughly have we all been brainwashed? Try the following word associations on friends or family members. Word association is a technique used by psychologists to evoke emotional responses from their patients in an effort to resolve psychological conflicts. When thought becomes strongly linked with emotions, an individual's ability to discern can become impaired.

For instance, what word do you associate with the word depression? Prozac maybe, an anti-depression drug that gets tons of publicity?

If I say stomach problems, don't you think immediately of Zantac, Tagamet, or antacids?

If I say gallbladder, you think surgery, "get it out."

Isn't the term "disc problem" synonymous with back surgery?

Ear infections = antibiotics and tube surgery? Ritalin = hyperactivity.

I say headache. You think aspirin.

You get the point. At the first sign of pain, people have been conditioned not to think why the headache occurred but to rush, like automatons, to their medicine cabinet for an aspirin to snuff it out. It's almost as if the headache is the result of an aspirin deficiency.

Similarly, your cold is a Contact deficiency.

If you don't sleep well, it's a sleeping pill or tranquilizer deficiency.

The contemporary drug-and-surgical medical system has

created the medically-dependent consumer.

For our own good, we must start developing safer, natural word associations. Such as: Sore throats and vitamin C. Leg cramps and minerals. Back pain and spinal manipulation. Allergies? Maybe think echinacea, golden seal and pantothenic acid before antihistamines, decongestants or antibiotics.

We must expand this word association game so that people begin associating symptoms with underlying causes.

The ultimate association should be: Health. My responsibility.

PART TWO

The Gallagher Wellness Program:

Your Personal "Health Blueprint"

CHAPTER FIVE

Remaking yourself healthier –
The basics of 21st century medicine

"No doctor really cures his patients. Each patient carries his own doctor inside him, and comes to us not knowing that truth. We are at our best when we give the doctor who resides within a chance to work."

— **Albert Schweitzer, M.D.**

"Beloved I wish above all things that thou mayest prosper and be in health even as thy soul prospereth."

— **III John 2**

The best time to begin your journey to better health is right now. Don't procrastinate. Don't wait to make a new year's resolution. The sooner you start, the sooner you will feel better and the less time you will spend on the medical treadmill.

I always tell my patients about the great rewards of a healthy lifestyle. First of all a faith in God including prayer, fasting and meditation in God's word and then through natural means such as chiropractic, nutrition, herbal medicine and detoxification.

These methods empower you with the knowledge to better understand your body, why you become unwell, and how you can remake yourself into a healthier individual. Skilled health professionals are available wherever you live to provide the necessary healing techniques, programs and guidance to elevate you from poor health to good health. It's up to you though to follow through, on your own behalf, and be a health activist.

Most patients, once they see the results, don't want to return to a lesser level of health. They want to feel better. They want to feel energetic. They usually want to do what it takes to stay healthy.

To fulfill that need I have developed the Gallagher Wellness Program as a "health blueprint" for patients to achieve better health. We regard it as an enlightened model of health-care that focuses not on drugs and surgery but on the concept of "balance and wellness" and taking greater personal responsibility.

Health is not merely the absence of disease. Rather, it is a state of vitality and happiness in life based on physical, emotional, chemical, and spiritual balance. The steps in our health-care model attempt to strengthen these basic elements essential for optimum health. These building blocks of health are represented in the equilateral triangle below, referred to as the TRIAD OF HEALTH.

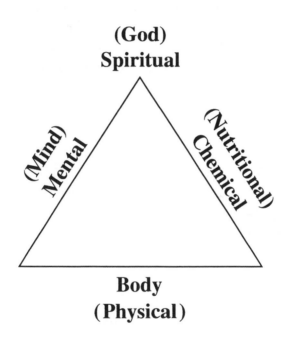

(God)
Spiritual

Body
(Physical)

When we violate the laws of nature

The problems of society, including our epidemic of poor health, stem from a violation of natural laws. We poison our environment. We poison our soil and food with chemical pesticides and fertilizers. We poison our bodies with unnatural foods, contaminated air, and toxic substances that include the medicines we are prescribed. We poison our minds with violent films. We overwork and don't rest enough, violating nature's most fundamental principle of balanced rest and activity. All such violations cause stress and imbalances in our individual bodies and in the body of society. The result is ''dis-ease'' — a sick body, a sick society.

Long ago, conventional medicine adopted the germ theory of Louis Pasteur and established a treatment dogma aimed at the annihilation of germs through powerful pharmaceuticals. The same dogma was applied later to cancer. They pour on the heavy artillery of toxic drugs to kill the bacteria, or kill the cancer cells. Of course they kill a lot of healthy tissue and poison other systems in the body in the process. The result is what we call side effects. Just like the original disease itself, side effects also maim and kill.

Interestingly, Pasteur, later in his career saw the mistake in his germ theory. He declared that germs do not cause disease unless the organism is in a weakened state. "The germ is nothing," he said, "the terrain is everything." The terrain is your body. Is it strong? Is it weak?

The pharmaceutical-based system is still locked in the germ mentality. That's where the money is. Looking for silver bullets that never come. Developing stronger drugs to kill the symptoms but never help to build up the terrain.

Alternative medicine is based on improving the terrain, that is, correcting and strengthening the entire body so that it is less vulnerable to the germs and imbalances that lead to malfunction and disease. In my practice, I achieve this by correcting misalignments in the spine, identifying and eliminating hidden food allergies, using nutritional supplements and homeopathy, and cleaning out toxic intestinal tracts. Our attempt is to bring an individual more into balance and harmony with the laws of nature that govern good health.

Daniel D. Palmer, D.C., the founder of modern chiropractic, wrote in great detail about the mind/body connection, the interplay between physical, chemical and mental influences. He described how vertebral subluxations (misaligned spinal vertebrae) block the flow of energy and messages in our nervous systems, which in turn lead to disease and loss of vitality.

Palmer referred to the field of energy within us as "innate intelligence." This, he said, was connected to a universal intelligence, another term perhaps for the laws of nature. The conduits for this "life force" are the spinal column and nervous system. Our "Innate Intelligence," or simply "Innate," as he called it, organizes our body into the miraculously complex, adapting, and growing organism that it is. Without this intelligence we would become "dust blowing in the wind," he said.

Doctors of chiropractic are uniquely trained to recognize the existence of this flow of natural intelligence within our bodies and to carefully evaluate each side of the delicate triad of health to determine a connection to health problems. We are trained to treat the "total person."

Structure: How misalignments lead to a malfunctioning nervous system

A nurse suffering from excruciating migraines was once brought to my office. She had to lay down in the back seat of a friend's car and then be carried into the clinic. She had had headaches for 30 consecutive days. She was totally disabled. If she sat up she vomited.

We did X-rays that revealed nothing significant. I then proceeded with a physical examination of her spine. At the first vertebra in her neck I found a misalignment. I adjusted her. She came back the next day the same way she came the first day — horizontal. I performed another adjustment. She returned again the third day. When I opened the door of the treatment room, there she sat with a big smile.

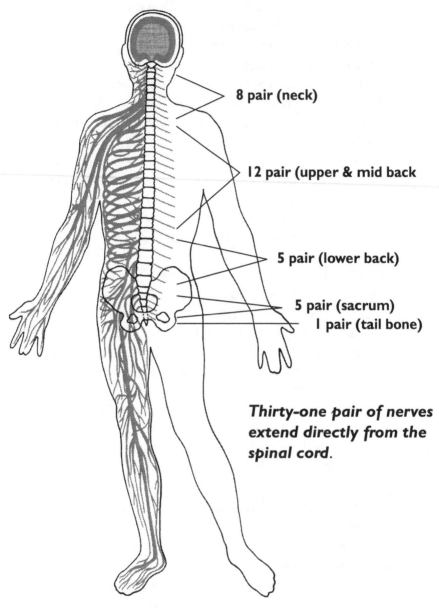

8 pair (neck)

12 pair (upper & mid back

5 pair (lower back)

5 pair (sacrum)
1 pair (tail bone)

Thirty-one pair of nerves extend directly from the spinal cord.

"The headache's gone," she said. "I can stand, sit, walk. I don't throw up. I'm fine."

The point of this story — and of many of the case histories you will read in this book — is that structure affects function in the body. In this woman's case, the constant pressure of a slight misalignment in her cervical (neck) spine was enough to interfere with the nervous system communications and energy flow and cause constant daily migraines. By readjusting and repositioning her neck, we removed the "glitch" in the nervous system and allowed her body to heal naturally.

To be healthy, you need a healthy functioning nervous system. The nervous system controls and coordinates the entire body.

The nervous system is comprised of the brain, the spinal column and spinal nerves. Up at the top, the brain is protected by the skull. Flowing down from the brain is the spinal cord of nervous tissue, sort of like the cables inside the walls of your house that contain the electrical wiring. Your main "electrical cord" extends down a central spinal column of 24 flexible bones, called vertebrae, to your tailbone. The column protects the spinal cord. All along the spine, between each vertebra, nerves branch out, just like a tree, to control and coordinate the muscles and organs of the body. The brain sends messages down the spinal cord and out to the organs, muscles and cells. Those body parts, in turn, send messages back to the spinal cord and from there back to the brain. It's a complete and wondrous communication system with feedback loops that we are only beginning to understand.

Starting with birth, and continuing through life, there are many ways the spinal structure can become disturbed. Trauma is an obvious way, but only just one way. Emotional, and nutritional stresses can also cause the vertebrae to misalign. A slight misalignment of one or more vertebrae is often enough to trigger malfunctions in the nervous system. In chiropractic, we often use the term misalignment or subluxation interchangeably. They mean the same.

Pain is just one of many possible symptoms

You might think that if your neck or back are misaligned you will have neck pain or back pain. That may or may not happen. Pain is really not the primary sign that your spine is out of line. This is one of the great misunderstandings about chiropractic.

The fact is that loss of energy and function, not pain, are the primary signs or symptoms of a mechanical misalignment. The specific purpose of chiropractic is to reposition or realign the vertebrae, or recreate motion where the vertebrae are locked, and allow the innate intelligence, the intelligence that made your body, now flow again to heal it and maintain it in a normal manner. We call this homeostasis.

One person with a spinal subluxation, like the nurse with the migraines, may have head or neck pain. Another may have back pain. Another with a subluxation in the same place may not have any pain at all, but rather a "silent complaint," that is, the blocked energy has impacted their digestive, reproductive, cardiovascular, immune or other systems.

The blockages can manifest in many ways:
- *arthritis*
- *headaches*
- *blurred vision*
- *ringing in the ears*
- *dizziness*
- *difficulty learning or concentrating, and mental "fog"*
- *chronic recurrent colds and sore throats*
- *ear infections*
- *cardiac irregularity*
- *chest pain that has nothing to do with your heart*
- *high blood pressure*
- *digestive upsets*
- *irritable bowel syndrome and ulcerative colitis*
- *ulcers*

The list may surprise you...and it is only a partial list. You may be surprised because you have been led to believe that chiropractic manipulation is solely a treatment for neck or back pain. But that narrow view is far from the truth, as you will learn as you read on.

Chiropractic physicians see the damage caused by a misaligned spine on a daily basis. I have been treating the misalignments for more than 20 years. If you could stand next to me during a typical day in my clinic you would be amazed at the variety of conditions that are related, either in part or in whole, to structural misalignments of the spine. From all that I have witnessed, I have come to regard misalignments as "silent robbers of health." They do so much more than just create back or neck pain.

If you could stand with me in my clinic and watch what goes on you would also be amazed at the remarkable effect that adjustments have on patients, many of whom have spent years on the medical treadmill, seen multiple specialists, taken drug after drug, and who have almost given up because they haven't been helped.

The role of spinal misalignment as a cause of unwellness is vastly unrecognized. Remember: the nervous system controls the entire body. If there is a misalignment in the bony structure that protects this system, you have the potential for many things to go wrong in the body. This is what is so missed. The structure-function connection. Your body is a structure. When something is out of line in that structure, things go wrong.

One day soon, I hope, people will realize this simple fact of life. I foresee a day when people will go to a chiropractor for a spinal checkup, just as you go to a dentist periodically to have your teeth checked. We aren't there yet. But I hope it will be sooner than later. It makes sense to treat our nervous system with at least as much respect as we treat our teeth. It could save a great deal of misery.

At this point I would like to invite you take the Chiropractic Challenge Test on the following page, as a measurement of possible mechanical stress that may be contributing to health problems.

The chemical-nutrition influence

The second part of the "Triad of Health" is the chemical/nutritional component. Healthy body chemistry requires a balanced interplay between our genetics, environment and diet.

Our genetic inheritance provides a basic blueprint for our lives and health, yet does not, in most cases, exert a rigid biological "dictatorship" on our existence. What we do and how we live has a great influence on our quality and span of life.

Many individuals feel doomed or limited by their genes. This is, in my opinion, a myopic view of human life that has been promoted by some medical geneticists.

Often we hear both health professionals and lay persons speak in terms of "family histories" of cancer, diabetes, heart disease or mental illness. For many, receiving a diagnosis along with the knowledge of a family history of disease is like receiving a "death sentence." Doomed, distraught and depressed, many people give up and begin to "live out" this misguided, self-fulfilling prophecy. There are even women who have their breasts removed "preventively" because of a family history of breast cancer. They fail to consider why breast cancer happens in the first place, that is, the nutritional factors and environmental toxins that have been shown to increase their risk.

I believe, as do other althernative practitioners, that although you may have a genetic susceptibility for a specific disease, and that there may be an incidence of that disease in your family, you can reduce your risks by lifestyle and dietary changes, overcoming nutritional deficiencies, and

CHIROPRACTIC

Scoring:	Good 0 pts	Fair 5 pts	Poor 10 pts
HEAD	Head erect gravity line passed directly through cente	Head twisted or turned to one side slightly	Head twisted or turned to one side markedly
SHOULDERS	Shoulders level horizontally	One shoulder slightly higher than other	One shoulder markedly higher than other
SPINE	Spine Straight	Spine slightly curved laterally	Spine markedly curved laterally
HIPS	Hips level horizontally	One hip slightly higher	One hip markedly higher
ANKLES	Feet pointed straight ahead	Feet pointed out	Feet pointed out markedly Ankles sag in pronation

Interpretation:

A score between 0-25 is suggestive of mild spinal stress with a low health impact. A score of 25-50 indicates moderate spinal stress often linked to early loss of function and intermittent pain. From 50-75 indicates severe spinal stress often associated with acute pain and organic illness. Finally, a score of 75-100 suggests complicated health conditions,

CHALLENGE TEST

Scoring: **Good 0 pts**   **Fair 5 pts**   **Poor 10 pts**

NECK

Neck Erect Chin in Head in balance directly above shoulders

Neck slightly forward. Chin slightly out

Neck markedly forward. Chin markedly rounded

UPPER BACK

Upper back normally rounded

Upper back slightly more rounded

Upper back markedly rounded

TRUNK

Trunk erect

Trunk inclined to rear slightly

Trunk inclined to rear markedly

ABDOMEN

Abdomen flat

Abdomen protruding

Abdomen protruding and sagging

LOWER BACK

Lower back normally curved

Lower back slightly hollow

Lower back markedly hollow

susceptibility to chronic illness, and disabling problems.

The Chiropractic Challenge Test does not replace the need for a direct chiropractic examination by a skilled professional. Only a chiropractic physician can determine if you have a structural misalignment.

chiropractic treatment to correct structural defects. You overcome genetic predisposition. You put yourself in control. You make yourself healthier.

This contemporary concept was developed more than 30 years ago by the late Roger Williams, Ph.D., a great scientist and pioneer of nutritional medicine at the University of Texas. He called his idea the "genetrophic theory of disease."

Williams postulated that people often become ill because their unique genetic makeup and need for specific nutrients were not being met by their diet or lifestyle. Such unmet needs could result in a variety of conditions, such as coronary heart disease, stroke, cancer, diabetes, high blood pressure, rheumatoid and arthritic disease, colitis and even certain psychiatric illnesses, he felt.

Williams used the term "biochemical individuality" to describe the unique nutritional and lifestyle needs each of us have. His studies demonstrated the wide variance among people and families in the anatomical size, shape and position of their organs. Since no two individuals have the same fingerprints or dental records, why should we expect their nutritional requirements to be the same?

Two Canadian physicians — Abram Hoffer, M.D., and Humphrey Osmond, M.D. — saw how this biochemical individuality related to mental illness. They pioneered the field of orthomolecular psychiatry, discovering that certain types of schizophrenia and depression responded to megadoses of vitamin therapy, especially B-3 and B-6. Reduced dosage of those nutrients would reinstitute the original complex of symptoms. The patients who responded, in other words, had imbalances in their individual biochemistry that could be corrected by specific nutrients.

Over the years, patients have told me of their concern about a family history of schizophrenia or depression. What they may have instead is a family history of eating bad food.

Research by George Watson, Ph.D., author of the best-selling book "Nutrition and Your Mind" (Harper & Row), goes deeply into the role of biological individuality and its relationship to brain function and mood. He identified different "psychochemical types," each requiring specific nutritional input to the brain. Without the individually correct amount of the right molecules, so to speak, the mind functions less than optimally. Providing the right food, the correct nutritional supplements, and optimum dosage, results in significant enhancements of mood, behavior, and emotional balance, according to Watson. This idea was also popularized by Linus Pauling.

Consider what happens to our bodies and our own unique biological individuality in the face of the notorious American diet. Some call it SAD for short — the standard American diet. Yes, it can be said that the way we eat may stress our bodies to death, and certainly helps account for the epidemic of poor health in this country.

As long ago as 1978, in a report entitled "Diet and Killer Diseases" compiled by the U.S. Senate Select Committee on Nutrition and Human Needs, the country's leading health experts concluded that the average American diet is responsible for the development of chronic degenerative diseases. Little has changed. We don't eat any better now than before.

In the past 60 years, Americans have shifted away from an agrarian culture that relied largely on fresh organic foods to a nutrient-poor and fiberless, processed diet.

Today, we consume on average 125-135 pounds of sugar per year and guzzle 220 cans of soda pop per person! We eat much more fat of all kinds now than we did at the beginning of the 1900s.

When you put it all together — empty calories, little fiber, too much animal protein and fat — you have discovered a primary reason for oncoming generations of unhealthy, nutritionally-deficient Americans experiencing varying degree of fatigue, confusion, headaches, stomach upsets, back pain, depression, poor resistance, low sex drive and a general sense of "I just don't feel well."

This loss of vitality and sense of well being is further compromised by poor air and water quality. A Greek philosopher once said that in order for a society to sustain itself it must have pure air, pure water and pure food. For sure, we don't have them. We have air pollution, pesticides and herbicides, chemical dumping, toxic metals, and water laced with parasites and toxins. Can we sustain ourselves on this? Already large numbers of mammals throughout the world are being poisoned, their ranks decimated by man's violations of natural law. Biodiversity on a global scale is being severely threatened.

For us, there is handwriting aplenty on the wall. But is anybody reading? According to a 1995 report from the Department of Health and Human Services, environmental toxins are responsible for 14 percent of annual deaths in America. A 1996 study by the Natural Resources Defense Council, a Washington D.C. environmental group, found that air pollution kills 64,000 Americans a year — a higher death than for auto accidents.

Pharmaceutical drugs, as I have already discussed, are not the cure-alls they have been touted to be and, in fact, contribute to chemical imbalances and new, often serious problems.

Most experts now agree that degenerative diseases such as heart disease, cancer, diabetes, and arthritis have nothing to do with germs. It's all about the terrain and how the lifestyle we lead contributes to premature aging, the early onset of illness, or a healthy body and mind. Smoking, drinking, recreational or prescription drugs, poor diet, air and water pollutants represent "chemical stressors" that can tip the triad of health in an unfavorable way leading to disease.

Developing a healthy lifestyle through proper nutrition, supplementing your diet with the correct and optimum nutritional supplements, and avoiding drugs, whenever possible, is a wise course of action. You may not be able to control what's out there in the environment. You can, however, take control over what you put into your body in order to keep your defense system at maximum effectiveness.

The mental-emotional Influence

The third part of the triad of health is the mental or emotional component. All of us become emotionally upset at one time or another. Some of us more than others. Emotional health, in fact, involves the recognition and expression of your emotional state, whatever it is at a given time.

Research in psychology has demonstrated that certain personality types express emotions differently. For instance, a type A personality is a person with an unrealistic sense of time urgency, an overly high set of expectations or goals, and a sense that the world is moving too fast for him or her. This personality type has an increased risk of heart attack and stroke.

The type B personality on the other hand has the tendency not to worry about time, be a procrastinator, and be less upwardly motivated. This individual has greater problems with intestinal disorders, low blood pressure and cancer.

From just these two examples of personality types you can readily understand the interaction between the mind and the body — the so-called mind/body connection. In reality, there is no separation between the you. You are not a mind and a body. You are really a mind/body entity. The two parts are not separated as some would have us believe. Every thought and emotion has a corresponding effect on the body and the body's stresses and reactions to outside conditions have a corresponding effect on the body. There are countless feedback loops between the two that bind them into a whole. What the mind perceives, the body feels, and what the body feels, the mind adjusts to.

This intimate relationship is being deeply studied by many scientists, including Candace Pert, a former National Institute of Mental Health researcher and now a research professor at Georgetown University. Her investigations are focused on neuropeptides, short strings of amino acids that cause physiological reactions when they lock into receptor sites located on the cell membranes of all the cells in the body.

In 1985, Pert and several other scientists published a pivotal paper in the Journal of Immunology describing how peptides constitute the biochemical foundation of a body-wide communication network triggered by emotions.

Pert believes emotions run every system of your body and govern the traffic of neuropeptides that dictate the state of the physiology, health, and the tendency toward disease. This is not a brain-centered system where the process starts in the mind and then trickles down to the body. The reality is "so weird," she says, "that after nearly 20 years of studying this she has only recently come to believe in it and experience it." The reality is that emotions are not limited to the head, but rather there is intelligence in every cell of the body. Every single cell has receptors on it. The emotional energy comes first and then peptides are released all over, not just in the brain or nervous system. Thus, she says, consciousness precedes and creates matter.

Her ideas find resonance in ancient philosophies, where wise men throughout the ages have always said that matter is secondary to consciousness. Her investigation explores the new field of quantum medicine that promises to "reconcile" Eastern and Western thought. Pert, in a 1990 Time Magazine article, described the inner world of neuropeptides and how they bind to receptors on a cell, beginning a cascade of biomedical effects, including protein synthesis and cell division. "It's like ringing a doorbell. All kinds of reactions happen inside," says Pert. The peptides, she says, are the "biochemical units of emotion." Exhilaration triggers certain neuropeptides, depression sets off others.

This is fascinating stuff: how we function down at the cellular level. You can begin to see how a stressed life can lead to distress and thus throw the triad of health out of balance. You can envision how emotions such as hate, fear, anger, anxiety, depression and jealousy can build up to toxic levels and create disturbance within our mind/body being and sow the biochemical seeds of disease. And you can also begin to understand how developing and encouraging the emotions of love, compassion, friendship, harmony and peace can promote the biochemistry of well-being.

The impact of stress

Stress comes in many forms. It can be psychological, nutritional, chemical or physical. It can come from anxiety, fear, overwork, surgery or its nature, has effects down at the neuropeptide level and many other levels.

The late Hans Selye, M.D., perhaps the greatest authority on stress in the 20th century, formulated what he called the "General Adaptation Syndrome," a description of how we humans experience a stressful reaction.

The first stage, he said, is the alarm reaction, which is a "call to arms" by our bodies. Here is when the nervous system recognizes a stressor and triggers your pituitary (master gland) to activate your adrenal gland (commonly called the stress gland). Your adrenal begins to "prepare" or "alarm" your body by producing extra adrenaline and cortisone. Your heart rate and pulse quicken. Your breathing becoming irregular. Your mouth gets dry. Your hands and feet become colder. You get butterflies in the stomach.

Your body then prepares you for the second, or resistant, stage of stress, also known as the "fight or flight stage." This is present whenever the stress is strong or prolonged. Your adrenals actually grow in size as you try to resist or flee the stressor. The third and final stage involves recovery in which the stressor is removed or neutralized and your body returns to homeostasis. However, if the stress is strong enough or long enough, this stage can become overwhelmed by exhaustion. In such cases, there is often an accompanying dizziness, anxiety, nervousness, low resistance and low sex drive. It may be associated with complex medical conditions, especially arthritis, ulcers, colitis, asthma, allergies, skin diseases, sinusitis, and most immune diseases.

Let's see how you stand on the stress scale. The following Stress Indicator Questionnaire, a classic test developed in 1967 by University of Washington researchers Thomas Holmes and Richard Rahe, assigns scores to different stressful events.

Here's how to do it: think of what has happened top you in the past year as you read through the list. When you encounter events that have affected your life, write down the associated value in the score column. When you finish, total the numbers in the score column.

Interpretation:

If your total score is 300 points or above, it indicates you are under heavy stress and you have a greater than 50 percent probability of being hospitalized during the next year.

If you total between 150 and 300 points, you are under moderate stress and have a 30 percent probability of being ill enough to miss work in the next year.

If your total is 100 or less, there is no indication stress is adversely affecting you.

THE STRESS INDICATOR QUESTIONNAIRE

Life event	Point Value	Score
Death of spouse	100	_____
Divorce	73	_____
Marital separation	65	_____
Jail term	63	_____
Death of close family member	63	_____
Personal injury or illness	53	_____
Marriage	50	_____
Fired at work	47	_____
Marital reconciliation	45	_____
Retirement	45	_____
Change in health of family member	44	_____
Pregnancy	39	_____
Sex difficulties	39	_____
Gain of new family member	39	_____
Business readjustment	38	_____
Change in financial state	37	_____
Death of close friend	36	_____
Change to different kind of work	35	_____
Change in number of arguments with spouse	35	_____
Mortgage over $10,000	31	_____
Foreclosure of mortgage or loan	30	_____
Change in responsibility at work	29	_____
Son or daughter leaving home	29	_____
Trouble with in laws	29	_____
Outstanding personal achievement	28	_____
Wife begins or stops work	26	_____
Change in living conditions	25	_____
Revision of personal habits	24	_____
Trouble with boss	20	_____
Change in work hours or conditions	20	_____
Change in residence	19	_____
Change in recreation	19	_____
Change in church activities	18	_____
Change in social activities	17	_____
Mortgage or loan less than $10,000	17	_____
Change in sleeping habits	16	_____
Change in number of family get-togethers	15	_____
Change in eating habits	15	_____
Vacation	13	_____
Christmas	12	_____
Minor violations of the law	11	_____
	TOTAL	_____

Stress is a necessary ingredient that stimulates each of us to reach our potential. But excess stress is linked with all diseases including cancer. That's when stress becomes distress. But it doesn't have to happen to you. **STRESS DOES NOT HAVE TO BECOME DISTRESS.** There are many measures you can take in your life to reduce stress and protect your health. This book will help you learn how.

The bottom line — obedience to God's spiritual and natural laws

Overlaying the triad of health is the spiritual component of life. If all sides of the triangle are in balance then we can more readily align ourselves with our spiritual nature (God). We become in harmony with His laws of nature that govern existence.

Since one of the primary distinguishing factors between man and animal is our ability to reflect, humans of all levels of accomplishment and pursuits have searched for the meaning of life. We have the unique ability to ask "who am I," "how did I get here," and "where am I going." This process endows us with fundamental choices — to do good or to do evil, to destroy or to transform. We talk of Peace on Earth and it does exist in the hearts of men. But there is also destruction on earth, and destructive tendencies in the hearts of men. Each person has the seeds of both within.

We see in our culture today the evolution of technology and the potential for nuclear meltdown or destruction through environmental poisoning. How is it then that we can achieve balance and live in harmony and unity? Fundamental to this, it would seem, is the recognition that God is fundamental, innate and supportive of all life.

Happiness and unity will never be achieved through technology, government, laws, religion, or war. True happiness, our intended purpose, will only be achieved through recognition and integration of the basic laws of nature. Since nature is infinitely diverse, then acceptance of each individual's uniqueness and rights is a critical stepping stone in our spiritual unfoldment.

A new century and a new millennium are at hand. To be present at such a great watershed in time should give us pause for reflection. We must think about where we are going. We must think about where we have been. We must learn what we all have in common. And we must learn profoundly who we are.

Prayer and meditation are primary conduits, given to us by God, to remind us of our true nature. Why not utilize God's natural remedies to heal ourselves and others?

How the Gallagher Wellness Program works

Mary Schesler's case

The case of Mary Schesler, 33, a hairdresser from Austintown, Ohio, is indicative of the potential that a wholistic approach offers. I will let her own words describe her transformation to better health:

> **The doctors said "the only thing that would 'cure' me...would be a heart-lung transplant."**

"I was born with a congenital heart problem known as ventricular septal defect as well as with a heart murmur. At the age of nine, I underwent open heart surgery to repair the hole in my heart. Growing up, I had no particular problems. I was able to live a normal life without medication and with very little restrictions. Until 1995.

"I had gone back for my yearly physical and at that time during my routine echocardiogram, the cardiologist found that my pulmonary pressure was elevated significantly from two years prior. Now my pressure was 100 percent higher than normal. As a result of that, I was tired and I wanted to sleep a lot. I was also tired when climbing stairs, dancing, and when doing just everyday activities. I could no longer exercise because I got tired and light headed quickly and at the same time feeling tightness in my chest. I really felt my life was going downhill and I had no energy or ambition to do anything. The doctors told me that the only thing that would 'cure' me for a while would be a heart-lung transplant.

"Right around that time, my father was having some problems and he began seeing Dr. Gallagher on a regular basis, who put my father on a special nutritional diet with supplements. I saw a significant improvement in my father's health and decided I had nothing to lose by trying that myself .

"Dr. Gallagher recommended a nutritional diet and supplements for my specific condition. That was in February 1996. Within two weeks, I felt like a new person. I was able to dance again with no tightness in my chest and hardly any shortness of breath. I feel really good about myself and my outlook on life is brighter. I have a lot of energy.   Before, I used to be so tired that I needed to be in bed by 9 p.m. Now I'm up until 11 p.m. and sometimes even longer without feeling fatigued.

"My diet comprises organic and wholesome foods. I want to continue on this program and am constantly on the lookout for new recipes that are good for my health. Since I started this program, I have been back to my cardiologist for my routine exam and as of today I am stable.

"He said that I look wonderful, that my color is good again and instead of returning in six months, I didn't need to see him for almost a year. "

For more than 20 years, I have been successfully treating patients such as Mary. Thousands of them by now. They often come with not just one but a variety of different chronic health problems. I try to help them with natural remedies and techniques.

Lynn Twaddle's case

One type of patient I frequently encounter is the individual who just never feels good. Our comprehensive approach works remarkably well in these cases. Lynn Twaddle, a 44-year-old house-wife from Salineville, Ohio, was one such patient.

> **She couldn't remember ever feeling good**

Lynn told me that she couldn't remember ever feeling good. Even as a child she was always sick. She suffered from menstrual problems, migraine and sinus headaches and bleeding hemorrhoids. She had under-gone numerous x-rays, CT scans, and taken seemingly a truckload of prescription drugs from Motrin to Percodan. The problems always came back and she was told by her doctors to "learn to live with them."

After evaluating Lynn's situation, we recommended chiropractic adjustments, particularly for the neck and lower back. We prescribed a detox diet to cleanse her body of toxicity and urged her to consume less coffee, sugary foods and refined carbohydrates and shift toward a more wholesome diet. We also put her on a program of herbals, nutritional supplements and exercise (in her case, walking 1 1/2 to 2 1/2 miles a day).

Lynn knew that not all these changes would be easy to swallow, as she put it.

But the effort was well worth it. "I can honestly say I have never felt so good," she told me. "My headaches are few and far between, and the ones I get are not as severe. My menstrual irregularities still continue, but the cramps are not as bad. Perhaps the most notable result has been that the hemorrhoidal bleeding has nearly stopped. In the two months since starting treatment, I have had only three episodes of rectal bleeding and these involved minimal blood loss."

In Lynn's words, "I feel so good that sometimes it's actually scary. When you are so used to feeling bad that you think it is normal. Feeling good, by comparison, is scary for me. I have so much energy I don't know what to do with it. I can actually clean house without a nap. I can walk up stairs without feeling like I am going to pass out. I have experienced nothing but positive changes since switching to this natural approach."

Alice Bevington's case

Many of my patients arrive at my clinic frustrated with so-called conventional treatment of endless pharmaceutical prescriptions that do not resolve the cause of their problems. They are exasperated by the side effects.

> **"More headaches.
> More allergies.
> More pills.
> No relief."**

Alice Bevington, 54, a housewife from Delmont, Pennsylvania, was thoroughly fed up when she came to see me in 1994. Her health problems had begun in her early twenties. Headaches. Colds. Allergies. And typically, onto the drug merry-go-round she went.

"The pills never helped, so I went back again for other pills," she told me. "Eventually I began getting allergy shots which I received weekly for many years. My doctor was a wonderful, caring person but he never really helped me. There was no really noticeable improvement. It was a cycle. More headaches. More allergies. More pills. No relief."

In 1981, Alice was diagnosed with breast cancer and underwent a double mastectomy. For one year after surgery, she followed a difficult course of chemotherapy.

"Now, in addition to headaches and just feeling lousy all the time, I had the problems of menopause and other changes associated with the chemo," she said. "The doctors told me at the time that they couldn't foresee the effects of chemotherapy 15 years down the line."

In 1994, nearly 15 years later, Alice was diagnosed with chronic bladder infections. She still had her daily headaches, often severe and of the migraine type. She was prescribed Fioricet, a drug used in cases of migraine and tension headaches. The potential side effects for this drug include nausea, vomiting, stomach pain, drowsiness, dizziness, lightheadedness, confusion, itching, skin rash, difficulty breathing, and yellowish skin or eyes. Too much of the medication can cause liver damage.

Alice worked her way up to nine tablets before noticing some relief. But her sleep was affected. She developed insomnia.

"I would sleep for a couple of hours, then have to get up for an hour," she told me. "Then sleep a couple of more hours and arise around 4 or 5 a.m., with a headache. I would start the day with three tablets, go back to sleep until 8 a.m., and wake up with a hangover. I went to an allergist for blood tests. He told me I had a deep-seated sinus infection and he put me on amoxicillin for a whole month. I broke out in a rash and showed it to the doctor. He never said anything about a reaction. He gave me some cream for it. I went to another allergist, who did more tests, including one for lupus, which I didn't have, and put me on other medication. I finally reached a point where I said, 'enough is enough. There has to be a better way.'"

Alice said she had heard me on radio and even though she was somewhat skeptical about chiropractors, she thought she would try my program. "I was in bad shape," she said. "I needed to do something."

"All of a sudden," she said, after starting on a chiropractic and nutritional plan, she began feeling better. Her improvement has continued. She hasn't taken a drug since. With our guidance, Alice learned how to take care of her body and pull herself out of a life of suffering and pain.

Mary, Lynn and Alice, as do all of my patients, follow individualized programs designed for their specific situation. Even though these programs are tailored to each patient's needs, there are certain fundamental steps we recommend for most people who come to us interested in overcoming ailments, finding their balance, and achieving optimum health.

The steps are summarized in the following chapters. I invite you to review them and learn how they can help you in your transformation to better health. Each is a tool to get well and stay well. The program has eight steps:

The Gallagher Wellness Program ══════════

Step I	**Detoxification**
Step II	**The "Biotype Diet"**
Step III	**Optimizing Your Digestion**
Step IV	**Food, Chemical and Environmental Sensitivity Identification**
Step V	**Exercise and Conditioning**
Step VI	**Nutritional Rehabilitation**
Step VII	**Relaxation/Stress Management**
Step VIII	**Chiropractic evaluation and manipulation**

CHAPTER SIX

Detoxification – Cleaning up the toxic dump inside you

Karen Smith's case

S t e p

O n e

Karen Smith, 51, an executive secretary from Irwin, Pennsylvania, hadn't been feeling good for weeks. A flu bug, she thought.

Now it was the night before she and her husband were leaving for a summer vacation at Cape

> "Amazingly," she said, "the evening of the first day on the detoxification program I was actually able to sleep without pain for the first time in months."

Cod. During the packing, she became so exhausted that she stopped and decided to finish up early in the morning before departing. In the morning, however, she could hardly get out of bed. She struggled to finish packing and slept through most of the trip.

The vacation turned out to be an ordeal. She started getting cramps. She became constipated. She had continual fatigue.

After returning home, the cramps became severe in her lower abdomen, so bad at times that she was unable to sleep. She developed diarrhea.

Convinced she had a stomach virus, Karen went to see her physician. He prescribed an antibiotic. It did not help. He prescribed another antibiotic. The pain grew worse.

Routine chores and activities became major challenges. She had to rest after even the smallest exertion. It became an effort to perform her daily job. This went on for months.

"One night, I found myself sitting on the edge of my bed clutching my pillow and thinking to myself that I must have a tumor the size of a grapefruit to be in this much pain," Karen said. "I called my gynecologist, who examined me and told me there was no tumor. She said I must see a gastroenterologist. I knew I couldn't get through one more day of pain. I got a prescription for Donnatol, a relaxant."

Karen was on the medical treadmill. She saw several doctors but her problem persisted and even worsened. Nothing was found. In such cases, the level of distress and anxiety accelerated, as it common in such situations. People often become convinced they have cancer or some serious debilitating disease that no one can find.

Karen found her way to our clinic and we were fortunately able to help her. We diagnosed her with colitis and candida (yeast infection). Her painful problems had apparently started months before after she received an antibiotic for a dental problem. She then received other antibiotics for the complaints that started emerging. As a result, she developed an intestinal yeast infection and became intolerant to foods.

We immediately attended to the intestinal chaos. We recommended a 10-day detoxification diet of almost exclusively fruits and vegetables, along with colon cleansing supplements to remove impacted toxins and plaque from the intestines. She also started a beneficial bacteria supplement to restore balance to her intestine. She underwent a deep cleansing of her colon with colonic hydrotherapy.

Karen's condition began to stabilize immediately and reverse. "Amazingly," she said, "the evening of the first day on the detoxification program I was actually able to sleep without pain for the first time in months."

The neglected environment — inside your body

Like many people, Karen's intestinal environment was out of balance.

Environmental issues are of major public concern. We are VERY concerned about the environment we live in. However, we never think about the living environment inside our bodies. We often ignore our inner environment until the alarm of pain and symptoms warns of a problem.

It wasn't always this way. Many ancient natural healthcare systems recommended a seasonal cleansing treatment to eliminate excess wastes collected in the body.

In "A Woman's Best Medicine: Health, happiness and long life through Ayurveda," (Tarcher/Putnam), physicians Nancy Lonsdorf, M.D., and Veronica Butler, M.D., describe how these purification procedures open the bodily channels for optimum functioning of the individual. They point out that these channels allow the flow of our natural biological intelligence. Remember, we talked about the intelligence of the body in the last chapter, intelligence being those laws of nature that govern good health.

The authors describe the purification concept thusly: "If there is an obstruction to the flow of biological intelligence — if some information doesn't arrive where it is needed — part of the body gets cut off from the whole, and this can lay the groundwork for disease: a carcinogen gets trapped in the breast glands, the immune cells cannot reach a virus lodged in the lung tissue, bacteria start to proliferate in the bladder, etc. A biology of disorder caused by blockages takes over the biology of orderliness."

The first step in the Gallagher Wellness Program is purification, or as it is more commonly called, detoxification. Unlike traditional western medicine that focuses on the obliteration of symptoms by the use of drugs, the natural approach strives to cleanse the body and restore balance by "allowing the organism to discharge."

An example of this basic principle is the role of fever in overcoming infections. Although conventional medical doctors prescribe drugs to suppress fever, the elevation of your internal thermostat activates your immune system to naturally fight infection. Mucus secretions, increased urination, diarrhea, sweating, coughing and sneezing are all inborn mechanisms designed to strengthen your body and remove toxins.

Our core program frequently begins with a ten day detox diet. If you follow a standard American lifestyle featuring sugar, white flour, colorings, dyes, pesticides, food additives, soda pop, alcohol, tap water (if you drink water at all!), caffeine, and cigarettes, the cleansing program is a radical shift for your metabolism. If you stick with it, results are profound.

Is your body a toxic waste dump?

Why profound results? Over the years I have found there is a common cause underlying many conditions and symptoms. The cause is something you would never think of yourself. Nor, unfortunately, would your physician. Simply put, your body may be a toxic waste dump, the result of accumulating contaminants and impurities from the air you breath, the food you eat and the liquids you drink. Eventually, this "stuff" reaches a level high enough to interfere with normal functioning. And unless you properly cleanse your body of the toxins, they will continue to build up and increasingly erode your health and vitality.

> "There is only one disease, and that disease is auto-intoxication, the body poisoning itself."
> — V.E. Irons

All of us are toxic to some degree. Others more. Others less. It depends on what we eat and drink, where and how we work, and where we live. Some things we can control. Others we can't.

Marshall Mandell, M.D., a pioneer in environmental illnesses and allergies, believed strongly that many of the conditions he treated were the result of chemical proliferation.

"For hundreds of thousands of years during the course of human development, changes occurred much more slowly in man's natural environment than they do in the rapidly changing chemicalized and polluted world of today," Mandell said. "When organic chemistry began in the 19th century, a whole series of combinations of chemicals were created that were never found naturally in the environment. Pesticides, herbicides, insecticides, waxes, preservatives, colorings, and additives, although they did the jobs they were designed for, they contaminated the environment and filled man's body with residues that were totally alien to the human system."

Add to that the contamination from automotive fuels, jet fuels, and oil and coal burning industries.

"In short," Mandell said, "everything man eats, drinks or inhales is now polluted with chemical agents that are foreign to his bodily chemistry, and he is suffering the consequences of possessing a body that is incapable of handling the byproducts of his amazing chemical technology."

Doris Rapp, M.D., another leading practitioner of environmental medicine, says the problem of chemical proliferation is compounded by the inadequacy of our eating habits.

"Unless our nutrition is good we can't hope to detoxify these things," she says. "But our nutrition has deteriorated over the last half-century and we are no longer the robust, hardy people we used to be. We never had as much cancer as now. We never had Alzheimer's. We didn't see babies you couldn't breast feed. Teachers will tell you they never had the behavioral problems years ago they are now having. The food we eat is processed, pesticided and poor in nutrients. What we drink is full of chemicals. The result is that our bodies have indeed become toxic dump sites."

Any part of the body can become affected, says Rapp. "If you have weakened or damaged areas in the body, those areas or related-functions can be affected. If you have allergies, you'll be more prone to a wide variety of symptoms because you already have a weakened immune system."

The Journal of the American Medical Association has acknowledged that the proliferation of drugs and chemicals used in food, agriculture and industry is so widespread that it is contributing to an alarmingly increasing number of people "who are allergic to everything."

Joseph D. Beasley, M.D., a former professor of population sciences at Harvard University who has thoroughly studied the state of American health, says the problem is so widespread that physicians should approach diagnosis with the assumption that "all patients, regardless of their symptoms, are at risk of environmentally induced sensitivity and toxicity."

Adds Beasley: "Most emerging research and physicians' reports are linking a wide variety of syndromes and symptoms — allergies, rashes, gastrointestinal disorders, fatigue, migraine, 'vague' but persistent complaints, and a number of mental and behavior disorders — to a range of environmental triggers, with increasing evidence that the responses of susceptible patients are neither neat nor predictable."

Now you have an idea why detoxification is so important to me and why it is the first step in my program.

My detox plan is fairly simple.

The 10-day detoxification plan

• *For nine days you eat a diet of raw vegetables and fresh fruits (water fruits are preferable), vegetarian soups, juices, distilled or mineral water (one to two quarts), and herbal teas.*

• *On the tenth — and last — day, you fast with distilled or mineral water (one to two quarts). For 24-hours, you drink water only.*

During this process I recommend a number of different detoxification products designed to clean out the intestines and restore them to good health. They include:

• Colon Cleanse

A unique detoxification product featuring ground psyllium husks and liquid bentonite. Psyllium is hydrophilic (attracts water) and expands ten fold in size in your intestinal tract. Bentonite, a type of clay mined in the western U.S., also swells and has the ability to remove toxins, parasites and yeast colonies out of your colon. The two combine to serve as a powerful intestinal broom.

How to use Colon Cleanse: Add 1 tablespoon each of the psyl-

lium and bentonite to 4-6 ounces of orange juice. Mix. Take before
bedtime.

• *Herb Lax*

A herbal stimulant that increases the motility of the colon, encouraging the removal of encrusted mucus and plaque.

How to use Herb Lax: Take 1-2 tablets before bed.

• *Nutri Tox*

A nutritional supplement that binds and removes toxic metals (such as lead, aluminum, cadmium and mercury) from the body.

How to use Nutri Tox: Take 3 tablets before bed.

• *Nutri Zyme*

A combination of the anti-inflammatory plant comfrey, to soothe the intestinal linings; bromelain, an enzyme from pineapple that aids digestion and combats inflammation; and cabbagin, also known as vitamin U, that acts as a natural gut repair and anti-ulcer factor.

How to use Nutri Zyme: Take 2 capsules after meals 3 times a day.

• *GFS*

A green food supplement high in antioxidants that stimulates the immune system, enhances cellular nutrition, and implants healthy bacteria in the intestine.

How to use GFS: Take 2 capsules after meals three times a day.

Caution: Although this program is safe and effective for most people, it is not for everyone. Individuals with serious health conditions, or who are heavily medicated, should consult a qualified natural health care practitioner before starting. For some people, the program should be undertaken only with medical supervision.

I have witnessed remarkable recoveries from serious illnesses with this program. But often it involves some hard going during the first part of the detox.

Many patients will go through what is called a Herxheimer reaction. This reaction involves withdrawal symptoms created by the rapid release of stored toxins into your bloodstream. This "healing crisis" usually occurs in the first three days of the detox. During that time our office often hears from patients who are having a difficulty time. Detox symptoms include severe headaches, nausea, and flu-like symptoms.

Those with the strongest addictions, particularly to caffeine and sugar, will usually experience the most difficulties. However, once your body dumps the toxins and you pass through the "healing crisis," you will soon start to feel remarkably better.

Invariably, your energy will rise. Chronic pain will diminish or even disappear. Headaches will dissipate. Digestive upsets will stabilize. Skin rashes begin to clear. Overall, you will feel a general sense of well-being and rejuvenation.

This is what patients typically tell me. Some go through light symptoms of detoxifying, others heavier. It just depends on each individual situation and toxicity load.

After the detox

After the 10 day detox, it is very important to follow some basic guidelines so as not to nullify your good effort.

Continue with raw and cooked fruits and vegetables.

Continue with Colon Cleanse.

Gradually over a week's time, you can reintroduce whole grains (such as brown rice, millet, and oats), raw nuts and seeds, as well as starchy fruits (bananas) and vegetables (corn, peas, beans, tofu, and potatoes).

Animal protein and 100 percent whole grain pastas can commence the following week, if indicated.

Drink one to two quarts daily of the best quality water you can obtain. Make this a permanent habit. Water helps clean your system.

Colon Hydrotherapy

For individuals who require more sophisticated detoxification, our office provides colon hydrotherapy. Performed by certified colon therapists, this unique detoxification method removes hardened plaque from the colon through a series of in-office treatments. These treatments often help restore normal stool transit time (12 hours), improve immune function, reduce food and chemical allergies, and a host of other problems.

I was introduced to this unique technique by another chiropractic physician who had become severely ill for unexplained reasons. He began experiencing extreme fatigue, sore throats and swollen lymph glands, and had muscle and joint pain throughout his body. Almost forced to retire from his thriving practice and unable to find the cause after a litany of medical tests, he finally traced his illness to a cleaning agent used by a drapery company at his home the day before the mystery illness began. He subsequently began colon hydrotherapy and completely regained his health and overcame the chemical illness.

A final word

The role of toxicity as a major cause of illness, despite the warnings and evidence, is pretty much ignored by most doctors. Did your doctor ever advise you to clean up the mess inside your body? Instead, you are likely to have received a pharmaceutical prescription — another chemical — to combat a particular symptom. In my opinion, that often just adds more toxicity into the body without getting to the cause of problems.

Without cleansing your body first, even taking vitamins and minerals may be ineffective because of the accumulated toxicity. Most people who are nutritionally-minded concentrate only on what they put into their body and NOT ON WHAT COMES OUT. So inadvertently they are just clogging their insides more. Delivering nutrition to trillions of cells may not be enough unless you dump the garbage first. If you are overflowing with toxicity and you take handfuls of supplements, you may get some help but probably not the big relief you are seeking. Your body utilizes vitamins much more effectively once you detoxify.

I can't really emphasize detoxification enough. You shower or bathe regularly to keep your exterior clean. What have you done for your insides lately?

CHAPTER SEVEN

The Biotype Diet –
Much More Than Just Losing Weight

S t e p

T w o

Just have a look at what people are putting in their supermarket shopping carts or in their mouths at greasy spoons and you can understand — at a glance — why fatigue and poor health are so rampant. Without doubt, the standard American diet (SAD) sets you up for the illness treadmill.

At the turn of the century, only 10 percent of our diet was processed. Today, nearly 90 percent is processed, meaning that most of our food is manufactured, devitalized and chemicalized.

We consume large quantities of "empty calories" — foods that are poor in nutrition, and high in fat and sugar — that drain nutrient reserves from the body to digest the junk.

We eat too much fat, too many wrong kinds of fats, too much salt and refined sugar, and too many chemical additives and contaminants. Along with that we eat too little of what is good for us — fiber, vegetables and fruits, essential nutrients, complex carbohydrates and fresh, unprocessed food.

Nutritional research overflows with studies revealing the consequences of these eating habits. Yet the public at large doesn't seem to be getting the message...or if people do, they don't care.

Too much fat in the diet, for instance, leads not only to a higher incidence of heart disease but also cancer. Studies conducted throughout the world make that amply clear. Neal Barnard, M.D., president of the Physician's Committee for Responsible Medicine, says that "if all environmental risk factors, particularly diet and fat consumption were removed, a woman's risk of breast cancer would be cut by probably 80 percent." Despite much research, he adds, public awareness is "dismal."

Many studies demonstrate the benefits of anti-oxidant compounds, natural chemicals found in vegetables and fruits that can strengthen the immune system and combat disease. But only nine percent of Americans eat enough of these health-giving foods. Research shows that countries with the lowest fruit and vegetable intake are generally in poorer health and have higher rates of cardiovascular disease and cancer.

Avoidance of fruit and vegetables appears to develop early in life. According to the U.S. Department of Agriculture's 1989-91 Continuing Survey of Food Intakes by Individuals, young children consume about one serving of fruit daily and teenagers a half of a serving. Only 20 percent of children eat the recommended five or more servings of fruit and vegetables. The favorite vegetable of youngsters? You guessed it — french fries. Fries account for fully one quarter of their vegetable intake. The consumption of dark green and yellow vegetables, the source of many important nutrients, averages 0.1 to 0.3 servings daily.

The bottom line is that we don't eat enough of the right food and eat too much of the wrong food. There is no doubt that we are an overfed but undernourished nation.

Over-eating — viewed by history

"A full belly makes a dull brain," said Benjamin Franklin.

That's because heavy meals, particularly those high in fat, condemn your body to hours of hard, energy-sapping labor.

Over-eating generates more than just dullness, according to modern and ancient experts alike. It is hazardous to your health.

The words of Maimonides, the great Spanish physician of the 12th century, ring as true today as in his day: "Most maladies afflicting humanity result from bad food or an excess of food that may even have been wholesome."

Consider also these anonymous sayings:

"There are more gluttons in hell than drunkards."

"Eat to live — don't live to eat."

According to the most ancient dietary wisdom known to man, the advice is simple — eat to the point of satisfaction and not to fullness.

Diet and Individuality

Nourishment is the reason for eating. Yet for most people the goal of dietary awareness concerns the struggle to stay thin, the result of a lifetime of media bombardment with the "thin is beautiful" message.

Health depends on what we eat. If we just concentrate on the most nutritious diet our weight would tend to take care of itself, and normalize. Yes, a diet lower in fat is healthier for us. However, a healthy diet is not necessarily a low fat diet. If you fill your low fat diet with "junk" you are not accomplishing much. And this, unfortunately, is often the case. In search of low weight and body fat and reinforced by food advertisers, most people believe low cholesterol, low fat eating is healthy and nutritious. All too often, the low fat diet consists of "fat free" pasta, bread, cakes and other processed foods. Although these "foods" are indeed low in fat, they are usually seriously lacking proper amounts of vitamins, minerals, fiber and enzymes essential for longevity and well being.

In my wellness program, the second step to health is a diet specially designed for each person. I call it the Biotype Diet.

The Biotype diet recognizes the unique genetic and individual nutritional requirements necessary for ideal health. For instance, consider that native Eskimos eat a diet that is among the world's highest in animal fat, yet they have the lowest incidence of heart disease. Certain indigenous tribes, found in Africa, whose diets consist of only raw potatoes and water, have no evidence of western diseases.

Also consider that once the Eskimos began cooking their food and eating more carbohydrates, their rate of heart disease and other "modern diseases" began to accelerate. Similarly, when individuals of African descent move to the U.S., and begin eating the American diet, they develop osteoporosis and other diseases at rates similar to the rest of the population.

Along these same lines, it is interesting to note the discoveries of Weston A. Price, a California dental researcher, who traveled the world during the 1930s and found that native peoples displayed little facial and dental structure degeneration and cavities when they ate their traditional diets. But when they began eating more of a Western, refined diet, there was a rapid appearance of degenerative changes.

The reality is that there is no one single diet ideal for everybody. We are biologically unique, each of us, even though we share many similar characteristics. That is why the 2,500 year old words of Hippocrates are as true today as they were then: "what is one man's feast is another man's poison."

Each person's body type is like an individual blueprint of nature's guidelines on how people should live. By knowing the strong and weak points of our body types and then following the appropriate guidelines, we can achieve balance and optimum health. Diet is one aspect of achieving balance.

For the person who desires to eat healthier and get away from the standard American diet, proper guidance is important. That's why at our clinic we developed a comprehensive and modern approach to optimizing individual diet. First, we incorporate each patient's unique genetic requirements and physical characteristics. Then we conduct tests to determine sensitivities and allergies, digestive strengths and weaknesses, and nutrient shortfalls. Based on this information, we can make individualized recommendations.

In general, the plan reduces the percentage of processed, nutrient-poor food in the diet and accentuates whole foods in the form of raw and cooked vegetables, fruits, grains, nuts, and seeds.

We follow a system of metabolic typing, as formulated by nutritional cancer specialist Dr. William Kelly years ago. The system recognizes ten distinct metabolic classifications of individuals and provides a nutritional prescription for each. These prescriptions can vary from a strict vegetarian diet to one emphasizing animal protein foods.

To get an idea of how this works, following are several examples of Biotype diets we formulate for different patients and conditions:

Biotype diet # 1

• Patients of northern European descent

• Patients with a history of low blood sugar, and who are easily subjected to mood swings, fatigue, irritability, depression and dizziness.

Traditionally, people of northern Europe have eaten a high animal protein and low carbohydrate diet. Both types of people generally respond well to small, frequent meals consisting of meat, eggs, fish, poultry, nuts, seeds and little carbohydrate and dairy. Fruits should be raw, but limited. Grains, such as 100 percent oats and brown rice, can be eaten but on a limited basis. This type of diet tends to stabilize the blood sugar in carbohydrate-sensitive individuals and provide them with more energy and mental clarity.

Biotype diet # 2

• Patients of Indian and Asian descent, whose traditional diet was predominantly vegetarian.

• Patients who suffer from degenerative diseases, especially cancer, heart disease, arthritis, and ailments of the liver and kidneys.

A modified vegetarian diet usually works well for these types of patients. The usual diet overloads and overwhelms the liver and kidneys with animal protein. Medications can damage the ability of these organs to perform their detoxification activities. This plan emphasizes fruits, vegetables, nuts, seeds, and primarily plant-based proteins such as legumes, tofu, and brown rice.

Biotype diet #3

• Certain allergic patients with rheumatoid arthritis, irritable bowel syndrome, ulcerative colitis, depression and even schizophrenia, who have genetic sensitivities to gluten products.

Removal of wheat, rye, oats and barley from the diet will often improve their conditions. Similarly, some may also be sensitive to the nightshade family of vegetables, plants such as peppers, tomatoes, potatoes, and eggplants.

Biotype diet #4

• Patients genetically predisposed to diabetes, who have sensitivity to certain foods and who may be consuming excess animal protein and refined carbohydrates.

This group does well on a high complex carbohydrate diet emphasizing raw fruits and vegetables, plant-based proteins including lentils, kidney beans, black beans, brown rice and tofu. Identification and elimination of food allergies/sensitivities is critical for optimum health.

Optimize your digestion

S
t
e
p

T
h
r
e
e

You are what you eat, they say, which goes a long way to explain why we have such poor health in this country. But there is more to it than just that. The Gallagher Wellness Program takes it much further. We believe you are what you eat, digest, absorb and eliminate.

If you look at current statistics and illness trends, you see that the average American suffers from some form of digestive affliction. Stomach ulcers, reflux, constipation, hiatal hernia, irritable bowel syndrome, diverticulitis, colitis, parasite and yeast infections and intestinal cancers of all types abound in our society.

By and large, we do these things to ourselves by what we eat and how we eat, and then compound our problems on the medical treadmill.

Our digestive tract is a 15-foot long tube that starts at the mouth and ends at the anus. Food enters, gets ground up, churned, broken down by countless chemicals and digestive bacteria, and transformed into small molecular units. Those units are absorbed through the walls of the intestines and into the blood for delivery, as needed, to the tissues of the body. The unused and undigested parts of the food are also processed and eliminated at the far end of the system — the colon. This is how nature designed our digestive system.

A key to ensuring this system works well is fiber, also known as roughage. Man's primitive diet consisted of whole foods, that is, foods containing fiber. The basis of such fare is complex carbohydrates — whole grains, whole grain breads and pasta, seeds, nuts, natural fruits, beans and vegetables. The normal stool transit time of a man living in a primitive society eating these kinds of traditional foods is about 12 hours. Transit time refers to the time it takes from eating to passing the waste products.

Here, in America, it is a different story. We generally eat refined carbohydrates — white bread, white rice, pastry and pasta made with enriched flour, and sweets. On our typical diet, the average transit time is three days! The consequences, in terms of cost and human suffering, is beyond measurement.

Not just important nutrients are missing. Also missing is fiber.
The processing or refinement of food removes the fibrous components of
plant food. Even though this material is not digested by the body and
absorbed, it still plays an essential part in good digestion.

Fiber absorbs moisture, increases in size, gives the intestines something to grip on, makes the stool softer, and acts as a natural laxative.
Fibrous food speeds up bowel transit time and facilitates elimination, thus
providing relief against constipation and reducing intestinal exposure to
cancer-causing chemicals, putrefying food residue and other waste material.

If you could journey into your digestive tract and look with a
microscopic eye at the lining of your intestines you would see what resembles a shag rug landscape. You'd see countless numbers of tiny fingers
— called villi — projecting out toward the middle. Down at the cellular
level on the surface of the villi, the minute components of food that have
been broken down through the digestive process are absorbed through the
lining and into the bloodstream.

If your intestinal tract is unclean, this fundamental process doesn't
work well. The villi can become buried under a growing paste of mucus
and waste products, inhibiting their capacity to absorb nutrients. If the
situation is widespread, a deficiency of nutrients can result and many
toxins become absorbed into the body, resulting in a wide range of both
psychological and physical symptoms.

Autopsy findings

Remember what I said earlier about the toxic waste dump many of
us carry in our intestines? Autopsies often reveal colons to be just that.
The colon is the large intestine where unused food and waste products are
prepared for elimination. According to medical examiners, many colons
are found to be blocked up to 80 percent with waste material! When we
think of blockages in the body we usually think of clogged coronary
arteries. But blockage can occur, and with severe consequences in our
bowels as well.

With our typical diet, an average person may have six to twelve
pounds of food residue in the intestines. Some of this slow moving bulk is
enveloped in layers of mucous that narrow the passageway, or is buried
into the countless folds of the colon lining. The collected material grows,
putrefies, promotes pathogens and a ripe terrain for parasites. Some becomes absorbed into the bloodstream to trigger toxic effects elsewhere in

the body. No wonder it is often said that "death begins in the colon."

A diet rich in fiber solves the problem. In our clinic we strongly recommend that our patients eat a diet of whole foods rich in fiber. Over the years, I have learned that an ounce of fiber is worth a pound of any cure — or a ton, for that matter. It's such a simple tool for good health because it acts like an internal broom to keep the intestinal environment clean and the digestive process moving.

It's simple and proven by time.

Back 2,500 years ago, Hippocrates was telling his ailing countrymen, "You people, complaining of your health, should pass large and bulky motions after every meal, and that to ensure this, you should eat abundantly of whole meal bread, vegetables and fruits..."

Fiber worked then. It works now. Many physicians tell their patients to eat more of it in their diets. Alas, the incidence of bowel dysfunction in our society indicates that few people are listening.

In America, the consumption of fiber-containing fruit and vegetables has dropped about 20 percent since the turn of the century. Intake from whole grains has dropped in half. A 1987 study by the National Cancer Institute indicated that Americans consume about 12 grams of fiber a day, a figure "considerably lower" than even previously thought. Compare that to the 20-35 grams recommended by the American Dietetic Association and you get an idea of why we have such widespread digestive disorders.

During the 1970s, Denis P. Burkitt, M.D., determined through years of research that native, rural Africans rarely suffered from intestinal disease because their traditional diets contained 25 to 30 grams of fiber daily. The renown British physician contended that our Western diet, lacking adequate fiber, was the reason we experience a growing incidence of intestinal disorders.

Diverticular disease was rare before 1900. Today, it is the most common illness of the colon, and especially affects people over age 50. Abram Hoffer, M.D., a Canadian expert on nutrition, says this disease is still "very rare among people who still eat a high-fiber diet, but its incidence goes up quickly when they adopt our low-fiber, sugar-rich diet."

In diverticulitis, the typically small, hard stools of a fiberless diet pass with difficulty through the intestines. We strain our intestinal muscles, creating repeated pressure that over time produces sac-like herniations in the inside lining of the lower colon. These sacs become filled with fecal matter and over time, similar to an appendix, develop swelling, inflammation and pain. A high fiber diet is now widely used in the treatment of this condition.

Toxins that build up in the intestines are a danger to the whole body. That's because they can become absorbed into the bloodstream. This danger was apparent in a study of 1,481 women at the University of California. Among the group, individuals with severe constipation tended to have abnormal cells in the fluid extracted from their breasts, suggesting that these women had an increased risk of cancer.

The art of eating

Optimum digestion depends not just on what you eat but how you eat as well. Earlier I talked about emotions and how they affect health. Emotions also affect digestion.

In a 1987 study at Temple University's School of Dentistry, researchers reported that deep relaxation appeared to be the single-most important factor contributing to optimum digestion and subsequent absorption of complex carbohydrates, the most important food for high energy. Participants in the study attained deep relaxation through prayerful meditation.

When deep relaxation was combined with thorough chewing, the process of digestion was enhanced even more.

Throughout the ages, families have sat down to eat and expressed gratitude for their food. In addition to the spiritual nature of this ritual, there appears also to be a digestive benefit as well. The moment of silence or thanksgiving serves to calm the nervous system, which in turn allows a more efficient digestion and absorption process to take place.

You don't have to do relaxation techniques to get into a properly calm eating state, but think for a moment how your eating environment and activities may interfere with digestion.

Do you sit down to eat?

Do you eat while working or discussing business? Or reading or watching television? By not paying attention to what you are eating, you are very likely to overeat and underchew.

Underchew?

I'll bet nobody ever advised you about the importance of chewing. Maybe your mother did when you were a kid. But you probably didn't pay attention.

Chewing is a fundamental mechanical act that grinds mouthfuls down into smaller, more digestible pieces while at the same time mixing the food with saliva. The saliva contains enzymes which begin breaking down the food, particularly carbohydrates and starches, and lubricates the mix for a smooth drop down into the stomach. It is also here in the oral cavity that your body recognizes whether food is friend or foe by "tagging" the food with specific antibodies to enhance utilization. As the chewing starts, the stomach begins to produce its own lubricating and breakdown juices that further enhance the digestive process.

The late Arthur L. Kaslow, M.D., a nutritionally-oriented California physician, always asked his patients about their eating habits and found that if they weren't busy talking, they were often reading or watching TV. In short, not paying much attention to chewing.

Kaslow determined there was a strong connection between improper chewing and indigestion, gas, constipation and diarrhea. He even developed a special stool examination that could tell, among other things, if a person chewed well or not.

"What we often find are incompletely digested food particles and evidence of improper chewing," he said in a magazine interview. "These people usually have a lot of gas, a lot of bowel problems, a lot of difficulties, and they may even be in what we call secondary malnutrition. They may be taking good food into their mouth but don't get good nourishment out of it.

"I tell these people that I can take care of your digestion, I can give you digestive enzymes, I can take care of the gas-forming bacteria, but nobody else but you can take care of the chewing. That's your job and nobody else can do it for you."

The message is clear. Get your digestion off to a good start. Chew!!!!

Trouble in the tummy

After swallowing, your liquefied food drops down the esophageal tube and into your stomach where it gets an acid bath. Hydrochloric acid (HCL) is a critical part of the digestive process. The acid prepares food for absorption in the small intestine — the next stage of digestion — by breaking down protein and acidifying food.

If you have insufficient HCL or too much of it, you have trouble in the tummy.

Too little HCL (hypochlorhydria):

It's common. As we age, HCL production diminishes. Up to 40 percent of adults are, in fact, deficient and asthmatic children are frequently short, too. Ten percent of all people have no stomach acid at all.

Signs of HCL deficiency include bloating, heavy full feelings, constipation and diarrhea. Many autoimmune and chronic health conditions are now associated with low HCL, including cancer, diabetes, rheumatoid arthritis, adult acne, osteoporosis, food and chemical allergies, thyroid disorders, skin problems, lupus, yeast infections, and chronic fatigue syndrome. Up to 80 percent of all gallbladder disease cases involve deficiencies. Inflammatory and irritable intestine conditions may also result.

When protein isn't broken down adequately in the stomach, large protein molecules enter in the small intestine and then pass into the bloodstream. Instead of entering as sand particles, so to speak, they come in as stones. They are treated as foreign proteins and trigger a variety of allergic, inflammatory and irritating reactions throughout the body, depending on an individual's weaknesses.

Too much HCL (hyperchlorhydria):

Now you have a situation where the stomach produces too much acid, often resulting in stomach or duodenal (small intestine) ulcers. You experience heartburn, burning or pain over the stomach, intense hunger sometimes relieved by eating, and pain when laying down or in the middle of the night.

Major contributors to excess HCL include low fiber and high fat diets, milk, carbonated beverages, fried foods, chocolate caffeine, sugar, alcohol, smoking, aspirin, non-steroidal anti-inflammatory drugs (NSAIDs) and many other pharmaceuticals. A type of bacterium, called heliobacter pylori, has been found in the stomach lining of a majority of ulcer patients.

The conventional medical approach to ulcers varies: antacids, bland diets, surgical cutting of the cranial nerve that controls acid production, stomach surgery, anti-ulcer drugs such as Tagamet, Zantac, Prilosac, and antibiotics. Although some of these approaches can be effective on short-term basis, relapses frequently occur along with multiple side effects. I will be talking more about this in the ulcer chapter, and also detail how we treat the problem.

The HCL Test — What's your HCL level?

Many of my patients perform this hydrochloric acid challenge test below to determine whether they have insufficient HCL and need to supplement. If you have allergies, malabsorption problems, chronic fatigue, yeast infections, adult acne, this is a particularly useful test. There is a good chance you are deficient. If you are older, too, it is likely you may not be producing enough HCL.

1. To perform the test you need to purchase HCL tablets at your favorite health food store. Begin by taking one tablet or capsule containing 10 grains (600 milligrams) of hydrochloric acid with your next large meal. The hydrochloric acid should be bound to betaine or glutamic acid. Betaine hydrochloride is a popular supplement. The formation should also include at least 150 milligrams of pepsin, another gastric secretion important to digestion.

2. Pay attention to any side effects you may feel. Do you have gas, a burning sensation or pain? If there are no side effects or aggravation of symptoms, begin increasing your dose. This indicates a deficiency. At every meal of the same size after that, increase your dose by one more tablet or capsule. For instance, increase by one at the next meal, two at the meal after that, then three at the next meal.

3. Continue to increase the dose until you feel a warmth in your stomach, or other side effects. Do not use more than seven tablets. A feeling of warmth in the stomach means that you have taken too many tablets for that meal. If you have this sensation, take one less tablet for the next meal of that size. It is a good idea to try the larger dose again at another meal to make sure that it was the HCL that caused the warmth and not something else.

4. Once you have found the largest dose that you can take at your large meals without feeling any warmth, maintain that dose at all meals of similar size. (You will need to take less with smaller meals.)

5. When taking a number of tablets or capsules, it is best to take them throughout the meal, and not in one swallow.

6. Supplementation sometimes restores the ability to produce the amount of HCL needed to properly digest food. The sign of this quiet healing will be the warm feeling in your stomach. When you feel this, cut the dosage. Continue to reduce according to the degree of your stomach's regained ability.

Are your intestines breaking down food or breaking down?

From the stomach, food continues its digestive journey and moves on to the small intestine. The major breakdown of foodstuffs takes place here. The food mass is processed into basic components for absorption into the bloodstream and nourishment of the tissues. Those components are vitamins, minerals, fatty acids, sugars, and proteins.

Among the chief chemical ingredients secreted into the small intestine for food processing are bile, made in the gall bladder, and enzymes, made in the pancreas. The production of these substances normally slows down with age, but can also be affected by poor diet, viruses, and drugs. Just as with insufficient HCL, insufficient bile and enzymes lead to problems. Among them may be digestive disorders, constipation, diarrhea, malabsorption, systemic toxicity, lower abdominal bloating and pain, respiratory ailments, allergies, arthritis, and cancer.

In our clinic, we use digestive enzymes and bile extract to facilitate absorption.

Is your diet causing gallstones?

Gallbladder disease is so rampant in our culture that even 15-year-old American teenagers often show evidence of gallstones on radiographic studies. Could that be in part a result of excessive consumption of sugary sweets and soda pops? Nutritional researchers have found that sugar intake increases cholesterol synthesis in the body and the risk of gallstone formation.

A half-million Americans undergo gallbladder surgery every year even though their difficulties are largely avoidable or treatable with natural remedies. Most cases of gallbladder problems are not caused by gallstones, rather they are generated by "SAD eating," the standard American diet loaded with sugar, fat and fiberless food. Food allergies are another source of gallbladder difficulties. The removal of the gallbladder is unnecessary and can often lead to more complicated digestive problems.

Who is winning your bacterial war?

No discussion of digestion is complete without mentioning the friendly bacteria who colonize our intestines and help keep us healthy. That's right. Bacteria that keep us healthy.

Most of us regard bacteria as dangerous, microscopic lowlife that reproduce wildly and inflict deadly disease on us. However, not all bacteria are disease-producing. Many, in fact, render life-sustaining service to man. The bacterial benefactors that live in our intestines are known as friendly flora or probiotics, a word derived from the Greek which means "for life."

Your intestines may be host to some 400 different species — the most famous of which is lactobacillus acidophilus, the bacterium found in yogurt. Individually, there are billions of bacteria. In return for the space and the food your system provides them, they do great work for you.

It is no understatement to say that you live or die at this microscopic level of existence. And you have lots of energy or little of it depending on who has the upper hand in the intestinal battle of bacteria.

On the one side there are the pathogens, those dreaded bacteria associated with death and disease. They grow strong and spread their toxic influence whenever the body's immune system is weak or whenever the army of beneficial flora is depleted.

On the other side fighting for you is your bacterial army, which combats the pathogens and aids the body's defense system by producing natural antibiotics that are known to counteract harmful microorganisms.

Bacterial benefactors: ═══════════════════════
What beneficial bacteria do for you

• *The production of enzymes that digest our food. Lactase is one such enzyme, essential for the digestion of milk and dairy products. Dairy allergies can result from inadequate lactase.*

• *The manufacture of vitamins, such as biotin, niacin, pyridoxine and folic acid, members of the B complex family.*

• *Promoting healthy bowel function.*

• *Filtering and elimination of toxins, including preventing the formation of cancerous substances.*

• *An array of anti-viral, anti-fungal, and even anti-cholesterol properties.*

Normally, we are totally unaware of the bacterial comings and goings in our intestines. However, when we are not digesting our food well, experiencing a wide variety of health problems, and not efficiently eliminating wastes, the problem could very well be a problem among our bacterial allies.

Such disturbances are commonly caused by the use of antibiotics, stress, a meat-rich diet, not enough stomach acid, and acute diarrhea from food poisoning or infection.

Let's consider the impact of antibiotics. Scientific research has clearly shown that virtually all antibiotics taken orally cause changes to the balance of the bacterial flora in the colon. Even as little as one course of antibiotics may damage the protective population of beneficial bacteria. This can upset the balance between healthful and unhealthful bacteria, and reduce resistance to illness. For instance, the antibiotic ampicillin is often associated with a condition called Pseudomembranous enterocolitis, where the harmful microbe Clostridium dificile overruns the large intestine and causes ulceration, bloody diarrhea, pain and major weight loss.

Many people who think they are allergic to foods may in reality be simply eating inappropriate food that is mixing with unhealthy bacteria. The result: allergic-like reactions from an unholy combination.

One common result of antibiotic treatment is an overgrowth of Candida albicans, the yeast microorganism normally held in check by friendly bacteria. Candida can set off a wide array of seemingly unrelated symptoms such as allergies, vaginitis, bloating, heartburn, constipation, diarrhea, premenstrual difficulties, loss of alertness, chronic fatigue, skin disorders and fungus infections. Approximately a third of all persons around the world above the age of 12 — and mostly females — are suffering from yeast-related illness, according to the summary of a British symposium on Candida. I will talk more about yeast infections in a chapter dedicated to that problem.

Many physicians fail to address the problem of intestinal bacteria imbalances. This is tragic because of the potential for serious consequences. Unhealthy intestinal bacteria and yeast can migrate to other areas of the body and promote the development of fibromyalgia, breast cancer, arteriosclerosis (hardening of the arteries), chronic fatigue, migraine headaches, depression and mental illness, rheumatoid arthritis and many autoimmune problems.

Signs of beneficial bacteria bankruptcy

- *chronic fatigue*
- *frequent diarrhea*
- *frequent intestinal gas*
- *frequent constipation*
- *extended food transit-time (the time it takes between food ingestion and waste product elimination; the longer the transit time, the greater the opportunity for toxins of stagnant waste matter laying in the bowels to be reabsorbed into the body).*

- *poor immune responses to common infections*
- *chronic bladder infections*
- *chronic vaginal infections*
- *Candida infections*
- *allergies*
- *rashes and other skin conditions*
- *rapid onset of osteoporosis*
- *high cholesterol levels*
- *vitamin B deficiencies*
- *dairy product sensitivities*
- *increased menstrual complaints*
- *chronic bad breath*

You can aid your intestinal health through supplementation with food products rich in beneficial bacteria — foods such as cultured yogurt, whey, kefir, and sauerkraut.

These foods may be enough for general prevention. However, if you have any of the signs and symptoms of ill-health above, or you have had a course of antibiotics, or have a high stress load, than you may need a probiotic product. In our clinic we often use different combinations of multi-strain probiotics, anti-parasitic Chinese herbal medicines (MFP herbal), colonic hydrotherapy with herbal implants, and intravenous Vitamin C with HCL to rid patients of insidious, debilitating infections.

Defusing your intestinal time bomb

Most Americans experiencing digestive disorders become caught on the medical treadmill. They undergo elaborate and often invasive diagnostic tests, yet often feel frustrated by the inability of modern technology to discover the cause of their problems. Medications are prescribed to suppress symptoms. The drugs often create new symptoms while the cause of the problem is still at large and continuing to have its disruptive effect.

Our approach is different. We look for the cause. We conduct functional testing that includes digestive stool analysis, parasite and candida blood antibody tests and liver detoxification assessments. We feel these approaches, performed routinely in our clinic, are effective in helping us determine hidden health problems.

We also try to provide our patients with "intestinal education" and help them develop dietary and lifestyle habits to support good digestion. A lack of this awareness is deadly. You become a risk to yourself with a time bomb ticking in your intestines. Our approach is to defuse the bomb before it's too late.

CHAPTER NINE

Food, chemical and environmental sensitivity identification

S
t
e
p

4

Environmental medicine is a growing branch of medical specialty practiced by more than 2,500 physicians. Their main idea is that many behavioral, emotional and physical problems, conditions that are not conventionally accepted as being due to an allergy, can indeed be caused by sensitivity to different factors in the environment or diet. My clinical experience over the years has overwhelmingly demonstrated the validity of this concept.

Doris Rapp, M.D., a leading authority on environmental illness, has extensively studied the difficulties encountered by youngsters due to food, dust, mold, pollen and chemical sensitivities. Many children who are labeled with hyperactivity or learning disorders, and even the teachers who teach them, may be suffering in reality from chemicals found in their classrooms — substances such as chemical cleaning solvents, magic markers, or gasses emitted from new synthetic carpets.

Rapp's important message has been picked up by the media. She has appeared on the Oprah Winfrey Show and many other top talk shows. Recently she published her eye-opening findings in a must-read book for parents and educators: "Is This Your Child's World: How You Can Fix the Schools and Homes that are Making Your Children Sick" (Bantam Books, 1996). This is a book that I highly recommend.

"Children may not just develop your typical allergic reactions such as asthma, hayfever, eczema or hives," says Rapp. "They may instead have complaints not usually recognized by allergists and physicians as being related to allergies. This could include headaches, leg aches, muscle aches, hyperactivity, irritability, fatigue, depression, belligerence, silly behavior, temper tantrums, disturbed sleep, bed-wetting, digestive upset and learning difficulties."

Are such cases rare or extreme? No way, says Rapp. She sees them daily in her clinic and has received thousands of letters from people seeking help for their children and themselves.

"It is said that allergies affect 10-15 percent of the population, but I believe this kind of illness is much more common," she notes. "In schools, for instance, if you ask teachers who have been teaching for 20 or 30 years, they will tell you there is no comparison to how children were before and how they are now. I believe the reason for these increased problems is the vastly larger amount of chemicals in our lives today that are damaging our immune systems.

"These problems don't necessarily end with childhood," she adds. "The dis-ease inside little bodies continues and you eventually have an irritable, repressed, and fatigued adult, who doesn't live up to his or her potential, who can't form a good relationship with the opposite sex, or who can't hold a job."

Allergies can strike anywhere on or in the body, and affect the emotions, according to experts such as Rapp. When the nervous system and brain are affected, people experience a wide variety of psychological and behavioral problems. They may become violent, depressed, suicidal, exhausted, or unable to learn, talk or write coherently.

At the Advanced Metabolic Imaging Center in North Dallas, Theodore Simon, M.D., says that with imaging techniques "we can see objective, physical changes in brains. We have any number of patients who come in with very minimal or no findings at all, and are then exposed to the material that makes them clinically sick. Afterwards their brain image looks dramatically abnormal."

At the Anderson Laboratories in West Hartford, Vt., a facility that specializes in evaluating indoor air quality, testing shows that exposure to carpeting material is capable of causing adverse health effects. Lab manager Mark Goldman says that the use of carpets in schools "should make people nervous" because of the fumes they emanate, as well as the mold, tracked-in dirt, dust mites and dust mite feces they harbor.

Chemical sensitivities can open a pandora's box known as "the spreading phenomenon." From an initial chemical sensitivity, individuals often become sensitive to — and react to — other chemicals that didn't cause them problems before. Suddenly a person may develop symptoms when exposed to perfume, after shave, fabric softener, laundry detergent, or gasoline fumes. Says Rapp: "The potential is created for literally any odor to trigger symptoms."

One big unanswered question is how long can symptoms endure. Much depends on the body's defenses and how strong they are, the degree and frequency of exposure to offending substances, and lifestyle factors that either strengthen or undermine resistance.

The barrel concept

Why does one person become affected at a certain time and not another? Think of your body as a barrel that can hold a certain quantity of stress and pollution. Each person's barrel has a different genetic capacity. In addition, our lifestyle can either shrink or enlarge that capacity. You can hold so much and the next person so much — maybe less, maybe more.

Symptoms start any time your individual barrel overflows. Reactions may last a few moments or re-occur over years. Damage to the body may be temporary or permanent.

The treadmill fallout

The illness treadmill brings many patients into my clinic suffering from chronic allergies and bewildering combinations of complaints. They have often withstood allergy shots, steroids, decongestants, and antibiotics. Many have received prescriptions for psychiatric drugs because physicians regarded their problems as psychological. These patients have been on everything. Maybe they have had some degree of symptomatic relief. Or maybe their treatment has created a new problem — a side effect to deal with. Maybe they haven't been helped at all.

Millions of Americans are not getting relief for a wide variety of problems related to undiagnosed hidden food, environmental and chemical sensitivities. Such sensitivities may cause your typical allergy symptoms of hayfever, hives and asthma, sinus disorders, itchy eyes and scratchy throats, but they can also provoke a countless number of conditions you would never think had anything to do with allergies.

Before the 1920s, allergies were broadly defined as reactions to something present in the air, food or environment in a concentration or quantity that did not affect most other people. Then, medical researchers discovered immunoglobulin E (IgE), an antibody manufactured by the body against airborne allergies (such as pollen, dust and animal dander). As a result of that discovery, allergists adopted a narrower view of allergies as reactions involving an IgE response. The IgE response is what physicians look for when they do skin testing (the prick test or the patch test) and the IgE RAST (radioallergosorbent test) blood test.

With time, and more knowledge, it has become apparent that allergies do not fit into this tidy, compact definition.

Food allergies, for instance, may not cause a skin response or even necessarily an immediate reaction. They can activate different antibodies and chemicals in the body, and aggravate any system, organ, or tissue in the body, not just a limited few, and trigger a limitless combination and severity of emotional and physical responses.

A massive headache, painful joints, or crankiness may occur a few hours or even a couple of days after eating an allergenic food. Even more confusing is the fact that individuals usually aren't sensitive to just a single food. More than likely, they have problems with 5 to 15. Individuals with IgE allergies, on the other hand, are usually affected by only 1 or 2 substances.

Many, if not most traditional allergists, still operate according to the IgE principle. I believe it's a clinical straightjacket that limits them to recognizing fewer than 10 percent of food allergy problems. It's the equivalent of an ice cream parlor only recognizing vanilla and chocolate when there are dozens of other flavors out there.

Fortunately, there is growing acceptance among the public and professionals alike of major advances in the treatment of hidden food allergies. Mountains of research, numerous international medical conferences, and the extensive clinical experience of thousands of physicians, have resulted in effective ways to identify sensitivities, relieve symptoms, and eliminate the allergies.

One ironic byproduct of this progress is that when people eliminate their food allergies they often become less affected by their airborne allergies! I see this frequently in my practice. One striking example involved a female patient who told me that four days into her detoxification diet her husband's asthma condition cleared up.

"But he's not a patient," I replied.

"No, but when I started the detox program for my condition he went along with me," she said.

Her husband had had a 15-year-history of bronchial asthma, allergy shots and daily inhalers. He had always believed the asthma was related to environmental allergens. Now, with restricted food intake on the detox program, he stops eating his regular food and his symptoms clear up. Later, as a patient, we determined which foods were contributing to his problem and had him eliminate them from his diet.

The natural approach

You have no doubt heard of the "Sick Building Syndrome." I see people all the time in my practice who tell me they are sick because of sensitivity to the chemicals, dust or air in the building they work in. Once we get them healthy they experience fewer or less intense reactions in the building or none at all.

Individuals with allergies and sensitivities need the assistance of alternative medicine to help them confront the following question: Am I really allergic or is my body defenseless?

We frequently find that allergic conditions are actually the result of reversible weaknesses and vulnerabilities present within the body. Medication, poor diet, intestinal toxicity and disorders, and spinal misalignments can all undermine the body's defenses — overload the barrel, so to speak — and set the stage for allergic-like reactions and illness.

In our clinic we routinely check for internal causes creating vulnerability. Our approach, therefore, is two-pronged. First, we utilize revolutionary methods in an effort to effectively identify sensitivities.

One of them is Applied Kinesiology, a unique muscle testing technique discovered and developed by George Goodheart, D.C., more than 30 years ago. In this method we place minute extracts of different substances — such as wheat, dairy, dust, and pollen — under the tongue and test for a reaction using muscle resistance. If an individual is sensitive, an associated muscle will become weak. Once the reactive substance is positively identified, a neutralizing treatment can be applied to counter the reaction. We have expanded this method at our clinic to include testing of hundreds of foods, chemicals, environmental factors, and even vitamins, minerals, herbs and homeopathics.

We also use sophisticated laboratory blood tests to identify potentially harmful substances that may generate reactions days after exposure.

Secondly, we attempt to repair and strengthen the body. We do this wholistically, through each of the elements in the Gallagher Wellness Program. We improve the function of the nervous system with chiropractic manipulation. We boost the immune system. We clear out toxicity and enhance digestion, and strengthen the liver so it can perform its critical job of processing foods and chemicals.

Our approach is extremely successful in clearing up or reducing symptoms. Even patients who regard themselves as "allergic to everything" become more compatible with their environment. They don't have to settle for a life of "chemical imprisonment."

As an example, I treated a 67-year-old woman with multiple sensitivities. In the supermarket she couldn't go near the aisle with detergents and bleaches. If she did, she might develop a nosebleed, dry mouth, itchy eyes, dizziness, or a spacey feeling.

Through chiropractic examination, I determined she had spinal misalignments affecting her immune function. Through Applied Kinesiology, I also found weaknesses in the liver, spleen and thymus.

All her previous conventional blood tests were "normal." For one month we administered a series of chiropractic adjustments and placed her on a number of herbal and glandular supplements to strengthen weakened organs. At the end of the month, she returned to the supermarket and marched down the detergent aisle with no problem.

Joan Ross' case

Joan Ross, 53, a housewife from Greensburg, Pennsylvania had severe allergies and bronchial asthma. Exposure to household chemicals, grass, mold, car fumes, perfumes, carpets, animals and dust caused her to experience fogginess, blurred vision, choking, and coughing.

> "I refuse to live in a bubble."

" Since 1982, I have been on daily inhalers and antihistamines for allergies," she told on the occasion of her first office visit in 1996. "This has made me very hyper. I've had anxiety, constipation and periodic yeast infections. Sinus infections in the spring and fall. My bones were starting to ache as were my joints and back. The pain was so intense I was able to sleep and walk for only short periods.

"I have also been taking Ibuprofen/aspirin/Motrin for arthritis and back pain. I was also diagnosed as having irritable bowel syndrome and the doctor prescribed daily medicine for that as well."

Joan said she was fed up. "I refuse to live in a bubble," she said. "I have been getting no relief on my medicines. My body is still aching."

Joan started a program of chiropractic adjustments and avoidance of certain foods. Her improvement was dramatic.

"I no longer need painkillers, inhalers, allergy medicines, or irritable bowel medicines, in fact, I take no medicines at all anymore," she told me during a subsequent appointment. "I haven't had yeast infections. My sinusitis has cleared up. I can walk by freshly cut grass. I am tolerating household chemicals. I am able to care for my daughter's dog in my home. My husband and I went camping with my daughter and son-in-law for the first time in two years and I was able to tolerate mold."

CHAPTER TEN

Exercise and conditioning

S

t

e

p

5

Wouldn't it be wonderful if you could swallow a pill that could:
- increase your energy and sense of well-being,
- decrease your risk of heart attack, high blood pres
  sure, low back pain, and indigestion,
- strengthen and enlarge your heart,
- eliminate psychological and physical tension,
- help you deal with daily stress,
- promote muscle relaxation and better sleep,
- give you a more youthful appearance and a hardier,
  stronger, better-looking body,
- help prevent osteoporosis,
- relieve depression and anxiety,
- enhance immune function,
- help you lose weight by burning fat,
- and improve your self-image and self-confidence.

Alas, nobody has invented the WONDER PILL as far as I know. "But as many gerontologists and researchers have found, exercise is the closest thing to an anti-aging pill that exists," says Ronald Klatz, D.O., and Robert Goldman, D.O., in their 1996 book, "Stopping the Clock" (Keats Publishing).

A regular program of physical activity indeed does all the wonderful things mentioned above. In fact, research suggests that adequate exercise along with a healthy diet "can recapture youthful vitality by slowing or reversing many of the physiologic changes that are associated with aging," say Klatz and Goldman.

Exercise as a longevity elixir was the focus of a widely-publicized 1986 study published in the New England Journal of Medicine. The study compared the exercise habits and longevity among some 17,000 Harvard alumni. The findings, according to Ralph Paffenbarger, Jr., of Stanford

---

"A man falls into ill health as a result of not caring for exercise."
— Aristotle

University, showed that "people who are active and fit can expect to live a year or so longer than their sedentary counterparts. For each hour of physical activity, you can expect to live that hour over — and live one or two more hours to boot."

This potential for life extension may have something to do with the very nature of the human body. It was built, after all, for movement. And when you don't move it, that's when trouble starts. "Use it or lose it" the saying goes. A sedentary life results in a rapid shrinkage of muscles and a loss of response to normal everyday challenges. This debility is called disuse atrophy of the muscles.

Every year in America, the death of up to a quarter-million people is related in part to a lack of regular physical activity. "An inactive lifestyle only places extra strain on the body, increasing risk for cardiovascular problems, cancer, and many other diseases," Klatz and Goldman say.

Moreover, research shows that the beginning of obesity comes with a sudden decrease in activity level.

In a 1996 analysis of physical activity and health, the prestigious British Medical Journal made the consequences of sedentary living quite clear. "Studies suggest causal associations between regular physical activity and reduced rates of coronary heart disease, hypertension, non-insulin dependent diabetes mellitus, osteoporosis, colon cancer, anxiety and depression," the journal said.

In particular, "the most persuasive proof" relates to heart disease. Regularly active individuals have half the risk of couch potatoes. An estimated one-third of annual deaths from coronary heart disease (about 160,000) in the U.S. are linked to a lack of physical activity.

Tips for exercising...and staying with it

• **What's the best exercise for me?**

Most of us are not interested in peak performance and getting into the athletic record books. Our concern should be finding forms of physical activity and exercise that we enjoy. Exercise should not be boring. It's the boredom that turns off many people after an enthusiastic start.

• **When should I start?**

Whatever your age, there is no time as right now to start exercising. Nobody ever proved that fitness is the monopoly of the young. And, as Mae West said, "you're never too old to become younger."

• **How much do I need?**

Once you select your type of exercise, you need to go out and do it.

Twenty minutes at least three times a week is the recipe for big health and fitness benefits. Make sure that whatever you do increases your heart rate to about 60-70 percent of maximum capacity.

Don't think you have to go out and run miles every day to get fit. In fact that may be detrimental to your health. The streets are full of joggers huffing and puffing polluted air and incurring joint injuries from too much pavement pounding.

> "All things in excess bring trouble to men."
> – Platus,
> Roman writer

Ron Lawrence, M.D., president of the American Medical Athletic Association, points out that indeed too much exercise may indeed bring trouble to men. Increased susceptibility to illness is one common form of trouble.

"No doubt in my mind that it's dose related," says Lawrence, who practices in Agoura, California. "Exercise done at a non-exhausting level enhances the immune system. Too much, and you hurt it."

• **What if I haven't been active for many years?**

Then it is essential to start your exercise program very slowly and gingerly. The body must be brought slowly back into use because even slight exercise for some people can cause muscle aches and pains and sometimes permanent damage.

Some exercise ideas to get you going

Below are a few simple start-up suggestions that work for many people. In all cases, start out slowly and gently. You can use this program as a springboard to aerobics classes, walking, hiking or bicycle groups, or even gym membership.

• A brisk walk — not window shopping, but striding out. Gradually build up intensity. Under no circumstances, should an obese person try running. It is too hard on the joints.

• Exercise bicycles or the running/walking treadmill. (That's the only treadmill I recommend!!)

• Experts regard a combination of conditioning and strengthening exercises (aerobics and weight training) as the most effective exercise. Weight training with light weights is highly efficient for weight loss and exercising the main muscles of the body —the legs, chest, upper back, shoulders and midsection.

You will be amazed at the results. A tiny bit each day begins to reverse the effects of muscle disuse. Your muscles begin to grow slightly larger and firmer. When they do, they burn far more calories.

All you need to get started is a barbell, a few light weight plates, and a flat bench, something like a patio bench. Or you can join a gym and do it. If you have any doubts about physical problems and your ability to do these exercises, check with your physician.

Start these exercises very gently, even with just one repetition if that's all you can do. You'll soon develop your own pace of repetitions and sets.

Legs

Hold the back of a chair with one hand for balance. Your feet are flat on the floor, shoulder width. Do a deep knee bend or as far down as is comfortable. Then come back up again. Climb a flight of stairs . When you feel comfortable, you can start adding weight. Maybe 10 pounds or so to start. Go up and down 4-5 times.

Chest

Lay down on the bench, face up. Take a barbell with 10 or 20 pounds on it, or a light dumbbell in each hand. Press upward away from your chest multiple times. An alternative is modified pushups. Lean into a wall and just push away. Back and forth multiple times.

Upper back

Fold a towel into a pad and place it on the edge of a table. Take a barbell and place it on the floor in front of the table. Bend down and rest your forehead on the pad. This will take any strain off your lower back. Lift the barbell in your hands up to your chest. As you do so, your elbows will rotate outward. Lift and lower the weight multiple times.

Midsection

Forget doing sit-ups. They can cause lower back problems. Your best bet are modified crunchers.

Lay on your back with your knees up. Your feet are flat on the floor close to your buttocks. Bring your shoulders up off the floor and reach for your knees. Hold for a count of 3. Relax back down and count to 3. Then reach for your knees again. By raising your shoulders you are bringing your ribs closer to your pelvis and exercising the abdominal muscles.

Variation # 1: Both shoulders off the floor at the same time and reach with both hands.

Variation # 2: Spread your feet 2-3 feet apart. Your knees are still up. Reach for one knee and then alternately for the other.

Fitness and health are not synonymous

Joe Weider, the famous guru of bodybuilding and weight training, once offered the following perspective on the importance of taking care of all aspects of one's health, not just physical fitness:

"Old school bodybuilders used to believe that exercise 'plugged all the leaks' in your system — you could go without sleep, eat anything, abuse your body with substances, but as long as you exercised, you'd stay healthy as a bearcat. Hah! Exercise may be the simplest, most effective and cheapest way to preserve your health, but it can't counter all the bad effects of unhealthy habits."

Gina Zazac's case

Fitness, as Weider so correctly points out, is a wholistic proposition requiring integration into a supportive lifestyle including family, career, outside interests, adequate rest and good food. A case in point is Gina Zazac, a marketing manager from North Versailles, Pennsylvania, has been a patient of mine for years. When she first came to my office in 1986, at the age of 24, she was extremely fit. Ever since she was a teenager she had followed a vigorous daily routine of aerobics, weight training, and flexibility exercises. She danced and biked and enjoyed life. Nevertheless, she was full of medical complaints: heartburn, severe menstrual cramps, and urinary tract and yeast infections. She had occasional back and neck pain.

The medical doctors she had seen for her problems prescribed drugs that caused side effects and failed to give her relief. When I first saw Gina I asked her about her diet. It was high in fat, refined sugars, and dairy products with minimal fruits and vegetables. The diet, she told me, was similar to that of her mother and two sisters, all of whom had died of cancer at an early age.

We transformed Gina's diet, added a nutritional supplement program, and from time to time, give her a chiropractic adjustment. Today, at age 35, she says she feels better than ever. She exercises three times a week to maintain her fitness and ideal weight. She has no more heartburn or infections and says she rarely gets a cold or flu. Her menstrual cramps and back pain have improved significantly.

Gina is most proud about the health of her two young children. Throughout her pregnancies she stayed on her healthy lifestyle program along with chiropractic adjustments. She had completely natural and drug-free deliveries and breast-fed both infants until the age of three.

Rehabilitation and conditioning

Many of the people who come to see me have been hurt on the job, in automobile accidents, or through athletic activity. They have seen physicians who prescribed anti-inflammatories, muscle relaxants, and exercise. But they have ongoing pain and wonder why. "I am taking the pain pills," they say. "I'm doing the exercise. But how come I'm still hurting?"

The reason for the continued hurt is that the joints are misaligned as a result of the injury or trauma. The chiropractic approach is to restore normal joint movement and decrease pain naturally and then start the rehabilitation and exercise program to strengthen the tissue around the injured joint. If you have an injury, you need to have your joint checked for alignment, and realigned if necessary. Then exercise.

In my opinion, the healing process should be chiropractic first and then exercise. Not drugs and then exercise. The conventional medical model is to drug it and then exercise it. In our clinic, we prescribe Cybex exercise rehabilitation for many patients. This is a specific technology that identifies weak or deconditioned muscles and joints that can contribute to impaired function and chronic pain. With the use of computerized programs, our sports medicine specialists and rehab therapists are able to measure the degree of weakness of your trunk, shoulder, wrist, hip, knee, back or foot and can prescribe a strengthening program to rehabilitate injured areas or post surgical problems. This computerized technology is currently employed by the National Football League, the National Tennis Association and many professional and amateur athletic teams.

We also use a functional rehabilitation program developed by Craig Liebenson, D.C., director of rehabilitation at the Los Angeles College of Chiropractic. The program incorporates chiropractic mechanical realignment of the joint structures followed by specific rehab activities that are fitted into a person's daily routine. If you are a competitive athlete or a computer programmer you will obviously receive different rehab exercises. The effect is a healing integration of the nervous and musculoskeletal systems directed according to a patient's needs.

As an example, if you sit for long periods of time at your job, we would first determine the alignment irregularities in your back and then correct them. Once completed, you would receive a series of exercises that are task specific for you. This would rehabilitate the weaknesses that have developed posturally in your spine. This kind of program is highly effective in preventing recurring pain and impaired mobility.

CHAPTER ELEVEN

Nutritional rehabilitation

S
t
e
p

6

Most Americans fail to eat properly. As a result, many are deficient in nutrients vital to health. About half of us, in fact, are at least marginally deficient. Government surveys repeatedly show many of us literally malnourished in our land of plenty, with <u>gross</u> deficiencies in essential nutrients such as calcium, iron, zinc, magnesium, and vitamins A, B-1, B-2, B-6 and C.

Here are some of the reasons this is happening:

• Intensive farming and long-term use of chemical fertilizers and pesticides have caused serious loss of nutrient content of agricultural crops.

• Canning, cooking, storage, freezing and preparation cause major nutrient loss. Frozen vegetables have 25 percent less of the major vitamins than cooked fresh vegetables and the canned varieties have two or three times fewer than even frozen.

• Fast food, the symbol of the modern American diet, is notoriously deficient in vitamin A, several of the B vitamins, iron, and copper.

• We are the world's leading consumers of painkillers, antibiotics, anti-inflammatory and tranquilizing drugs. In addition to their side effects, pharmaceutical drugs undermine nutritional status. To some degree, all interfere with basic metabolic processes.

• Aspirin, perhaps the least toxic of painkillers, increases the bodily needs for every known nutrient, including oxygen, and speeds up the urinary loss of calcium, potassium, the B vitamins and vitamin C.

• Long-term use of antibiotics cause immune system suppression and rob the body of potassium, calcium, iron and vitamin B-12.

• Oral contraceptives, used by an estimated 10 to 18 million American women, deplete vitamins B-2, B-6, B-12, C, E, folic acid, and zinc.

• Any type of stress, whether physical, emotional, or due to illness or injury, drains the body of important nutrients, particularly vitamins C and B complex, and the minerals zinc and magnesium. According to Mildred Seelig, Ph.D., of Emory University, if the body is deficient in magnesium to begin with, the added depletion of magnesium from stress actually intensifies the body's reactions to stress. "Without adequate magnesium, and the life-supporting activities it contributes to in the body, events can dramatically turn life-threatening," she says.

> **Deficiencies should not be taken lightly. They can and do create health problems leading straight to the medical treadmill, the emergency room, and the cemetery. As Harvard researchers Meir Stampfer and Walter Willett point out, the scientific evidence "strongly indicates" that "low intakes are associated with serious health consequences."**

Given the reality of widespread deficiencies and American eating habits, it never ceases to amaze me that many conservative nutritionists and registered dietitians still argue that you don't need vitamin and mineral supplements as long as you eat a "balanced diet."

Just who is eating a "balanced diet?" Surveys show that not many of us are.

Michael Colgan, Ph.D., a leading nutrition researcher, scoffs at the idea that even a good mixed diet is insurance for supplying adequate nutrition. In his highly-informative book, "Your Personal Vitamin Profile" (Quill Books, 1982), Colgan says this concept may have been true when people grew much of their own food or bought it from local growers. "But with modern methods of storage and process-ing," he says, "our food comes from all over the world and may be years old before we get to eat it. Such food can be completely devoid of nutri-ents and may also contain harmful chemicals that have no business in the human body."

In "The Vitamin Revolution in Health Care" (Arcadia Press, 1996), the very first words by nutrition expert Michael Janson, M.D., are these: "Your health may be at risk if you believe the current medical and food industry myths that assert that you do not need extra vitamins and minerals if you eat properly (what is called a balanced diet)."

For many years, nutritionally-minded health professionals like Colgan and Janson have successfully used nutritional supplements in their treatment strategies. In my own practice, supplements have been a major part of my wellness program from the start. I have found them to be an effective healing tool for many conditions.

Live longer and healthier with supplements

Although most of the 60 million or so Americans who take vitamins do so for "health insurance" against an inadequate diet, most of them still resort to drugs when their health is threatened. We are conditioned by advertising and the medical PR machine to do so. It's the word association game I described at the end of chapter four. We are programmed to think Prozac for depression, Zantac for ulcers, Tylenol for headaches and Motrin for arthritis. Most patients are unaware that specific megadoses of vitamins and minerals and other nutrients, when taken either orally or intravenously, represent a safe and effective strategy for overcoming serious health problems without the undesirable side effects associated with drugs. Nutrients can also do things that pharmaceuticals can never hope to do. Take vitamin C for example, an important antioxidant, natural detoxifying and painkilling agent, and key ingredient of the body's connective tissue.

UCLA researcher James Enstrom, Ph.D., carefully analyzed the dietary and lifestyle habits of 11,000 people and found that men who consumed at least 300 milligrams of vitamin C from food or supplements were 41 percent less likely to die during a 10-year period compared to those with an intake of only 50 milligrams (The U.S. Food and Drug Administration's recommended daily allowance is 60 milligrams). Women experienced 10 percent less deaths during the same timeframe.

The findings were consistent with the theory that high levels of antioxidant vitamins, such as vitamin C, increase the body's defense system against free radicals and reduce the risk of arteriosclerosis, Enstrom wrote in a 1992 issue of the journal Epidemiology. (See the explanation later in the chapter on free radicals).

In a later article, Enstrom said his research indicates that higher consumption of vitamin C translates to longer life. A 35-year-old man, for instance, could expect to live 5.5 years longer than expected. A 55-year-old man, 5 years longer. A 35-year-old woman could live 2.3 years longer and a 55-year-old woman 1.3 years longer with higher vitamin C, he projects.

Do you know of any drug that can do the same?

Imagine how much money we could save Medicare alone just by promoting a major vitamin C campaign among the elderly, who are consistently found to be deficient.

Supplements vs. heart disease

Let's look at one major health problem — heart disease — and consider the potential of nutritional supplements. For years, Americans have been told to lower their cholesterol, eat a low-fat diet, exercise, cut out smoking, and try to control weight and stress. Yet many who do not smoke, have no history of heart disease in their families, who are not overweight, overstressed or hypertensive, and who exercise routinely, still suffer from cardiovascular disease.

The solution to this mystery may be the vitamins and minerals that are deficient in our diets.

Previously, vitamins and minerals were regarded in a narrow perspective by most physicians. They were seen as necessary elements found in food that prevent clear-cut nutritional deficiency diseases such as scurvy, beriberi, rickets and pellagra. The medical establishment's position has focused on the "balanced diet" myth and the belief that we get all we need from our diet. In this view, supplementation has been regarded as unnecessary. It just creates expensive urine, a conventional doctor would tell you if you asked about vitamins. For decades, only a relatively few nutritionally-minded physicians championed the use of supplements.

Since the beginning of the nineties, a flood of solid research has eroded the conventional viewpoint and, in my opinion and the opinion of many experts, rendered it utterly obsolete...and dangerous. Study after study indicates that individual nutrients at doses higher than those usually found in the diet, have a substantial preventive and therapeutic effect for serious diseases, including cancer and heart disease.

In a January 1993 cover article, Medical World News, a periodical read by many doctors, said that new studies on the role of vitamins are shifting the foundations of nutrition research, policy and public health in this country.

Consider some of the findings on supplements against cardiovascular disease:

• People with the highest intake of beta carotene (the top 20 percent) reduced their risk of heart disease by 29 percent. Among the smokers in the high intake group, there was an even greater effect: a 70 percent reduced risk compared to individuals with low intake.

• Anti-oxidant vitamins C and E and beta carotene team up to reduce the oxidation of LDL cholesterol, the so-called "bad cholesterol," that forms fatty deposits and accelerates the buildup of plaque on arterial walls.

• Vitamin C helps elevate HDL, the "good cholesterol."

• After an evaluation of 3,000 Swiss workers, researchers determined that individuals with low blood levels of vitamin C had twice the risk of heart attack, and quadruple the risk for stroke, than those with normal levels.

• An adequate intake of certain B complex vitamins — folic acid,

B-12 and B-6 — will prevent the creation of homocysteine, a toxic break-down product of the amino acid cysteine. An elevated level of homocysteine is now being regarded as a potent indicator of cardiovascular disease.

• Forty percent less disease among people with the highest intake of vitamin E compared to those with the lowest intake, according to a Harvard University study of 120,000 men and women.

• Vitamin E markedly reduces arterial plaque build-up.

• Sufferers from chest pain (angina) report less pain if they take vitamin E.

• Numerous studies show that magnesium deficiency can contribute to heart irregularities, heart attack and sudden death. Canadian and Israeli researchers demonstrated that when magnesium was added to standard critical care treatment for heart attack patients, the death rate dropped by 66 percent.

• Co-enzyme Q10, a vitamin-like substance naturally produced in the body, facilitates oxygenation of cardiac tissue and cellular energy output. Heart patients are typically deficient. Given as a supplement, CoQ10 significantly benefits cardiac patients, including improved long-term survival. At the University Hospital in Copenhagen, researchers concluded that CoQ10 offers an "effective breakthrough" in heart failure therapy.

• Garlic helps prevent platelet stickiness, lowers blood pressure and has a beneficial effect on cholesterol metabolism.

• Supplements of omega-3 fatty acid, an essential fatty acid, helps prevent damage to coronary artery tissue following balloon angioplasty.

You have to wonder why aren't cardiologists prescribing supplements for their patients. Most, however, usually prescribe drugs and surgery. They tend to ignore or be unfamiliar with nutritional options. The result, I believe, is a serious omission for patients.

Cardiovascular health depends on more than just avoiding fat and salt. The research gives us immense potential for impacting the nation's No. 1 disease killer. For sure, this and other serious illnesses are affected by our poor intake of essential nutrients.

Looking for the pieces to the puzzle

Many of the patients who come to my clinic are caught in the vicious cycle of the medical treadmill. They have seen numerous physicians and received numerous prescriptions but never had their nutritional status analyzed. The disregard of something so absolutely fundamental as nutritional intake amazes me.

Some patients come with shopping bags filled with vitamins, tapes, books and health magazines. They have heard advice from friends, or people at the gym, or read something somewhere. They are desperate to help themselves and escape the treadmill. They feel that if they take vitamins, that will cure their condition.

Often these individuals have not been helped. One woman with chronic migraines had previously gone to the health food store and bought Feverfew after a friend told her that the herb could help her condition. Despite studies showing it is frequently effective, it didn't help her. She still had the pain.

Men will sometimes call into my radio show and say they are taking zinc for their prostrate but are still up three or four times a night urinating.

These cases are examples of pharmaceutical thinking, that is, taking one drug to suppress a symptom. There are multiple reasons why people are unhealthy and many ways of approaching it. The problem can be mechanical problems at the base of the back requiring chiropractic manipulation. Another person might have a toxic bowel that is putting pressure on the prostate. Another person may not have enough essential fatty acids or vitamin C in their diet. Or they are drinking alcohol which inflames the prostate.

I encourage the use of vitamin and mineral supplements, particularly in this age of depleted food. However, one particular vitamin, mineral or herb may not completely address one particular problem. And typically, when one nutrient deficient exists, there are others as well.

Unless you locate the missing pieces to the puzzle — there may not be just one —— you may likely remain ill.

Each of us is uniquely individual. From every standpoint. Personality. Structure. Ability to eat certain foods. Ability to handle stress. Requirements for certain vitamins and minerals.

At our clinic, as in other wholistic practices, careful assessments of all patients are made in order to find the missing pieces to the puzzle. Nutritional detective work is an important part of our sleuthing for the answers and our investigation produces an individually- tailored diet best suited for the needs of each patient and specifically to help them recover from their health problem.

One common denominator is the recommendation to eat the freshest, least-processed foods available. For us, this is the basis of any good nutritional program.

Then, on that good foundation, we fortify the diet with nutritional supplements — specific vitamins, minerals, amino acids, enzymes and herbals. Again, an individualized program is designed to help patients escape from the medical treadmill and to achieve optimal health.

It is worth emphasizing the importance of developing a sound diet as the basis for any good nutritional program. Eating junk and gobbling down vitamins, as many people do, is like trying to build a house on quicksand. Nutritional supplements are often the first step a person takes in the direction of alternative medicine, but they are not a substitute for nutritious food.

Our supplement program starts with a high-quality multi-vitamin and mineral formulation. To determine the best possible supplement program for you, we recommend consulting with a nutritionally-oriented physician.

We will usually also recommend extra vitamin C plus antioxidants such as vitamin E, selenium, co-enzyme Q10, grape seed extract and other naturally-occurring plant compounds. These are significant nutrients to counter the harmful effects of free-radical activity in the body. In case you haven't heard about free radicals, let me take a brief moment to explain them.

Free-radicals — molecular terrorists inside the body

The trillions of cells throughout the body utilize oxygen to produce energy to fuel their widely varied functions. As a by-product of this ongoing process they generate free radicals, highly-reactive and unstable molecular combinations of oxygen and other atoms with a fierce appetite for robbing electrons from surrounding atoms or molecules. Unless free radicals are kept to a tolerable level by the body's own natural anti-oxidant and repair mechanisms, they can set off a destructive blitz of oxidation that over time takes a heavy toll on healthy cells and bodily function.

The effect of free radical oxidation in the body is similar to how oxygen spoils food, turns butter rancid, and rusts metal.

Compounding the natural pace of free radical activity in the body are our lifestyle habits and the world we live in. Both conspire to generate free radical opportunities galore. Stress, smoking, alcohol, excess exposure to sunlight, chemical contaminants, pesticides, chemotherapy and pharmaceutical drugs, and processed, smoked or barbecued foods — all increase the production of free radicals and create dangerous overloads in the body.

"These free radicals become terrorists in our physical bodies," says Hari Sharma, M.D., an expert on free radicals at Ohio State University.

"They can attack DNA, leading to dysfunction, mutation and cancer. They can attack enzymes and proteins, disrupting normal cells activities. They can attack cell membranes, producing a chain reaction of destruction; such membrane damage in the cells that line our blood vessels can lead to hardening and thickening of the arteries and eventually to heart attacks and strokes. Free radical attacks on the protein in collagen (connective tissue) can cause cross-linking of protein molecules and a resulting stiffness in the body. Excess free radical activity in the skin, caused by radiation from the sun, can reduce skin suppleness and increase wrinkling."

Free radicals are involved in MANY diseases ══════

- *Cancer*
- *Vascular and heart disease.*
- *Strokes*
- *Emphysema*
- *Maturity onset diabetes*
- *Rheumatoid arthritis*
- *Ulcers*
- *Cataracts*
- *Crohn's disease*
- *Senility*

To help protect us against these conditions it is important that we eat a diet high in foods containing antioxidants. The best are fruits and vegetables. For extra health insurance or to help combat specific conditions, our nutritional program always includes antioxidant supplements, such as vitamin A, C, E, selenium, co-enzymeQ10, and bioflavonoids.

Comprehensive therapeutic approach

Oral supplementation is just one part of a comprehensive nutritional therapeutic approach offered at our clinic. Among our other practices are the following:

- intravenous infusions of Vitamin C and HCL are often prescribed at our clinic for patients suffering from chronic fatigue syndrome, flu symptoms, upper respiratory infections, arthritis and depressed immunity.
- intravenous infusions of magnesium, Vitamin B-6 and B-12 are often used for patients with cardiac irregularity, arrhythmia, hypertension,

asthma and depression.

- injections with homeopathic remedies, a popular form of therapy in the European medical community, is often used in cases of chronic pain, bursitis, tendonitis, viral infections and immune dysregulation.

- natural hormones such as DHEA, the anti-aging hormone, and estrogen and progesterone, derived from plants, are frequently prescribed. Taken orally or transdermally (rubbed on the skin), they are able to help in the treatment of PMS, menstrual migraine, menopause, low libido, impotence, osteoporosis and depression.

Chelation therapy

We also administer chelation therapy, a procedure in which a man-made amino acid (EDTA) is infused intravenously during a series of painless office treatments. EDTA removes toxic metallic agents involved in the buildup of arterial plaque and the free radical process.

In more than 400,000 clinical cases and many published studies over a 30-year period, chelation therapy has demonstrated a significant improvement in blood flow and symptoms. The effectiveness and safety record of chelation therapy for arteriosclerosis, angina, circulatory disorders, hypertension and diabetes is overwhelming. According to current drug safety standards, aspirin is about three and a half times more toxic than EDTA.

Chelation therapy is much less expensive than conventional medical treatments (such as bypass, carotid artery operations) and does not require hospitalization.

Despite the evidence and the cost, medical insurers, including Medicare, will not cover this procedure! Obviously, there are forces within the medical community that do not want to see their lucrative operations economically challenged, even if the results of these procedures are dubious. Thirty to 50 percent of bypass surgery cases involve a recurrence of symptoms within the first year due to the fact that the underlying disease has not been addressed. As one expert says, they just modify the situation "with a piece of pipe."

In "Forty Something Forever: A Consumer's Guide to Chelation Therapy and Other Heart-Savers," Harold and Arline Brecher point out wisely that chelation "does not 'cure' old age and its symptoms. It does give the body a reprieve — a chance to regenerate."

This reprieve offers a critical opportunity. It gives motivated patients the chance to get a handle on their conditions and reverse the underlying disease process with a broad program of diet, nutritional supplementation, exercise and other wholistic methods. In clinics such as ours, all these supportive elements go along with chelation treatments.

Fannie Nadle's case

Fannie Nadle, 67, is a housewife from Pittsburgh who had a stroke in 1990 that affected the right side of her body.

> In about a month's time, she was able to eat an entire meal with her right hand

"My right arm felt like a 2 by 4," she told me. "It's solid, unmoving and unfeeling. I had to wear a sling to protect my shoulder from the damage that would occur due to the dead weight of the arm.

"My vocational therapist used an electric vibrator to stimulate my arm. It took six sessions before my arm started to react. During the year that followed, physical therapists worked on my arm and back, massaging the back muscles which led to my arm. At home, my husband regularly exercised my fingers three times a day. I squeezed plastic clay with my right hand to strengthen it. After two years of unrelenting work, I finally was able to raise my right arm over my head."

Fannie started treatments in our clinic in 1992. Through chiropractic and other means we were able to help her walk better but hadn't achieved much help with her arm.

In December of 1996 she began chelation therapy. Her right hand still was not working well.

"It is very difficult for me to use it for eating because I can not articulate the fingers well, and my hand tires quickly," she said at the time. "I have been forced to become left-handed."

Chelation treatment made a rapid difference.

In about a month's time, she was able to eat an entire meal with her right hand. She was able to hold a pencil in her right hand as if she were about to write something. She hadn't been able to do that since the stroke.

"I still can't write yet, but I'm looking forward to the day that I can," she said.

CHAPTER TWELVE

Relaxation and stress management

S
t
e
p

7

Research makes it clear that stress is a major cause of illness. In fact, 44 percent of all Americans suffer from stress-related health problems, including anxiety, hypertension and heart disease.

We all experience stress at one time or another throughout life, the kind of stress that causes butterflies in your stomach, your heart to race, your blood pressure to elevate, your mouth to get dry, your hands to become cold, your muscles to tighten and your breathing to become irregular. Such symptoms actually represent a natural mechanism essential to protect the body from sudden intense stress or low grade prolonged stress.

But when stress becomes excess in life, it can breakdown our natural coping mechanisms, causing "distress" and health problems.

Stress is not necessarily just the pressure of work, a tyrannical boss, or a divorce. Stress wears many faces. Noise, light, weather changes, food and poor diet, chemicals, worry, bickering kids, and countless other things in life have the potential to overwhelm our coping mechanisms.

In our mad headlong plunge for success, many of us ignore or forget the importance of rest and relaxation. I believe these must be part of any good healing and anti-stress program. Note the first four letters of r-e-s-t-o-r-a-t-i-o-n.

Research has shown that effective stress reduction is a means to actually prevent illness and thereby reduce the need for medical services. Some examples of stress management techniques used in our clinic include breathing exercises and progressive muscle relaxation. Since stress usually leads to irregular breathing patterns and increased blood pressure, learning to control your breathing is essential to well-being.

Breathe out your stress

Try the following breathing exercise, which we recommend to many of our patients. It can be done by anyone.

- Sit upright in a comfortable chair.
- Close your eyes.

- Turn your attention to your breath.
- Slowly breathe in through your nose to a silent count of four.
- Hold your breath to a silent count of four.
- Breathe out through your mouth to a silent count of four.
- Continue this process for 15 to 20 minutes. When you find your mind drifting off to thoughts, very gently return your attention to the breath. Over time you can progress to counting to five or six or whatever works well for you.

Although this method is well-suited for individuals with hypertension, anxiety and panic disorders, and other stress-related conditions, it is also an excellent preventive method.

Rest — Are you getting enough?

Former football running great Jim Taylor of the Green Bay Packers was once fined $25 by Vince Lombardi, his coach. Taylor's crime: sitting on the edge of his bed in his socks and shorts at 11:01 p.m. Lombardi wanted his players in bed — horizontally — at 11. Lombardi considered rest absolutely vital for his athletes.

Long before Vince Lombardi, ancient healers put great value on rest as a balance to activity. As an example, we have the yin and yang of Chinese medicine in which rest, recovery and nutrition are yin, while competition and activity are yang. In the original Chinese medicine text, The Nei Jing (300 BC), it is written: "Physical activity is necessary to harmonize the flow of vital energy and blood to develop strength. Exessive labor, however, can strain the ability of the spleen to produce energy, and this causes deficiencies. The body must rest."

Often ignored, but critical to stress management is deep, restful sleep. Robbing from the sleep bank leads to a condition called sleep-deprivation. Many illnesses can be traced to lack of sleep or irregular sleep patterns. In our modern, often-intrusive world, closing our eyes for prayer and meditation and establishing consistent rest and activity cycles are part of a healthy, fulfilled lifestyle.

Are you a "drowsy American?" A 1990 Time Magazine cover article revealed that

- Millions of us are sleep-deprived, trying to get by on six hours or less.

> "Most Americans no longer know what it feels like to be fully alert."
> – William Dement, director of the Stanford University Sleep Center

● A third of Americans have trouble falling asleep or staying asleep.

● Human error, in which lack of sleep is a major factor, causes between 60 percent and 90 percent of workplace accidents.

● The U.S. Department of Transport reports that up to 200,000 traffic accidents a year may be sleep related.

The status of sleep-deficient Americans apparently has gotten worse since the Time Magazine article. A 1997 article in the New York Times Magazine informed readers that many sleep researchers believe that sleep deprivation is reaching "crisis proportions."

This is a problem not just for serious insomniacs, but for the populace at large, the article said, and added: "People don't merely believe they're sleeping less; they are *in fact* sleeping less — perhaps as much as one and a half hours less each night than humans did at the beginning of the century — often because they choose to do so."

The power of prayer

Is there real healing power in prayer and faith? Yes, according to 99 percent of doctors polled at an October 1996 conference of the American Academy of Family Physicians. The survey was conducted among 269 attending physicians and reported in the December 1 issue of Parade Magazine. Three-quarters of the doctors also said they believed that the prayers of others can help a patient's recovery.

Herbert Benson, M.D., a well-known Harvard expert on stress and relaxation, notes: "We've seen that belief is powerful in conditions including angina pectoris, asthma, duodenal ulcers, congestive heart failure, diabetes, all forms of pain. We see it all the time, and we can't deny it."

One interesting study that tested the power of prayer to heal involved some 393 patients with heart failure in the coronary care unit at San Francisco General Hospital. These individuals were divided up and randomly assigned to two groups. The patients in one of the groups were prayed for each day by home prayer groups, who were given only the first names of the patients and a summary of their condition. There were no fixed criteria for praying. Rather, the participants prayed in whichever way they understood prayer.

When the study was concluded, the patients who were prayed for were five times less likely to require antibiotics and three times less likely to develop fluid backup in the lungs, a result of heart failure.

In addition, none of the prayed for patients needed endotracheal intubation, a life-support procedure in which a tube is inserted into the windpipe and connected to a ventilating machine. In the group that was not prayed for, 12 patients needed intubation.

Brian Rees, M.D., M.P.H., an expert in natural medicine, commented that "the magnitude of these changes is significant; if a drug or surgical procedure had accomplished these, it probably would be standard therapy in corony care units all over the country."

CHAPTER THIRTEEN

Chiropractic — Much more than just treating back pain

The amazing case of Leslie Lockerman

Step 8

If you are a physician and you see people like Leslie Lockerman enter your office, you take a deep breath and pray with all your heart that you have the ability to help such a person. In the summer of 1995, Leslie, then 30-years-old, was escorted into my clinic by her devoted mother Barbara.

Leslie was born with extensive physical defects. She saw the world at a 90 degree angle, the result of her neck being bent to the right, locked in a position so that her head practically rested on her shoulder. It was impossible for her to bring her head to a normal upright position, and at any given time, her head could roll forward involuntarily.

Leslie always required assistance when walking. She walked up on her toes, her body bent forward at the waist. From her angle of sight, it seemed as if she was always walking uphill. She would often fall and injure herself. On several occasions, she had fractured her feet and toes.

Leslie can hear, but she cannot speak. She lacks the fine hand coordination with which to use other than the simplest of hand signs. With the help of her mother, who carries a portable computer and printer with her wherever they go, Leslie has been able to "communicate" better with the world around her. She points to letters of the alphabet on a large pad as her mother types the sequence of letters into words, sentences and thoughts.

A few months after she was born, Leslie began suffering from

"When one or more vertebrae of the spine go out of place, they are likely to produce serious complications and even death, if not properly adjusted."

— Hippocrates,
the "Father of Western Medicine"

seizures that would convulse her entire body. She was on three different anti-convulsive medications at the time of her first appointment with me.

Leslie was also sensitive to chemicals and electromagnetic energy. She suffered from hives over her entire body. She experienced frequent infections, headaches and menstrual problems. She was always constipated and required routine daily warm water enemas throughout her life. She urinated only once a day. She drooled from the mouth continuously. She could never drink water while standing up.

Leslie didn't sleep like you and I do. She would sleep continually for a few days at a time. Then she would remain awake for the next few days.

Over the years, Leslie had been given varying diagnoses, including cerebral palsy, autism and mental retardation. She had been treated with allergy shots, physical therapy and heavy drug therapy.

"All this had little or no beneficial effects," Barbara Lockerman told me.

During my physical evaluation of Leslie, I found multiple and severe spinal misalignments. I felt she could benefit from chiropractic adjustments, as well as nutritional supplements and elimination of certain foods from the diet.

Leslie's response to adjustments was nothing less than amazing. After one single adjustment on her neck and lower back, the following things happened:

- Her head straightened to an upright position for the first time.
- She walked unescorted out of my office.
- She was no longer constipated.

Leslie continues to be treated and improve. Her head is upright. She walks on her own — without any assistance — and no longer on her toes. Although she cannot yet fully bring her heels to the ground, she is getting close. She is more sure-footed. She no longer falls. The hives are long gone. She sleeps normally. She can stand on her own and drink a glass of water. The infections and headaches are rare. She urinates three or four times daily. Her menstrual cycles are becoming more normal with less pain. Her seizures have lessened dramatically and she has been able to stop the anti-seizure medication.

Far from being retarded, Leslie is a very bright human being with a sense of humor. With the help of her mother on the computer, she told me after one particular treatment: "Ha! Ha! I'm not retarded. I'm not autistic."

On another occasion, she said: "I feel better. I eat better. I see better. The adjustments make powerful changes."

With time and continued weekly adjustments, her mother says,

Leslie's fine and gross movements have improved. The adjustments are lessening the severity of lifelong spinal subluxations and accompanying distortions in her musculature. With continued perseverance, effort and a focus on wellness, I am confident this long-suffering woman will continue to make progress in the direction of better health and physical function.

I have had many successes using chiropractic on challenged individuals. When you stop and think about it, doesn't it make sense that such individuals, who often have severe misalignments, would benefit from chiropractic manipulations?

I recall the case of an autistic child of kindergarten age. By the end of the school year, after a series of adjustments, the boy was so improved that he made a "graduation" speech on behalf of his classmates. His mother, a registered nurse, had considered chiropractic as unscientific, but chose to try it because she had no conventional options.

Another dramatic case involved an 18-month-old girl whose left arm was paralyzed. The girl's pediatrician sent her to a neurologist who said nothing could be done. A second neurologist prescribed physical therapy. After a year of therapy there was no change and the condition was described as permanent. We performed one adjustment on a misaligned fifth vertebra in the neck. A few days later she was starting to move her arm. After a second adjustment, the arm was free. She has had no problems ever since.

Why do I mention these particular cases? How do I explain these recoveries? Are they just rare or lucky occurrences?

Absolutely not!

Spinal misalignment is more than just back pain

Countless millions of us live our lives in various states of impairment because of a malfunctioning nervous system caused by spinal misalignments. Unless we have back pain, we generally tend to ignore our spine, the flexible, bony column that runs down the backside from the skull to the tailbone and protects the nervous system "wiring" operating the entire body. Yet the evidence is becoming clear that much of the pain and suffering we experience in our lives may be due to spinal neglect.

In studies here and abroad, chiropractic has been scientifically-validated as the most effective <u>and</u> cost-effective treatment for back pain. But don't let this fool you into believing that chiropractic is just for back pain.

Research is increasingly confirming what I and other chiropractic physicians have observed for many years in our practices — that manipulations are beneficial for many conditions of infants, adults and seniors, including fever, anxiety, bronchitis, asthma, allergies, arthritis, digestive disorders, disc problems, migraines, PMS, and memory loss.

Chiropractors long ago learned that you can't determine whether something is wrong with your spine just because you have pain. Pain, in fact, is not the only sign of spinal problems, or even the best.

I have personally treated many patients with kidney, bladder, bowel, and sexual organ dysfunction who did not have neck or back pain. While many people with misalignments do have pain, most do not. They have painless subluxations that impair normal nerve and blood supply to target organs. The effect is gradual loss of vitality and function, and the generation of a wide array of neck, back, nervous system and organ problems. I refer to these misalignments as "silent robbers of health." Unattended, they create symptoms that develop into dis-ease and eventually into disease.

Misalignments of the cranium — your skull — can produce a variety of behavioral and mental disorders that might never be pinpointed or corrected without chiropractic evaluation and treatment.

Misalignments in the neck can produce not only neck pain and headaches but make you vulnerable to ear infections, memory loss, mental confusion, depression, anxiety, dizziness, and hearing and visual difficulties.

Misalignments in the upper back can produce functional disorders in the lungs and even create symptoms that mimic the chest pain associated with heart disease.

Misalignments in the lower spine and sacroiliac joints can, of course, produce severe pain in the back and legs, but also pain in the abdomen and pelvic regions. Such stress can interfere with bladder function and sexual potency.

Many of the long-term health problems we have as adults are, in fact, the result of untreated misalignments that develop in infancy or childhood. Some of the health and behavioral problems of children are related in part or in whole to misalignments.

How many people are affected? It's hard to say. But in one study conducted more than 30 years ago at Prague's Charles University, researchers estimated that more than half the population in Czechoslovakia suffered for certain periods of time from conditions caused by spinal problems. Although not currently documented, spinal misalignments are probably more common than cavities.

Spinal facts

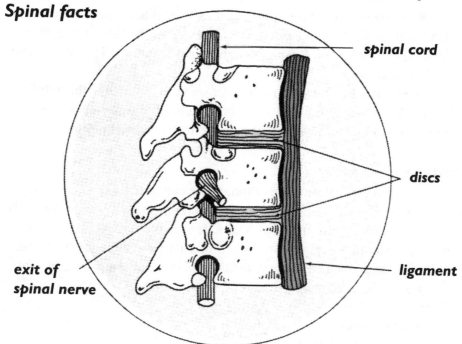

Your spinal column, extending downward from the skull, consists of 24 spinal bones, known as vertebrae. Each has a hole in the center that houses and protects the spinal cord. Branching out from the cord, between each vertebra, are the spinal nerves that supply the extremities, organs, muscles and tissue of your body with the electrical commands generated in the brain.

The spinal column also serves to support the head, ribs, shoulders and hips, and acts as an anchor for the muscles.

The column consists of :

• 7 cervical (neck) vertebrae. The uppermost (C-1) is called the "atlas." It supports the skull. Below it is "axis" (C-2), which allows the head to tilt and turn.

• 12 thoracic (mid-back) vertebrae. The ribs connect to all of them (T-1 to T-12).

• 5 lumbar (lower back) vertebrae. These are the biggest and strongest and carry the weight of the whole spine.

• Below the fifth lumbar vertebra is the sacrum, a triangular-shaped structure made up of five fused vertebrae. The sacroiliac joints connect the sacrum to the hip bones on both sides. The sacrum and hip bones make up the pelvis.

• At the bottom of the spinal rung, attached to the sacrum above it by ligaments, is the tailbone, or coccyx. Seen from the side, it resembles the beak of the cuckoo bird, which is how it got its name. The Greek word for cuckoo is kokkyx.

The cervical, thoracic and lumbar sections give strength, stability and flexibility to the spine. Between the vertebrae of these sections are gelatinous discs that act as shock absorbers for the spinal column.

Misalignment facts

A misalignment (or subluxation, as we chiropractors call it) simply means a bone or joint that is out of its normal position. Any joint in the body can become misaligned — the hips, knees, feet, hands, and the skull bones — but especially in the spine. But right now let's concentrate on the spine. Misalignments can happen in many different ways, and at any time of life:

• at birth, as a result of cesarean section, difficult breech, an obstetrician's error, or forceps delivery
  • from falls
  • athletic or work injuries
  • car accidents
  • sitting at a desk with your neck bent forward for long periods of time
  • over-using one side of the body
  • poor posture, even poor sleeping posture
  • if one leg is shorter than the other
  • weakness in the spine that makes you more susceptible to subluxations
  • long-term anxiety, emotional stress or unexpressed tension
  • overwork
  • poor diet
  • sedentary lifestyle

Misalignments can occur in the cervical (neck) part, or in the upper, mid or lower part of the back, or at multiple locations along the spine.

Each vertebra is a flexible joint that can move in distinct ways — forward bending (flexion), backward bending (extension), side bending (lateral flexion), and rotation. Any vertebra can misalign or lock in any of these motions, resulting in pain, loss of function, or both. If untreated, degeneration of the joints and disc develops.

Misalignments cause a major or minor disruption in the nervous system depending on the degree of subluxation, and the location. This generates a loss of normal communication between the brain and the organs, systems and cells that are supplied by the affected nerves.

The following can result from misalignments:

1. Painful joint or muscle problems.

2. Loss of organ and bodily functions, a silent eroding away of your health over years usually without you ever realizing the cause. I call such misalignments "silent robbers of health."

3. Loss of energy.

4. Degeneration of tissue.

3. All of the above.

Only a skilled chiropractor can tell if you have a misalignment.

Also, don't be lulled into believing that your children have a normal spine just because they pass the annual school scoliosis test. Nurses and medical doctors are not chiropractors. They have no training in spinal alignment or manipulation.

Your neglected spine

Modern research is making it clear that regular chiropractic evaluation — beginning from infancy — can be a powerful tool for regaining or maintaining optimum health. Think about it, you brush your teeth daily. You see a dentist regularly even though your teeth may not hurt. You may even have your teeth straightened for purely cosmetic reasons. You have regular eye examinations, gynecological examinations, blood pressure evaluations, cardiovascular checkups and yearly physicals. But did you ever have a chiropractic spinal checkup?

The truth is that your spine and nervous system are probably the most neglected parts of your body, and yet misalignments may be the cause of your ongoing health problems. Back pain is the No.1 cause of disability, not cavities.

Unless you suffer a traumatic injury, or experience pain, your joint misalignments are usually not recognized or diagnosed. You carry them with you over the course of your life. The price you pay for this neglect is high: degeneration and loss of health. It takes chiropractic evaluation and treatment to determine the presence of misalignments... and then correct them.

Your medical doctor usually won't recognize the spinal connection to health because he or she has received scant training in problems of spinal alignment. Moreover, most people aren't aware of the preventive or therapeutic value of chiropractic other than its role in the treatment of back pain, whiplash or injuries. This has to change — for the sake of your health. We are achieving remarkable results for conditions you would never imagine would be helped by chiropractic manipulation.

What is chiropractic?

Chiropractic is a philosophy, a science, and an art.

The philosophy: Chiropractic physicians recognize that innate intelligence supports and maintains all of life. We are dedicated to treating the whole body rather than just an isolated symptom or part, and in the process promote the body's innate intelligence and ability to heal and self-regulate, including, but not limited to, times of physical injury or mental and environmental stress.

The science: Chiropractic is a method of locating spinal and joint misalignments and reducing their impact on the nervous system and the organs of the body. As in other health professions, continual research is aimed at explaining how and why this healing method works. Scientific studies have clearly validated chiropractic treatment for back and neck pain, for vertigo, migraines and other disorders. Research will eventually catch up with the benefits that millions of patients already experience.

The art: A professor at my chiropractic college once said that to become a great chiropractor, you have to integrate your head, your heart and your hands to heal others. And so it is that chiropractic adjustments or manipulations are expressions of that complete integration of mind, body and compassion.

Researcher Tedd Koren, D.C., explains chiropractic in this way:

"Chiropractic adjustments are administered to relieve the body of the vertebral subluxation complex, a serious interference to life and health, a major stress in the body.

"Chiropractic is not a treatment for disease, nor do chiropractors claim to cure disease.

"Our natural healing ability, although potentially powerful, is often interfered by...(this) spinal nerve stress. Chiropractors remove spinal nerve stress, thus permitting us to tap into our reservoir of wholeness and healing.

"While no one can guarantee the healing, or curing, of disease, people who are ill need subluxation relief to maximize their ability to heal. It may make the difference.

"Research studies indicate the correction of the...subluxation can have a beneficial effect on health."

In a few words, chiropractic uniquely treats the systemic effects on health and function that subluxations cause.

The first modern adjustment

Knowledge of spinal care and adjustments is very old. Even in Hippocrates' time, 2,500 years ago, the benefits were known. Adjustments have been practiced for thousands of years throughout the world — in the Americas, China, India, Japan, the Pacific islands, the Middle East, and in Europe.

The "discoverer" of modern chiropractic was an Iowan, Daniel David Palmer (1847-1913), who performed his first adjustment on a deaf janitor in 1895. The deaf man, Harvey Lillard, worked for Palmer, a successful practitioner in natural healing methods. One day, Palmer asked Lillard how he had become deaf. The janitor replied that his deafness had started 17 years before when he heard something "pop" in his back.

Palmer was curious. He examined the man's spine and found what he believed was a misaligned vertebra. With Lillard's agreement, Palmer placed his employee face down on a table in his study. He then pressed his hands over the spine and carefully thrust downward. Lillard stood up, turned to Palmer, and smiled. He could hear again after 17 years.

Palmer at first suspected he might have found a treatment for deafness. But then a man with a heart condition came to see him. Palmer examined the spine and once again found a spinal abnormality. In this case, he reasoned, the misalignment might be causing interference with the spinal nerves that energize the heart.

"I adjusted the vertebra and gave immediate relief," he later wrote. "Then I began to reason if two diseases, so dissimilar as deafness and heart trouble, came from impingement, a pressure on nerves, were not other diseases due to a similar cause?"

Palmer soon began seeing and helping a wide variety of patients with his spinal technique. Word spread of his successes with asthma, skin problems, digestive disorders, headaches, pain and many other problems.

Chiropractic: "done by the hand"

One of his early patients was a scholar who coined the term chiropractic. The word stems from the Greek "cheir," meaning "hand," and "praktos, meaning "done by." Thus, chiropractic literally means "done by the hand."

Palmer, meanwhile, began researching and refining his new healing system. Eventually, he established the Palmer College of Chiropractic. His son, Bartlett Joshua, further developed the new profession, and expanded a teaching program for chiropractors that attracted thousands of students.

The medical profession ridiculed Palmer's treatment and "cure" of Lillard's deafness, as well as his other work. Nevertheless, similar positive results were later achieved by other doctors of chiropractic and a number of medical doctors interested in spinal health. J. F. Bourdillon, M.D., one of the few medical manipulators in the world, wrote extensively about his clinical findings. He, in fact, verified Palmer's work on deafness.

For many years, chiropractors worked in a hostile climate designed to eliminate their profession as competition to medical doctors in the U.S. health care system. This unlawful situation endured despite the positive results achieved by thousands of chiropractic physicians and a growing body of scientific research.

Clear-cut validation of chiropractic care emerged during the anti-trust suit filed by chiropractors against the American Medical Association and other medical organizations (Wilk et al vs. AMA et al., 1987). In 1990, following more than a decade of litigation, a federal appellate court, and then the U.S. Supreme Court, upheld a ruling by U.S. District Court Judge Susan Getzendanner that the AMA had engaged in a "lengthy, systematic, successful and unlawful boycott."

In her decision, Getzendanner cited scientific studies which implied that "chiropractic care was twice as effective as medical care in relieving many painful conditions of the neck and back as well as the related musculo-skeletal problems."

In 1991 the AMA agreed to publish a statement explicitly stating that medical doctors and chiropractors could associate professionally. Following the court decision, increasing numbers of medical doctors, hospitals and health care organizations in the U.S. have discovered the value of chiropractic care and began including the services of chiropractors.

For patients primarily, this is a most welcome development. No single method can possibly have all the answers for every condition. No single profession of physicians or health practitioners can possibly treat all sickness and disability. We must cooperate and work together, not for economic advantage, but for the ultimate good of the patient. Each practitioner must have the liberty to do what he or she does best, whether we are medical doctors, chiropractors, osteopaths, acupuncturists, doctors of oriental medicine, naturopaths, or ayurvedic physicians.

> *Salus aegroti suprema lex*, says a most relevant Latin phrase: "The welfare of the ailing is the supreme law."

For back pain — the treatment of choice

In recent years, government agencies and researchers have conducted scientific studies, based on many thousands of cases, that clearly demonstrate the benefits of chiropractic treatment. The Manga Report of 1993, funded by the Ontario Ministry of Health in Canada, overwhelmingly endorsed the efficiency, safety, scientific validity, and cost-effectiveness of chiropractic for low back pain. In addition, it found higher patient satisfaction compared to medical treatment.

"Evidence from Canada and other countries suggests potential savings of hundreds of millions annually," the Manga report states. "The literature clearly and consistently shows that the major savings from chiropractic management came from fewer and lower costs of auxiliary services, fewer hospitalizations and a highly significant reduction in chronic problems, as well as in levels and duration of disability."

In 1994, the U.S. Government's Agency for Health Care Policy and Research endorsed the use of spinal manipulation as a first line of treatment for low back pain.

For more details, see the chapter on back pain.

Who are chiropractors?

Chiropractic students begin their educational process by following a standard undergraduate pre-med curriculum. Afterward, they undergo a rigorous 4 1/2 year program in chiropractic school. Here, the basic and clinical sciences that are taught are identical to medical school. The unique difference is that the chiropractic student, unlike the medical student, receives extensive training in manipulation, physical therapy and nutrition.

In order to graduate as a doctor of chiropractic (D.C.), a candidate must pass a National Board Examination. Subsequently, new doctors apply to governmental or professional licensing boards and pass other challenging tests before being permitted to practice.

Following graduation, many new doctors of chiropractic opt for specialization in orthopedics, nutrition, acupuncture, neurology and other areas of expertise.

In my case, I obtained an additional master's degree in biology and nutrition. I have taken or taught postgraduate courses that include clinical nutrition and assessment, whiplash, head and spinal trauma, infectious diseases, obesity, inflammatory bowel diseases, radiology, orthopedic evaluation, and physiological therapeutics.

The educational process never ends for a chiropractor.

Chiropractic — vital statistics

- *Chiropractic is now the third largest primary health care profession in the western world after medicine and dentistry.*
- *There are approximately 50,000 chiropractic physicians in the U.S., 10,000 in Japan, 5,000 in Canada, 2,500 in Australia, 1,000 in the United Kingdom, and up to 500 in other European countries, South Africa and New Zealand.*
- *One in 15 Americans visits a chiropractor at least once a year and, according to a 1991 Gallop Poll survey, 90 percent of patients describe their treatment as effective.*
- *A 1989 study from the University of Toronto reported that a clear majority (62 percent) of family medical doctors refer patients to chiropractors and that 10 percent of medical doctors are themselves chiropractic patients.*
- *A comparative study of patients with low back pain found that individuals under chiropractic care were three times more satisfied with their treatment than care under family physicians.*
- *One study by a Washington D.C. health policies center listed chiropractic physicians along with osteopathic physicians and medical doctors as the only practitioners fully qualified to act as primary care providers by virtue of their education, licensure and health care focus.*
- *Chiropractic is currently the third largest primary health care profession in the Western world after medicine and dentistry.*

What is a chiropractic adjustment?

Chiropractors evaluate the motion of the spine to determine which vertebrae are locked and in which direction. An adjustment is the art of exerting a specific force in a precise direction or manner to a joint that is out of alignment, fixated, "locked up," or not moving properly. Adjustments reposition or restore normal movement to misaligned or restricted joints anywhere in the body and especially the spine. Although practiced worldwide by all health professions, chiropractors perform 96 percent of all adjustments.

Chiropractic adjustments take misaligned joints beyond their restricted barrier of movement to the "paraphysiological zone." It is in this zone that the greatest health benefits occur. In addition to increased range of motion, better movement, less pain or better pain tolerance, chiropractic adjustments restore the disturbed communication in the nervous system, allowing the brain once again to connect normally with vital organs and the rest of the body. This cannot be achieved through exercise, diet, vitamins, drugs, surgery or trying to "adjust yourself."

It is worth repeating that chiropractic treatments can have a positive effect on many health conditions and not just merely "back" problems.

There are numerous types of chiropractic adjustments including cranial manual therapy, diversified, sacro-occipital technique, applied kinesiology, activator, muscle energy techniques, and many others. Some adjustments are rapid. Others require a slow and constant pressure. The pop or crack that you hear following one type of chiropractic manipulation is the mere release of a gas bubble from the joint surfaces, not unlike opening up a can of pop.

Some adjustments, for instance, those used for infants, are extremely gentle.

How safe are chiropractic adjustments?

If you have never consulted a chiropractor, you may be wondering if chiropractic adjustments are safe. One analysis of the research literature on complications from total low-back spinal manipulation between 1911 and 1991 indicated an average of less than one case a year.

In the landmark Manga Report in Canada on chiropractic treatment of low back pain, the researchers concluded there is no evidence "that chiropractic spinal manipulation is unsafe in the treatment of low back pain. Some medical treatments are equally safe, but others are unsafe and generate iatrogenic complications. Our reading of the literature suggests that chiropractic manipulation is safer than medical management of low-back pain."

A 1997 Scandinavian study reported in the medical journal Spine quantified for the first time the incidence of common side effects from routine chiropractic treatment. The analysis, funded by the Research Council of Norway, the Norwegian Chiropractors' Association and the Swedish Chiropractors' Association, involved 102 chiropractic physicians and 1,058 patients.

In 1993, David Eisenberg, M.D., a noted Harvard researcher, published his now-famous study in the New England Journal of Medicine on the popularity of alternative medicine. He found that during the previous ten years more than 60 percent of Americans visited alternative practitioners, a higher percentage than visits to conventional medical doctors. Among the types of alternative medicine used, chiropractic was one of the most popular.

The treatments included manipulation exclusively (38 percent), manipulation and soft tissue techniques (36 percent), and manipulation, soft tissue techniques and other methods (25 percent).

No serious complications were reported by patients. Three out of four side effects disappeared within 24 hours of treatment. Common reactions included local discomfort (53 percent of reported reactions), headache (12 percent), tiredness (11 percent), and radiating discomfort (10 percent).

How chiropractors diagnose problems

Chiropractic physicians utilize many conventional tests such as EKG, blood tests, X-rays, and MRIs. At the same time, many of us recognize the limitation of these tests.

For instance, you may have excruciating migraine headaches yet a CAT scan of your brain indicates everything is normal. You may be chronically fatigued but your blood test is unremarkable.

These results are typical for millions of patients treated in the conventional medical system whose real health problems are often dismissed as psychosomatic — "it's all in your head," "learn to live with it," etc. The problem isn't that your symptoms aren't real, but rather that the tests aren't subtle enough to pick up the sources of the problems.

As we enter into 21st century medicine, more patients will have the opportunity to receive chiropractic care. Chiropractic recognizes that subtle changes in the body can manifest as health problems long before you are diagnosed with disease.

One of the major methods of modern chiropractic care often enables us to detect these subtle changes. It is called Applied Kinesiology, or AK for short. It was discovered in the early 1960s by Detroit chiropractic researcher, George Goodhart, D.C. Goodhart theorized that physical, chemical or emotional imbalances could stress the body and cause disease. He subsequently began to identify in great detail how such imbalances could actually be evaluated or measured through a system of muscle testing. Ultimately, his investigations revealed a direct relationship between muscles and organs.

In other words, if your liver is weak or stressed, we can treat muscles in your body that are "liver related muscles." If the muscle is weak, based on AK evaluation, we can proceed to find out if it is due to a misalignment in your spine, a nutritional deficiency, a weakness in your acupuncture energy field, a toxic overload to your immune system, a sensitivity to a food or chemical, or any other of a number of possible malfunctions.

The therapeutic goal then is to bring the body back into a state of balance.

AK and many other chiropractic methods are part of the "New Functional Medicine," a global movement among health practitioners that seeks to determine why a person is losing function. Once the cause is found, preventive strategies are developed to correct the imbalances before degenerative disease takes over.

In a sense, AK and other chiropractic methods are "natural CAT scans." They are simple, inexpensive methods for pinpointing the origins of problems. Although other tests are certainly necessary and valuable for confirming a diagnosis, AK is often the missing link and may make the difference between living a healthy life and simply learning to live with a problem.

Your problem may be all in your head...
...but not how you think it is!!!!

Most of us are familiar with the classic Ink Spots tune that went: "Your head bone's connected to your neck bone, your neck bone's connected to your back bone, and that's the word of the Lord....."

The song really sums up the chiropractic idea. Everything starts with the head bone, which is connected to everything else.

And indeed, chiropractic physicians have long known, structural misalignments within the skull are frequently overlooked sources of problems.

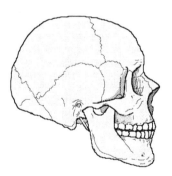 Your skull is not one solid piece of bone. Rather, it has plates that actually move, something like how the geological plates in the earth move. When you breathe in and out, for instance, the skull bones shift microscopically.

But if you have head or neck trauma, or you have cranial stress, your skull bones can lock along the suture lines — the "fault lines," so to speak — that separate the various plates of the skull. Inadequate pre-natal nutrition can cause misaligned cranial bones, as well as difficult delivery and incorrect application of forceps. Whatever the cause, there is a resultant loss of movement that creates neurological disturbances and stress, resulting in abnormal function and symptoms.

In youngsters, cranial misalignments commonly lead to ear aches, sinus congestion, vomiting, irritability and hyperactivity. In adults, it is more associated with constipation, headaches, anxiety, impotence, asthma, inflammatory conditions, pain, tendonitis, arthritis, interference with sensory function, and many chronic and non-specific conditions.

Cranial manipulation is often used for these conditions as well as in the treatment of strokes, cerebral palsy, spinal cord injury, and to improve overall body functioning.

In cranial manipulation, we apply a pressure point-type of treatment to unlock the sutures. This restores normal nervous system function. You don't hear the same kind of pop that you would with spinal or cervical manipulation.

Today, this form of therapy has gained acceptance by health professionals worldwide as a successful treatment modality. Cranial manipulation goes by various names, including sacro-occipital technique and craniosacral therapy.

"Brain hibernation"

In addition to misalignments in the head, misalignments in the spine can also cause typically misdiagnosed mental, behavioral and sensory problems. The mechanism for this has been explained in great length by Allen G. J. Terrett, D.C., of the Royal Melbourne Institute of Technology in Australia, who coined the term "brain hibernation" or cerebral dysfunction.

It works this way: There are arteries in your neck and head which carry blood and oxygen to your brain. If the blood is blocked or a clot occurs, a part of your brain can die. You have a loss of function related to that part of the brain no longer being supplied.

Compare this to a situation of severe or minor trauma to the head or neck resulting in misalignments causing a reduction of blood flow and interference of nerve impulses. The brain still functions, but underfunctions in varying degrees. Parts of the brain, in essence, are put into a "hibernating mode."

Research has documented that such misalignments set off a wide variety of symptoms, including dizziness, giddiness, difficulty sleeping, insomnia, excessive fatigue, depression, nervousness, disorientation, difficulty learning or concentrating, personality change, hyperactivity, "the whining child syndrome," temper tantrums, headaches, visual disturbances, auditory difficulties, mixing up words, losing track of conservation, and loss of interest in sex.

These conditions are often eliminated through manipulation. Normal blood flow and nervous system communication are restored. Adjustments remove the mechanical blockage. This allows the nervous system to function and the blood to flow normally.

Imagine a hose in your garden that has a pinched section. All the water isn't getting through. You unkink the hose and you restore normal flow.

In our contemporary medical system, most of these conditions I just mentioned are treated with drugs. You see a psychologist or neurologist and everything looks normal, so you are said to have a psychological problem. It's all in your head. And people go through life like this. Frequently, all that's wrong are undiagnosed misalignments.

Chiropractic — both a treatment and diagnostic method

Chiropractic is not just a method of treatment. It is also a method of diagnosis. If a patient's symptoms of vertigo, for intance, disappear after manipulation, then the true diagnosis is not vertigo. It is subluxation-induced vertigo. Just as you have drug-induced or viral-induced conditions, so, too, there are many conditions created by spinal or joint misalignments. It is important to understand this connection which is ignored by conventional physicians and even most alternative practitioners.

The expanding field of chiropractic research

Over the years, considerable research has been produced on chiropractic methods relating to many conditions. In recent years, the volume of research has grown dramatically. The following sampling of studies provides insight into the potential healing and helping role that chiropractic can play for young and old alike for problems other than back pain.

- **Improved brain function — chiropractic and the mind**

The theory behind "brain hibernation" to explain the many benefits of spinal manipulation was originally proposed by two Australian medical doctors: Eric Milne, a general practitioner, and Frank Gorman, an ophthalmologist. Each, with different training and a patient group complaining of a varying and large range of symptoms, realized that spinal manipulation generated multiple effects. They noted that after chiropractic treatment for headache, for instance, patients often commented that some other health complaint was relieved as well (such as tiredness, glare distress, and dizziness). Over time, they collected a growing list of conditions for which spinal manipulation was indicated. The mechanism they proposed to explain these post-manipulation effects was increased cerebral blood flow resulting in "hibernating areas" of the brain becoming functional again ("Chiropractic Medicine for Rejuvenation of the Mind," Academy of Chiropractic Medicine, 1983; Journal of Chiropractic Technique, 1992).

- **Manipulation improves mental function of a 14-year-old girl**

A 14-year-old girl with staring spells was unable to make eye contact. She rarely spoke and used only single words. Her left arm and hand hung flaccidly when she walked. She had been diagnosed with psychomotor seizures and degenerative neurological disorder. After upper neck manipulation began, her condition reversed. She started making eye contact. Within two weeks she was constructing sentences, standing straighter, using her arm and hand normally, and engaging in family conversations and activities. For those suggesting her improvement was a "spontaneous remission" unrelated to manipulation, chiropractors M. D. Thomas and J. Wood of the Palmer College of Chiropractic Clinic in Davenport, Iowa, reported that within six weeks of discontinuing treatment, she was unable to speak in sentences again. Following manipulation, proper speech was restored (Journal of Manual Medicine, 1992).

- **Chiropractic associated with better health in the elderly**

Elderly people under chiropractic care report better overall health, fewer chronic conditions, spend less time in hospitals, get around more, exercise more regularly, and are less likely to take prescription drugs compared to non-chiropractic patients. Those are among the findings of a 1996 study conducted by the Rand Corporation.

The study, conducted over a three-year period among 414 community-dwelling men and women 75 years of age or older, found that 87 percent of chiropractic patients described their health status as good to excellent. Only 68 percent of non-chiropractic patients said their health was good to excellent.

Of the total individuals in the database, 23, or 5.65 percent, were chiropractic patients. This percentage is similar to the number of geriatric chiropractic patients in the general population.

Fifteen percent more of the non-chiropractic group reported two or more chronic conditions, 22 percent more suffered from arthritis, and 21 percent more had been hospitalized during the previous three years (Topics in Clinical Chiropractic, 1996).

- **Short-term reduction in high blood pressure**

A significant short-term reduction in systolic and diastolic blood pressure was reported in this study of 21 patients with elevated blood pressure. Findings indicated that elevated blood pressure can be decreased on a short-term basis by chiropractic manipulation of the thoracic spine (Journal of Manipulation and Physiological Therapeutics, 1988).

- **Chiropractic treatment vs. Tylenol for neck pain**

Preliminary results of a 1996 study by the University of Colorado found that chiropractic adjustments are more beneficial than Tylenol (acetaminophen) for patients with chronic neck pain. In the study, researchers compared the effects of manipulation to 500 milligrams of acetaminophen taken four times daily. After six weeks, chiropractic patients reported significant improvements in neck pain and function compared to the medication group. In addition, they also showed a trend toward better range of motion and strength. The pill-takers had no such changes. A continuing follow-up was being conducted to determine if the results were long lasting (Family Practice News, June 1, 1996).

- **Chiropractic care may reduce menstrual pain without drugs**

Nearly half of all women suffer from primary dysmenorrhea (painful menstruation). The pain is so debilitating for 10 percent of these women that an estimated 100 million work hours are lost annually. One study of 45 women aged 20 to 49 showed chiropractic helped relieve the pain and distress associated with menstruation (Journal of Manipulative and Physiological Therapeutics, 1992).

In a 1979 study, women were divided into three groups. One group received chiropractic adjustments. The second received sham adjustments. The third was monitored only and did not receive any treatment. Eighty-eight percent of those individuals who received chiropractic adjustments reported reduced pain during their periods, while none of the other two groups reported improvement (Journal of Manipulative and Physiological Therapeutics, 1979).

- **Abdominal pain syndrome**

In a 1991 study of 36 patients with "abdominal pain syndrome," 30 individuals experienced improvement of symptoms as a result of chiropractic manipulation. The author reported that the success was due to correcting abnormalities of the nerve roots of the lower part of the back affecting the abdominal region (Klin Med, 1991).

- **Impaired hearing**

Nineteen patients with hearing deficits and cervical spine disorders were treated using chiropractic manipulation. Auditory tests showed that 17 patients responded to manipulation. The author concludes that it is possible to improve dull hearing by removing spinal interference in the upper part of the cervical spine (Vestn Otolaringol, 1987).

- **Sexual dysfunction and chiropractic**

J. E. Browing, D.C., reported the case of a 36-year-old female patient who "suffered from bladder discomfort, diarrhea, pain during intercourse, and an inability to experience orgasm. These symptoms had continued for 18 years, and were not resolved by numerous pelvic surgeries and other medical interventions. Although this patient never experienced low back pain, a chiropractic examination revealed evidence of a fifth lumbar subluxation with disc involvement. After four weeks of chiropractic care, bladder and bowel function were normal. All pelvic pain was gone within eight weeks, and by the time the paper was published, the patient was reportedly enjoying a normal sex life" (Journal of Manipulative and Physiologic Therapeutics, 1990).

An earlier article by Browning reviewed 10 cases. One involved a 41-year-old married woman with a 20-year history of urological, gynecological, sexual and bowel disorder. Following two weeks of chiropractic manipulation, bladder and bowel control returned to normal. The sexual difficulties resolved completely (Journal of Manipulative and Physiologic Therapeutics, 1988).

These studies are good examples of "silent subluxations," that is, spinal misalignments that cause problems other than low back pain.

• Subluxations of the spine common in children

Chiropractic is a vastly underused yet potentially powerful method to help the many ailments of infancy and childhood.

"Current research suggests that spinal health is particularly important for children. This applies from infancy, and extends far beyond back pain to prevention and general health," writes David Chapman-Smith, the editor of "The Chiropractic Report" and a Toronto attorney specializing in health law.

According to Philadelphia researcher Tedd Koren, D.C, who has played a major role in collecting research from around the world and making it available to clinicians such as myself, there is considerable evidence supporting the need for spinal care in infancy.

"Reports from Germany document what chiropractors have said for decades: that a significant percentage of newborns and infants have spinal misalignments," says Koren.

In one European study of 1093 newborns, 298 babies were found to have upper cervical (neck) subluxations and early signs of infantile scoliosis (an appreciable lateral deviation of the verticle line of the spine) (Rehabilitacia, 1975).

Karel Lewit, M.D., a Cezchoslovakian neurologist who has routinely used manipulation for decades, suggests that spinal misalignments in children may not necessarily generate spinal pain but rather create functional disorders such as sleep problems, loss of appetite, psychological disorders, and dysmenorrhea. In a 1970s book, Lewit cited research indicating that as many as 40 percent of otherwise healthy children reveal back subluxations with another 16 percent showing neck misalignments.

After manipulative treatments, problems rarely recurred ("Manuelle Therapie," J.A. Barth, Leipzig, 1973).

G. Guttman, M.D., another German medical doctor, has used chiropractic techniques for more than 35 years. From scientific studies and his own experience in treating more than 600 babies, he concluded that as few as 14 to 20 percent of children may have (autonomic) nervous systems in balance. He stated he has been "constantly amazed how, even with the lightest adjustment with the index finger, the clinical picture normalizes, sometimes gradually, but often immediately."

In a 1987 German medical journal, Guttman reviewed three cases to illustrate a misalignment disorder that has so far received scant attention — the atlas fixation syndrome — and which causes and perpetuates multiple problems in babies and infants. The atlas is the name for the first vertebra in the neck. When it is misaligned, the blocked nerve impulses can cause lowered resistance to infections, especially the ear, nose, and throat, insomnia, cranial bone asymmetry, retarded local motor development and linguistic development, conjunctivitis, tonsillitis, rhinitis, extreme neck sensitivity, curvature of the spine, delays of development, and seizures. "Chiropractic can often bring about amazingly successful results, because the therapy is a causal one," Guttman wrote.

In the same article, Guttman reported that an evaluation of 1,250 infants five days after birth revealed that a quarter of them suffered from vomiting, irritability and sleeplessness. Examination determined that 75 percent of these babies had cervical (neck) strain. Treatment frequently yielded immediate relief of symptoms, he said (Manuelle Medizin, 1987).

• **Health of children treated with chiropractic vs. conventional medicine**

Two hundred pediatricians and 200 chiropractors were randomly selected to determine differences in the health status of children raised under different health care models. Nearly 43 percent the medical children had suffered from tonsillitis, compared to less than 20 percent of the chiropractic children. Lower incidence of disease and less use of medication and antibiotics were reported in the chiropractic children. More than 80 percent of the medical children suffered from at least one bout of ear infections, compared to only 31 percent of the chiropractic children (Journal of Chiropractic Research, Summer 1989).

• **Asthma and bedwetting**

A 34-month-old boy with asthma and enuresis (bedwetting) had not responded to medical care. More than 20 emergency hospital visits for asthma attacks had taken place during a one year period. Three chiropractic adjustments were administered within 11 days. period. The asthma symptoms and bedwetting ceased for more than eight weeks. The symptoms recurred following a minor fall but disappeared after a new series of adjustments. At a two-year follow up, the mother reported no recurrence of either problem (Proceedings of the National Conference on Chiropractic and Pediatrics, 1991).

• **Visual recovery following chiropractic**

A 75-year-old man experienced a blow to his head in a fall. Headaches and dizziness followed and the next morning he woke up completely blind. Three months later, the patient was referred to a chiropractor who found subluxations in the neck. Following 11 manipulations over a three-month period, the patient's vision returned (Journal of Behavioral Optometry, 1990).

• **Pregnancy, labor and chiropractic**

Joan Fallon, D.C., reported that women who receive chiropractic care from at least the tenth week of pregnancy through labor and delivery have significantly shorter labor times compared to non-chiropractic patients. In first time pregnancies, the difference was an average of 24 percent less labor time. Women with previous childbirths averaged 39 percent less (Proceedings of the World Federation of Chiropractic, 1991).

• **Seizure disorders and manipulation**

A 5-year-old girl experienced up to 70 seizures a day. Following a series of chiropractic manipulations, the girl became seizure free. Subsequently, she underwent a spinal checkup every 2 to 3 months (Proceedings of the National Conference on Chiropractic and Pediatrics, 1991).

There have been additional reports in the chiropractic literature of reduced seizures as a result of chiropractic adjustments. One report described two children with petite mal (absent seizure) with potential for generating into grand mal. Upper neck adjustment reduced negative brainwave activity and frequency of seizures over a four-month period (Proceedings of the National Conference on Chiropractic and Pediatrics, 1992).

• **Paralysis improved with chiropractic**

An 11-year-old quadriplegic boy, injured in an accident, failed to respond to three months of conventional conservative hospital management, including steroid therapy. He made major improvements during a similar period under chiropractic care (Journal of Manipulative and Physiologic Therapeutics, 1993).

An earlier report involved a 24-year-old woman with myoclonus (uncontrolled spasms) of the inner thighs and abdomen. Her condition was triggered by a diving accident 17 years previous. She had not responded to conventional medical care. The condition was apparently resolved following a single chiropractic manipulation to relieve the subluxation in the thoraco-lumbar region (Journal of Manipulative and Physiologic Therapeutics, 1989).

• **Multiple sclerosis and chiropractic**

A 32-year-old male with fatigue, gait imbalance, double vision and numbness of his lower legs had a family history suggestive of multiple sclerosis (MS). The patient was evaluated by a neurologist who confirmed the multiple sclerosis based on examination and MRI. Following a single manipulation, the patient reported a complete absence of symptoms. Months later, the patient was still symptom free (Journal of Manipulative and Physiologic Therapeutics, 1993).

• **HIV patients benefit from chiropractic**

Five HIV positive patients were given chiropractic care, specifically upper cervical adjustments. Another group of five acted as controls and received no such treatment. After six months, the control group was found to have an average 8 percent reduction in CD4 (a measure of immune system function) count. The adjusted group experienced a 48 percent increase. The researchers suggested an association between correction of upper cervical subluxation and improved immuno competence (Chiropractic Research Journal, 1994).

What the future promises

As we move ahead into the 21st century, a greater spirit of cooperation is emerging between chiropractic and medicine that will redefine and expand the role of chiropractic in our lives. I believe that our profession will become an essential starting point to evaluate the relationship between structure (nervous system) and function (health).

Chiropractic is not a panacea but rather an integral part of an entire wholistic approach recognizing that health is not the absence of symptoms but rather a state of complete physical, nutritional, emotional and spiritual well being.

PART THREE

Natural Remedies For Specific Health Conditions

══ HOW TO USE THE INFORMATION ══

Charles Hodges, of Greensburg, Pennsylvania, thought his health was perfect. He never gave much thought to his diet, which included a typical breakfast of eggs, bacon, sausage and toast. Then he had a heart attack.

> **Charles Hodges —
> Proving his
> cardiologist wrong**

At the hospital, catheterization showed him to have a 95 percent blockage in a major coronary artery. He received angioplasty — the balloon technique — that reduced the blockage to 20 percent. His cardiologist said he would have to take heart medication for at least five years and probably would suffer another heart attack within six months unless he had a bypass operation.

Hodges, a 48-year-old accountant at the time, chose to go the natural route. He realized that his health was not as perfect as he thought.

At our clinic, we developed a therapy program that didn't just focus on his heart, but rather his whole body. It included detoxification of a lifetime of collected toxins, a change in eating habits, supplements to eliminate nutritional deficiencies, exercise, and chiropractic manipulation.

Now at age 51, some two-and-a-half years after his heart attack, Hodges is doing great.

"I believe I am in better health now than any time in my life," he told me during a recent checkup. "I feel like somebody 30-years-old. I work full time, do yard work, swim, walk, play ball with my son, paint the house, walk up steps, no limit."

Hodges never had the second heart attack. He never had the bypass surgery. The cardiologist said the operation wasn't necessary. Just keep doing what you are doing, the doctor told him. He no longer takes heart medication. He no longer regards the diet plan we gave him as a diet.

"It's just the way I eat now," he says. He lost 25 pounds.

His HDL cholesterol (the "good cholesterol) increased. His LDL cholesterol (the "bad cholesterol") decreased.

The diagnosis of heart disease for many is like a death sentence, synonymous with heart attack, stroke, severe debility and death. The combination of symptoms and fear is so overpowering that hundreds of thousands of Americans willingly submit to risky and questionable procedures.

Fortunately for Charles Hodges he decided to take the alternative medicine path and avoid the medical treadmill. He learned and experienced first hand that blockage and death are not synonymous.

Patients perceive heart disease and high blood pressure as causes of illness. They are not causes, but rather the effects of multiple systems in the body malfunctioning.

With alternative medicine, we can address those multiple defects, treat the whole body, and often are able to eliminate the effects, such as blockages and high blood pressure.

Few people realize it but chiropractic manipulation has the ability to help reduce blood pressure and improve circulation. Since the nervous system is the controlling agent in the body, spinal subluxations can impair circulation to the heart muscle as well as cause elevated blood pressure. Alleviating the spinal stress can reduce the interference in the lines of communication and help re-open blood supply to areas that have been shortchanged. Chiropractic manipulation offers great potential in restoring normal cardiovascular function.

Along with adjustments, Hodges began an exercise program to recondition his heart. Detoxification removed toxins from his body that can contribute to heart disease. Specific nutritional prescriptions and a new way of eating improved his nutritional status. The sum total of the treatment helped him establish a new network of vessels to circumvent the blockage.

Patients who become their own doctors

In a large sense, Charles Hodges — and thousands of other patients like him who I have treated — have become their own doctors. This is what the natural approach to health does for people. It awakens the doctor within. It educates patients. It engages them actively in their own self-healing process.

Usually you go to a doctor and you get a prescription. You don't learn much, except that you have disease X. You may get some relief for your symptoms but the underlying condition still remains. You aren't any healthier or wiser.

Many people are accustomed to think only in terms of surgery and medication. But as we have seen, this approach is limited and full of many risks. The natural approach has so many more options to offer:

- detoxification
- the broadened concept of allergy and sensitivity testing
- better nutrition
- supplements, herbals, and homeopathy
- and chiropractic care.

We have many powerful methods to restore balance and health to even the most seriously ill of patients.

Often patients who see me for the first time are taking multiple medications on a regular basis, a situation that may be compounding their problems. Our approach usually enables these individuals to function better on lowered doses or even without prescriptions. They learn why they are doing poorly and what they can do to improve their health and quality of life.

We treat, but more important, we try to inspire and encourage a process of self-healing. This is where the REAL health care reform has to begin. At the level of the individual. This is health empowerment. It starts with awareness of how we create our own ill-health and how we have the ability to create our own good health. This is what being in charge of one's own body is all about.

Think about it. Who should be in charge? You or a stranger called a doctor? It is up to you. We can only make recommendations and try to restore balance to your body. We are always there to help you maintain balance, but your lifestyle is what keeps you on the healthy path or puts you into a health nose-dive.

We can provide guidance and act as partners in the healing process. You MUST be the ACTIVE partner. And you must be faithful to the process.

Natalie Lauterbach's case

Natalie Lauterbach, 33, a housewife from Cheswick, Pennsylvania, suffered from multiple problems, including constant fatigue, environmental allergies, depression,

"Within three months, a new person emerged"

nervousness, confusion, severe menstrual cramps, lower back and leg pain, blurred vision, itchy dry skin, hair loss and white patches on her tongue. Over the years her doctors had treated her symptoms with conventional means.

"They gave me shots for my allergies, Motrin for my menstrual cramps, Flexeril for my back pain, steroids and Retin-A for my skin, counseling for my depression, and Rogaine for my hair loss," she told me. She said she also received a pamphlet on relieving stress.

As for the white patches on her tongue, that remained a "mystery" that lasted some 14 years.

When Natalie visited our clinic, we determined she had a systemic yeast infection, along with allergies to milk and wheat. In addition, she was deficient in many essential nutrients, tested high in toxic minerals, and had misalignments in her spine.

We put her on a detox program, followed by a diet free of milk, wheat and sugar. We prescribed a regimen of supplements. She received monthly chiropractic adjustments.

Natalie began feeling better. "Within three months, a new person emerged," she told me.

As she began feeling better, Natalie thought she would cheat on her diet. So she indulged in sweets and ate too many grains, which were taboo on her diet. She paid the price with a sore throat, stomach ache and sluggishness. She realized that in her case she was going to have to be faithful and follow the program. She became aware very quickly of how maintaining a certain kind of diet really worked for her.

"The key to wellness is proper nutrition, not the typical American diet," she told me. "I think of it as choosing life over half a life."

Today, Natalie has, in her own words, "more energy than ever. No back pain. No menstrual cramps. No depression. I am able to think and see clearly. My skin is much smoother. My tongue is improving. My hair loss is slowing down and my allergies are almost gone."

Natalie has become educated about her own health, on what it takes to keep her healthy. This is what we try to do with our patients. We give them the know-how, help them with techniques and natural remedies, and enable them to channel their determination for a healthier life into reality.

In part three, I will share some of these methods as they relate to different conditions. Much of the information you will be reading here you have not seen anywhere else. You will learn that there are many things you can do to improve your health. I will be covering some of the numerous conditions I treat and make general suggestions on how to overcome these problems and regain health. .

Remember: we are each unique

So many patients, like Natalie Lauterbach, have not just one, but many complaints. In fact, the patient in my practice with multiple problems is the typical patient. A patient will usually come not just with a migraine, but with a migraine, fatigue, poor digestion, allergies and perhaps other things. For that reason I have dedicated the entire next chapter to multiple symptoms. All the other chapters in part three focus on single conditions, but even in these situations many of the patients I see suffer from numerous complaints.

The material you will be reading includes relevant scientific studies, my clinical approach to problems and complaints, and answers to questions raised by callers during television and radio programs, or from the audience at lectures I have given. You will also read some very personal case histories, shared with me by my patients who expressed the hope that their own stories will inspire others to try a new healing path.

The blend of information here is not meant to suggest a protocol for treatment. My intent is to provide hope, ideas, practical knowledge, and inspiration to find an alternative to "learning to live with it."

Specific conditions and cases described here may be similar to yours. Nevertheless, each case should be viewed in terms of biological individuality, a theme I have talked about earlier. Each person brings a unique condition and background, and needs to be treated individually. Wholistic evaluation and treatment are always geared to the individuality of the patient. That means not just biochemical individuality but also structural individuality. If you were to take 10 patients with the same condition, not only will they have 10 different personalities, 10 different biochemical profiles but also 10 unique misalignment patterns. For this reason, one needs to treat the patient and not merely the illness.

For each condition, I will suggest a treatment and supplement prescription that always includes the Gallagher Wellness Program. This program is comprised of the eight steps described in the previous section of the book and lays the foundation for maximum healing. Some of the supplements I recommend are generic and widely available. Others I name by brand because my patients have responded exceptionally well to them.

If you are taking prescription drugs or have a serious medical problem you should always consult a qualified health professional. The natural remedies I recommend are not a substitute for medical care and treatment.

I welcome you to visit us at Medical Wellness Associates in Jeannette, Pennsylvania, just outside of Pittsburgh. In appendix A at the end of the book, I have outlined the many services we offer. For further information, you may call my clinic at (412) 523-5505.

If consulting with us is not convenient, then I encourage you to see a wholistic practitioner in your area. Refer to Appendix C for a list of some of the outstanding health organizations you can call for referrals.

MULTIPLE SYMPTOMS
REFUGEES OF A MEDICAL DISASTER

Patients often complain of multiple symptoms. Because of this, many run through medical hoops — going from one specialist to another — in an attempt to resolve what appears to be separate health problems. The process can be very costly and very frustrating. Moreover, when drugs are prescribed, the side effects from them can compound the misery and generate a whole new subset of symptoms.

The cases presented in this section speak for themselves. They are testimonies of a medical system gone awry. They represent typical patients in my clinic and the clinics of other alternative practitioners. They are, in essence, refugees escaping the madness of conventional medicine, where symptoms are drugged, masked, poisoned, burned, or cut out, and the causes of illness ignored.

These are typical cases. Not in the least bit unusual. These are the stories of patients who often come to my clinic out of desperation, frustration and confusion, almost as a last resort. For many of these patients, alternative practitioners are their last hope — a hope that there is indeed healing some- where in the healing profession they have long been led to believe in.

One of the great advantages of a wholistic or wellness program is that we treat the whole body, going to the core of the problems, addressing nutritional deficiencies, removing interference in the nervous system, and balancing the entire body. This means that frequently we can achieve across-the-board improvements and put at rest the troubled minds of patients whose multiple symptoms lead them to fear the worst.

Not every case is a success. Often we achieve great improvements. Other times, lesser degrees of help. A great deal depends on the willing- ness of patients to change their lifestyles and make an effort to become involved in their own health. When they do, results are maximized.

Sue Sloan's case

Since 1974, Sue Sloan, a housewife from Hopwood, Pennsylvania, had been treated by a long list of doctors. Each prescribed some new medication and by 1995 she was following a regimen of a dozen or so different drugs to deal with intestinal problems, stress, headaches,

> **Fatigue, depression, intestinal disorders, arthritis, infections and allergies**

arthritis, congestion, allergies, sore throat, and a fungal infection.

She told me she reached a point "where even turning over in bed was a cause of discomfort." Despite their best efforts, she was snared in a medical treadmill that wasn't helping her. In fact, she was getting worse and had reached a point of utter confusion and desperation when she came to see me in November of 1995.

"I just don't understand it," the 54-year-old woman said. "I have always been health conscious and have always worked hard to stay in good physical health by regular exercise, aerobics, and walking. I have tried to eat properly. Why am I so sick and weak?"

Sue needed to look no farther than her medicine cabinet at home for a big part of the answer. It contained 12 different medications. She took Premarin and Provera as hormone replacements, Axid and Bentyl for her stomach, Buspar for stress, Darvocet for headaches, the antibiotic Amoxil for sore throats, just to name a few. From her many years of taking continual medication, she was extremely toxic.

Sue's problem was also related to food allergies, nutritional deficiencies and multiple spinal misalignments. I told her I felt that we would be able to wean her off medication, reduce her pain and restore her health again if she followed the program. First of all I wanted to rid her body of accumulated toxins. We recommended the detoxification program. We also started her on a series of chiropractic adjustments and a regimen of nutritional therapy to improve liver and intestinal function. The first month was hard going for her as she slowly began to shed her dependency on medication. But in the second month, she said, she could tell definitely that her condition was improving.

"My daily headaches and pain are less," she told me. "My energy level is up. I know there is hope for me."

During the third month of treatment, Sue said the headaches were practically all gone and the depression as well. Today, she follows a wellness maintenance program that includes chiropractic checkups and nutritional supplements. She no longer is fatigued, depressed or in pain from arthritis.

John Lucy's case

John Lucy, Ph.D., a college professor, came to our office because of what he thought was arthritis in the lower back that he had suffered for years and which was increasingly

> **Arthritis, hypertension, gagging sensations, side effects from medication**

impairing his activities.

"The pain in my back and legs are preventing me from working around the house, something I really enjoy doing," he told me.

John had been on medication for the pain for more than three years. In addition, he had hypertension, and was taking medication for that as well. The anti-hypertensive drugs were causing trembling and impotence. He also frequently experienced choking and gagging sensations and had a difficult time swallowing both liquids and solids.

In May of 1994 John started on our comprehensive wellness program. He lost 40 pounds. He was able to cut out his hypertension medication and keep his blood pressure under control. After he stopped the drugs, the trembling and sexual dysfunction ceased.

His so-called arthritis problem in his back that had been causing him pain and limited motion, were spinal subluxations. With chiropractic adjustments, his back and leg pain diminished, his range of motion increased, and his gagging sensations and swallowing difficulties resolved.

John was able to return back to his "home improvement" activities, including some serious remodeling, all with much less pain. He visits the clinic for regular chiropractic "tune-ups" and makes a strong effort to follow his prescribed diet and supplement program.

"Anyone who knew me before is amazed at how much better I look and feel," he told me recently.

The Ryan Family

Linda Ryan, 39, of Pittsburgh, shared this report with me about her family: "Both my husband Tom and I were raised in the belief of conventional medicine. Tom has had chronic allergy and sinus problems since he was a teenager. For over 15 years he received allergy

> **Allergies, sinus infections, colds, bronchitis, ear infections, constipation, etc...**

shots and medication which he stopped using because they gave him very little relief.

"In his early twenties, Tom started getting sinus infections which were immediately treated with antibiotics. Over the next 10 years, the infections became more severe and more frequent and each medical treatment required a stronger antibiotic.

"Tom decided it was time to try another approach to treating his illnesses. He was missing valuable time at work and precious time with his family.

"Tom stopped using antibiotics to treat his sinus infections. He started changing his diet, taking vitamin and mineral supplements and getting regular chiropractic adjustments. When he did get a sinus infection he used natural remedies to get rid of the infection instead of medication. Before he used to get five or six severe infections a year. Now after four years of natural health care, he has only had one slight sinus infection.

"I also grew up with conventional medicine. As a teenager, I frequently had colds and bronchitis and was often treated with antibiotics. By my twenties, I was getting bladder infections and occasional yeast infections which were again treated with medication.

"By my early thirties, all my illnesses were snowballing. I had constant swollen glands and a sore throat. I also had bouts with sinus infections, pneumonia and mononucleosis. My immune system was being destroyed by antibiotics. My yeast level was four times the normal level because

> **"My immune system was being destroyed by antibiotics."**

the antibiotics were killing the good bacteria that keeps the yeast down to a normal level. As a result, my immune system was dangerously weakened. I felt tired and sick all the time and was unable to give as much time and energy to my family as I needed to give.

" So along with Tom I started using the natural approach. Just as he did, I changed my diet, took supplements, and got chiropractic adjustments. I quickly noticed an improvement in my energy level. I also had symptoms that disappeared without even trying to treat them.

"I had a rash on my back that I had unsuccessfully treated for months with a cream that was prescribed by a dermatologist. My rash was gone.

"Every year I look back to how I felt the year before and I know I am getting healthier and stronger. This is proof to me that we are heading in the right direction.

"Tom and I knew that a natural health approach would also benefit our three children. Our oldest son, Sean, now 13, frequently had ear infections the first five years of his life. Then he started getting a lot of colds and also had bouts with pneumonia and mononucleosis, but he most frequently suffered from severe headaches. The pain was so bad that he had to go to bed when the headaches occurred. By eliminating dairy products from his diet, taking vitamin supplementation and getting chiropractic adjustments, Sean's headaches vanished.

"Our other son, Devin, aged nine, has also benefited from our health care changes. He has had problems with constipation since birth and once again diet change, supplements, and adjustments greatly improved his condition.

"Caitlin, our five-year-old daughter, had a constant runny nose as a toddler which disappeared when we made our health care changes. When she had an allergic reaction that caused her lymph glands to swell up almost to the size of golf balls, we were able to resolve her situation with natural remedies instead of using medication.

"Our whole family has become healthier since we have chosen a natural approach to health care. The change has affected us in many positive ways. We spend less time being sick and more time doing things together as a family."

The case of Ryan and Jason Bonnet

Brothers Ryan and Jason Bonnet, of West Mifflin, Pennsylvania, were having more than their share of health problems.

> **Sinus infections, sore throats, allergies, immune deficiency**

Ryan had been taking prophylactic antibiotics because of what was termed by an infectious disease specialist as a genetic disorder of his immune system — specifically a failure to produce IgA, an antibody.

The boy had non-stop ear, nose and throat infections. His IgA count was almost zero.

In 1994, at age nine, Ryan was brought to see me. After starting on a program of chiropractic and nutritional care, he made a major improvement.

Over a three-year period, the youngster has rarely been sick. He was able to stop the routine antibiotics. According to Virginia, his mother, "he is a much healthier boy and now has a more normal antibody count." A recent blood test showed his IgA count at 35 His own natural internal pharmacy is now making what he needs.

His brother Jason, now 10, had always been a sick child. "One sinus infection after another and always on antibiotics," his mother told me when she first brought the youngster in several months after Ryan first came to the clinic. "He has had a very rough time with childhood illnesses."

Virginia hadn't had Jason's immune system tested. She thought he probably had the same defect as his brother and faced a lifetime of susceptibility to allergies and infections that would have to be controlled by repeated antibiotics.

We diagnosed Jason with an allergy to milk, which caused problems with his sinus, and a yeast infection due to repeated antibiotics. Like his brother, he started on a program of chiropractic adjustments, dietary and nutritional therapy. He, too, has improved greatly.

Many individuals with an immune system deficiency are locked into a lifetime of medications. The Bonnet Brothers can attest to the fact that there are better options. Both boys receive maintenance chiropractic and nutritional care instead of maintenance antibiotics. Each of them required an antibiotic only once since they started the program.

Catherine Marlene Palmer's case

This 58-year-old housewife from Ligonier, Pennsylvania, shared the following account with me:

> **High blood pressure, ulcers, chronic illness, loss of hearing and eyesight**

"I would probably already be dead if I hadn't found Dr. Gallagher's clinic.

"My blood pressure was up. I had stomach ulcers. I was continually sick. I had lost my strength. I couldn't pick up my one-year-old grand-daughter. I was losing my hearing and my eyesight. I had three eye prescriptions in three months. My memory was getting worse and I couldn't remember a phone number long enough to dial it. I was constantly in pain from my back. I was taking many vitamins but they did not appear to help.

"My medical doctor did not know what was wrong with me. He told me to go to a dietitian. Dr. Gallagher treated me nutritionally and performed chiropractic manipulations. Now my life is back to normal and I can do the things I used to do."

Catherine Marlene Palmer, like many people, tried to help herself by taking vitamins and following a better diet. However, she continued to deteriorate until she received the specific therapy and nutritional support appropriate for her individual situation. I determined she had chronic multiple spinal misalignments, low thyroid, and malabsorption. Her entire health picture began to change once her individual needs were met.

Ruth Cox's case

Ruth Cox, 59, is a homemaker from Washington, Pennsylvania, who developed circular skin lesions back in the late 1980s. Appearance of the lesions, called "granuloma annulare," prompted her to seek medical help.

> **Skin problems, neck and lower back pain, allergies**

According to Ruth, she spent several months under the care of two different specialists. Each said they didn't know the cause and had no cure for her. Both prescribed a very expensive strong cortisone cream and said to try it on a few areas. She had many spots.

"The treatment had no effect and I was beginning to feel hopeless and self conscious because I was getting more and larger lesions and also I knew my body was absorbing all this cortisone," she told me. "They gave me the option of taking steroids and I declined."

After hearing my Saturday radio program over a period of weeks, Ruth came to the conclusion that her problem could be solved internally, and not by external creams. She also suffered from neck and lower back pain, as well as allergies. Those problems, but particularly the skin lesions, prompted her to call for an appointment.

Testing determined that Ruth had a gluten intolerance. That meant she was allergic to the protein in wheat, oats, rye and barley. She couldn't handle rice either. Dairy was the cause of her constant sinus headaches. We first put her on a detox program and then a restricted diet. Ruth made rapid progress.

"By following the diet, I have lots of energy," she told me during one of her visits. "I used to be tired most of my adult life, and I thought it was natural for me. Now I know it's not."

Ruth's chronic skin problem has improved significantly. We have also helped her overcome depression that was related to low blood sugar. We have used diathermy, ultrasound, chiropractic manipulation and supplements to elevate her to a better level of health.

Diana Burch's case

Diana Burch, 48, a steelworker from Weirton, West Virginia, was in misery. She had colon problems, hives, carpal tunnel syndrome, and lower back pain. Her knees hurt when she walked up and down stairs.

> **Intestinal disorder, hives, carpal tunnel syndrome, lower back and knee pain**

By the time she came to see me in September of 1995, she had been to see six different medical doctors.

"I have been on prescription drugs for the last 10 years," she told me.

We recommended chiropractic adjustments for Diana, plus nutritional supplements and a strict diet.

Today, she reports, "I am no longer on prescription drugs. My colon problems have improved tremendously. My hives aren't as bad as they used to be. My finger isn't numb anymore from the carpal tunnel. My knees don't hurt.

"I decided to try natural health care because I wasn't getting anywhere with the medical doctors I had gone to. I am getting better everyday now. It's unbelievable."

Harriet Morring's case

Teacher Harriet Morring, 49, from New Alexandria, Pennsylvania, suffered from asthma, allergies, and sinus infections. She had headaches for 10 years and Epstein-Barr Virus for 7 years. She was taking a long list of drugs — antibiotics, Asthmacort and Ventolin inhalers, Theo-Dur, Prednisone at times, and vitamins.

> Headaches, fatigue, asthma, allergies, sinus infections, diarrhea

When she came to see me in November of 1995, she had been experiencing chronic diarrhea for 3 months.

"The doctors have done their best," she told me. "I just haven't gotten better."

We found she had a general yeast infection, parasites, and an allergy to wheat. We put her on a detoxification program, along with colonic treatments, and a restricted diet with yeast products, dairy and sweets. Instead of milk, she uses rice milk. Chiropractic adjustments helped to clear up her sinus problem.

Results? In her words, "I lost 39 pounds. Sinuses are clearer, nose is open, no diarrhea, seldom do I have headaches."

Harriett still has to use some medication for her asthma but we have brought her a long way. She has taken no antibiotics since starting natural health care.

Barbara Lockerman's case

This testimonial was provided by Barbara Lockerman, 60, of Washington, Pennsylvania:

> Systemic candidiasis, hypothyroidism, chronic cough, scoliosis, chronic diarrhea, reflux esophagitis

"I decided to try alternative medicine after I was admitted to the psychiatric unit of my local hospital as a result of a reaction to the third anti-hypertensive drug my medical doctor had tried on me. I had also spent days on intravenous antibiotics for three bouts of pneumonia and infiltrates in my lungs.

"I started treatment with Dr. Gallagher in the summer of 1994. At that time I had systemic candidiasis, hypothyroidism, chronic cough, scoliosis, chronic diarrhea, reflux esophagitis, with almost constant pain, headaches, chronic fatigue, some mental confusion, and, needless to say, depression. The recommended treatments included chiropractic adjustments, dietary supplementation, and elimination of certain foods from my diet, colonic irrigation and myotherapy.

"Two years later, my thyroid was almost back to normal and my many symptoms have been resolved or completely eliminated. My energy and endurance levels are better than ever."

Barbara originally consulted me for chiropractic treatment for back pain and then discovered that chiropractic care could do much more for her.

Wilma Martincic's case

So many people complain of general pain and just not feeling good. Wilma Martincic, a 71-year-old house-wife from Canonsburg, Pennsylvania, was one of them.

> **Joint pain, fatigue, overweight**

"I have had numerous health problems for probably 40 years," she told me on her first visit. "I need to sleep at least a couple of hours a day otherwise I am physically exhausted. My joint pain is awful. I have to walk with stooped shoulders because of the pain. And sometimes I have to go up and down steps on my fours. Years ago when I used to work and the weather was cold and damp I would have to sit on my hands to warm them up before I could start typing."

Wilma had arthritis and Paget's disease, a bone disease. She was also overweight. She went on a weight loss program we designed for her. She watched her diet, took supplements, and underwent a series of chiropractic treatments. Adjustments have enabled her to avoid carpal tunnel and hip surgeries.

Over the six years since she started natural health care, her condition has improved greatly. She currently receives maintenance care and has learned to become an activist for her own health. She knows what it is like not to be healthy.

Wilma avoids convenience, canned and frozen foods and any kind of junk food. "I don't buy any sweets when I shop," she told me proudly. She has even started to grow her own vegetables and shop at the local farmer's market.

"There is just a good feeling through my body and mind compared to when I first came to see you," she said. "I walk straighter with my shoulders back. And I have learned so much. My body tells me if I slide off the program. I get the message. And I just return right to the correct way of wellness."

ALLERGIES
AND CHEMICAL SENSITIVITIES

About allergies

Allergies and chemical sensitivities cause adverse reactions to food, chemicals and elements in the environment that most people find harmless.

Typical symptoms include:
- Headaches
- Fatigue
- Sneezing
- Watery eyes
- Stuffy sinuses
- Mood and behavior changes.

Conservative estimates suggest some 35 million Americans are allergic, however, allergy expert and author James Braly, M.D., believes a majority of Americans are affected, and particularly by food allergies.

When allergenic substances are detected, the body's initial responses are protective and defensive. Among the reactions is the production of a chemical called histamine. It is the release of histamine that triggers symptoms associated with allergies. Small blood vessels leak and ooze fluid, causing a swelling of tissue around them. The nasal obstruction in hayfever comes from leaky vessels and swelling in the nose. Leakage and swelling in the brain can lead to malfunction among nerve cells and possible changes in mood. This situation is called cerebral or brain allergy. Just as one might develop itchy eyes or scratchy throat from exposure to pollen, so, too, foods or chemicals can cause brain swelling and a range of symptoms such as depression, irritability, fatigue or migraines.

Histamine can also set off muscle spasms. In asthma, allergic spasms of the muscles of the bronchial tubes interfere with respiration, causing shortness of breath and wheezing. Similarly, spasms in tiny arteries of the brain can reduce the flow of glucose, oxygen and other nutrients needed by sensitive brain tissue, with resultant changes in memory or behavior.

Many sensitive people are intolerant to multiple substances. This can cause unique combinations of physical, mental, emotional and behavioral symptoms. As environmental illness expert Marshall Mandell, M.D., once described it, such people have "their own private syndrome of multiple symptoms affecting multiple systems in the body." In short, the brain can be affected, or the body, or both, in any combination and variety of intensity.

The conventional treatment for allergy involves anti-histamine prescriptions to neutralize the body's response. But these medications can cause side effects, including the production of more histamine by the body. Antibiotics, often used to counteract symptoms, may unleash a whole array of new problems and rebound allergic reactions.

Common offenders

• *Dust. In many buildings and houses, dust levels can become problematic due to inadequate ventilation or when ventilation ducts have not been properly maintained.*

• *Mold. A big problem in wet climates. Toxins made by molds are potent and can cause neurological and behavioral symptoms.*

• *Food. Offending food can change behavior, cause hyperactivity, or fatigue. The behavior of children often changes after eating a lunch containing sugar, junk food or offending ingredients.*

• *Pollen. Normally associated with hay fever and asthma, but can also affect how people think, feel and behave. In some states, pollen is a year-round problem.*

• *Chemicals. No escape from these. In households and schools, chemical odors are emitted from new carpets, carpeting glue, renovation work, painting, roofing, wallboard, plywood furniture, deodorizers, disinfectants, cleaning agents, pesticides and even magic markers.*

Raymond Benninger's case

In September of 1992, 12-year-old Raymond Benninger III, of Apollo, Pennsylvania, entered a new middle school.

> **Ray loved school but was allergic to his school building**

"The school building was only a few years old and clean and shining," his mother, Linda Benninger, said when she brought her son in to see me. "But during the first week he began to develop allergy symptoms: stuffy, runny nose, watery eyes, wheezing, and coughing. The symptoms continued, particularly a deep cough, and Ray often missed school as a result. When he entered the building the coughing would intensify. It was horrible and deep. Five minutes after he left the building, the coughing would stop.

"Our family doctor tried different antibiotics and antihistamines but none of them worked. A pediatric allergist we went to told us Ray was probably allergic to several environmental substances and would need allergy shots.

(Allergy shots are dilutions of substances that people are sensitive to. These can often cause reactions.)

"I told the allergist that I thought Ray was allergic to something in the building. He said that Ray was also allergic at home but reacted in school probably because he didn't want to be there. No, I had told him, Ray was an honor student and loved school. The doctor gave Ray more antihistamines and a new antibiotic for a sinus infection. X-rays indicated the lungs were clear.

"I tried to find out if any of the cleaning compounds being used at school might be causing a reaction, but the maintenance people insisted they only cleaned with water!

"Ray's ordeal at school continued. Schoolmates were starting to tease him and imitate his cough. Teachers would send him to another room when his coughing intensified. One even sent him to a storage room. Usually, I had to pick him up well before the school day was over. School officials were now saying that Ray had a psychological problem, that he didn't want to be in school.

"The school nurse suggested a psychologist and we went for a consultation. The psychologist said there wasn't any psychological problem. Ray did want to be in school. He felt our son should see another doctor with knowledge of chemical sensitivities.

"The new doctor did a battery of tests that revealed more precise information on Ray's sensitivity to chemicals. We now learned that the constant exposure to them had caused enough toxicity in his body to interfere with thyroid function as well as slow down his brain function. Cytomel, a medication for thyroid, was prescribed. A home study program with tutors was also prescribed. Sadly, Ray's learning ability had been significantly affected. One of his tutors did not understand the severity of the toxicity and suggested that Ray was not making enough of an effort and should be taken to a counselor. While home study removed him from the toxic exposure to school, his underlying problem was still not solved. He could, in fact, no longer sit down and read or do his homework."

It was at this time that Ray was referred to our clinic. His physical strength was poor. He had little muscle strength or tone. He was very overweight. I obtained chemical samples used in the school district and tested Ray through kinesiology. It turned out he was allergic to nine out of the 13 samples provided! Hair analysis revealed high levels of toxic metals, particularly lead.

I recommended a detox program, nutritional supplements, and a series of adjustments for a spinal misalignment that was pinching nerves and hindering function. I also suggested eliminating milk, white flour and refined sugar products from his diet.

Ray made good progress. A second hair analysis showed that toxicity levels were decreasing. As his system strengthened he became less sensitive. He lost body fat. He began rebuilding his muscle strength through a prescribed rehabilitation program in the clinic that utilizes Cybex equipment.

Ray is now 15. "He is tall, strong and healthy," his mother says. "He is rarely ill, has no coughing spells or allergy attacks. He needs no antihistamines, antibiotics or breathers. He follows a good diet, a nutritional program including herbs and vitamins, along with regular adjustments. His learning difficulties gradually disappeared and today he is once again back on the honor role. When I compare him now to the pale, fat 12-year-old who could not function in school, read, or hang out with friends because he was too weak and tired, it brings tears to my eyes."

Just imagine where Ray would be today if his mother had not found the persistence to guide him off the medical treadmill.

A note on chemical sensitivities: Ray tried three times to go back to his original school but showed signs of problems. That is the nature of chemical sensitivities. It is hard to say how long the vulnerability lasts. In the fall of 1995, Ray was enrolled in a private school where only natural cleaning products are used.

Michelle Morring's case

Student Michelle Morring, 9, of New Alexandria, Pennsylvania, suffered from earaches, allergies, and eczema. Several times she had been hospitalized with flu after vomiting and becoming extremely dehydrated. In the past she had received allergy shots, inhalers and antibiotics (which had caused severe diarrhea).

> **"I no longer need allergy shots. I no longer use the inhaler."**

In January of 1996, Michelle was brought in to see me by her mother, Harriett, who is also a patient. Testing showed the girl to be allergic to milk and wheat, the most common food allergies. She was recommended to start a vitamin program, substitute rice milk for cow's milk, limit wheat and sweets, avoid food products with yeast, and undergo a series of chiropractic manipulations.

"I no longer need allergy shots, only homeopathic drops. I no longer use the inhaler," says Michelle.

Harriet, her mom, is grateful that Michelle found relief through the natural approach early in life. She didn't want her daughter to go through the same treadmill ordeal she had experienced for asthma and other health problems.

"Previously, an allergist had said Michelle has a genetic condition," Harriet told me recently. "Well, all I can say is that she hasn't had to take a single antibiotic, steroid, allergy shot or decongestant since starting the program. She has developed a stronger immune system naturally. She uses apple cider vinegar topically for eczema (skin problems). She uses an herbal nasal spray for occasional sinus congestion instead of steroid drops. She expresses her gratitude by drawing pictures for the doctors and nurses whenever she visits your clinic."

About food allergies ━━━━━━━━━━━━━━━━━━━━━━

• *Food allergies are common as colds. Some 60 percent or more of the population is affected, both children and adults.*

• *These allergies are reactions to a nutritionally-depleted diet, to stress, drugs and alcohol, our chemically-polluted environment and food, and to genetic predisposition.*

• *The consequences of food allergies are serious, and often the unsuspected, misunderstood cause or contributing factor in many degenerative diseases and symptoms.*

• *Ninety-five percent of food allergies create delayed reactions — anywhere from an hour to three days.*

— James Braly, M.D., allergy expert

Foods that are craved or eaten with the most frequency are common causes of symptoms. A particular food eaten once every four or five days may be fine, but taken on a daily basis may cause symptoms because of a build-up effect. The amount consumed may also be a factor.

Wheat, milk, corn, soy, sugar and yeast are major food offenders. Sensitivities usually embrace all foods containing these products.

While some foods come out on top of the list because of heavy exposure, personal eating habits make a big difference. Marshall Mandell, M.D., recalls the case of one woman who ate asparagus every day and this caused her profound depression.

"Some people might eat a particular food perhaps only twice a week, but they are so sensitive to it that symptoms might smolder along indefinitely," he says. "Still others can be borderline sensitive to certain foods and under normal circumstances develop no symptoms. But if they undergo emotional or physical stress, become chilled or overheated, or inhale cigarette smoke or heavy environmental pollution, symptoms can suddenly break out.

"It is important to remember that food does not exist in a vacuum. We also drink, breathe, and are subject to all kinds of stresses and chemical contaminants. All of these factors can play a role. A food allergy can be terribly aggravated by cigarette smoke."

How we treat allergies

Q *"Every spring and every fall, I get allergies. It seems that when ever the trees bud or when ragweed comes out, I get in trouble. My nose starts to run, my eyes get itchy, my throat gets sore and I even get some colitis problems. My husband says it is hayfever and my doctor calls it 'allergic rhinitis.' He wants me to take some type of cortisone drug but that scares me. I have been thinking about vitamins but where do I start?"*

A Although some allergy sufferers are genetically reactive to certain food or environmental allergens, the most common cause is the body's inability to handle foreign proteins or substances. The net result is what we refer to as the accumulative "allergy load" (the barrel concept I mentioned in chapter nine).

Your nervous system has to work optimally so that your immune system can recognize and neutralize foreign substances. Your digestive system has to be able to break your food down into small compatible molecules while your liver and kidney must be equally efficient at filtering toxins and removing waste products. If the burden becomes too heavy for your body, the capacity to handle the allergens in your life is exceeded and you develop symptoms.

A low hydrochloric acid level, commonly found in asthmatic children and post-menopausal women, is a typically unrecognized culprit in allergies. HCL acid is secreted by your stomach to digest protein and acidify your food. A shortage can lead to poor digestion, malabsorption and incompletely digested food particles that are treated as foreign matter in the bloodstream. Your body responds by trying to "get rid of" the "foreign proteins" by producing water and histamine. You can develop watery, itchy eyes, coughing, running nose, and itchy skin as a result.

All allergy sufferers should take the HCL test described in chapter eight. The exception is individuals with active ulcers. They should heal their ulcers first and then take the test.

Other measures we recommend include the following:

• Aged, deodorized garlic on a regular basis. It markedly reduces swelling and inflammation associated with allergies.

• Stinging Nettles, a European herb, is effective against allergic rhinitis (runny inflamed nasal passages).

• The enzymes bromelain and papain found in the fruits of pineapples and papayas, and pancreatic enzymes (Allerzyme), are also helpful for allergic rhinitis. They act as natural anti-inflammatories, reduce histamine without side-effects, and aid in the digestion of food often associated with allergies.

• Pantothenic acid (vitamin B-5) is crucial for most people with allergies. This important nutrient is involved with the production of adrenal hormones that help protect us in times of stress. Allergies are certainly a form of stress and depletes the body's stores of pantothenic acid and other B complex vitamins.

• Stress also depletes vitamin C. This important vitamin, along with bioflavonoids and other naturally-occurring antioxidants such as quercitin and pycnogenol, boost the immune system and act as natural antihistamines.

Help through homeopathy

Most of our allergy patients, including chemically reactive patients, take homeopathic liquid remedies for the substances they are sensitive to. Homeopathy, in case you don't know it, is a popular form of medicine practiced worldwide. The system is based on a concept called the "law of similars" in which remedies containing minute amounts of diluted substances are administered in order to stimulate the body's own defenses against specific symptoms and imbalances. These substances, if they were given in large doses to healthy individuals, would produce those same symptoms.

A homeopathic remedy for grass, for instance, will alleviate the symptoms of grass allergy. If you are allergic to grass, you can take the remedy orally as needed during the allergy season. I know personally how well this works because I am sensitive to grass. In high school I was a member of the golf team and during grass season my eyes would itch to the point of swelling. Often I would simply have to walk off the golf course. Doctors could only offer me anti-histamines and allergy shots. Later, in clinical practice, I became familiar with homeopathics and began using the grass remedy myself. I need to take it during the height of the grass season and it stops the problem immediately. I can even play golf now as long as I have my remedy handy.

There are literally hundreds of such helpful non-toxic remedies in our homeopathic "arsenal." The beauty of them is that they work — and without any side effects whatsoever.

Over the years I have seen these remedies help hundreds of my allergic patients, including the following:

Sensitivity to dairy

Recently, one patient who is dairy sensitive told me about an incident in a restaurant where the vegetables he was eating contained a hidden layer of cream sauce. In his case, dairy of any kind triggered a sore throat within 10 minutes. Sure enough, he soon started to feel something in his throat. He examined the food closely and found the sauce. Fortunately, he had a bottle of homeopathic dairy remedy in the car. He took the drops twice under his tongue in a 10-minute period and immediately felt the relief. The sore throat never developed.

Allergies to animals

Many people love pets and animals but can't go near them because of allergic reactions. They get itchy eyes and scratchy throat, among other symptoms. I have had excellent results with "Animal Mix," a homeopathic remedy. A mother and her son, who are patients, are severely sensitive to cats and if they go into someone's house with a cat, they feel as if their eyes are being pulled out. The remedy prevents the reaction and they now have no problems with cats.

Carpet sensitivity

Another patient, who is an artist, developed chemical sensitivities, and is particularly reactive to the chemicals and vapors of synthetic carpets. We provided her with a homeopathic remedy and she is no longer affected.

Cigarette allergy

One of my patients, a professional singer, used to develop migraines when exposed to cigarette smoke. Homeopathic nicotine drops have worked well for her and she can now perform without problems.

Beauty shop sensitivities

I recall the case of a beautician in her early 30s who became incapacitated in part from the dyes, sprays and chemicals used in her profession. She was chronically fatigued and depressed and had run the gamut of conventional medical treatments. I determined neck and back misalignments, causing weakness in her liver and spleen.

To counteract the chemicals in her beauty shop, I recommended "Beautox," a homeopathic remedy that helps the body to neutralize such overload. I started her on our comprehensive program, including chiropractic manipulation, and within two months she had regained her energy and no longer felt depressed. An additional benefit included resolving a chronic adult acne condition she had had for years. She now has a productive life again and a new lifestyle.

The chiropractic — allergy connection

> **"While other professions are concerned with changing the environment to suit the weakened body, chiropractic is concerned with strengthening the body to suit the environment."**
> **— B. J. Palmer, D.C.**

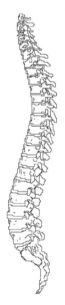

Chiropractic manipulations offer potentially great benefits for allergy sufferers. You can't activate your immune system without a healthy nervous system. Published chiropractic research is confirming the clinical experience of many chiropractic physicians, namely that adjustments enhance immune function, promote drainage, and the natural healing response.

Over the years I have consistently found allergy sufferers, particularly those who have eye, ear, nose and throat reactions, to have a second cervical (neck) vertebra misalignment. My files contain numerous cases of people, who, following a series of manipulations, developed greater resistance to sinus, throat and bronchial infections. Many individuals who think they are allergic are actually subluxated with impaired nerve function. Because this information is not widely known, such people typically wind up on the medical treadmill.

An accountant I treated a few years ago could never taste or smell his food because of chronic sinus infections related to allergies. Examination indicated cranial and second cervical misalignment. Following manipulation, his sinus ordeal came to an end. Cranial manipulation can be particularly beneficial in cases of allergies.

Natural Remedies for Allergies

- *The Gallagher Wellness Program*
- *Cervical (neck) manipulation*
- *Cranial manipulation*
- *Applied kinesiology (AK) to identify food and environmental allergies*
- *Betaine Plus (sustained-release)*
  hydrochloric acid .... 2 capsules, 3 times daily
  before meals (avoid with ulcers)
- *Allerzyme (10x pancreatic enzymes)* .... 2 after meals
- *Milk Thistle* .... 2 capsules, 2 times daily
- *Pantothenic acid* .... 250 milligrams, 3 times daily
- *Vitamin C* ....1000 milligrams, 4 times daily
- *Seasonal and food homeopathics as needed*

In Summary

We all know that the environment is toxic. We all know that we don't have pure air, pure water, pure food. But while many people blame their health problems on what is outside the body, our wellness program focuses on overhauling the internal environment. That means:

- Cleaning up the body's pollution through detoxification (see chapter 6).

- Revitalizing your organs with nutritional therapy (see chapter 11).

- Restoring your nervous system with chiropractic manipulation (see chapter 13).

This approach maximizes your body's ability to become compatible with what appears to be an incompatible world.

ANEMIA

About anemia

Taking place inside the many thousands of miles of blood vessels coursing through your body is a remarkable cargo operation that keeps you alive. Inside this "river of life," blood carries oxygen and nutrition to the billions of cells and takes away the waste products.

Within each red cell in the blood there are millions of large protein molecules called hemoglobin. And within these molecules are atoms of iron that bind with oxygen, picking it up in the lungs and then releasing it where needed among the cells of the body.

Anemia is a condition in which not enough oxygen reaches the cells of the body. This situation occurs from a loss of hemoglobin and/or a reduction in the number of red blood cells. When the oxygen supply falls short, carbon dioxide, a waste product of cellular metabolism, accumulates in the cells and interferes with the efficiency of their normal activities. You may then experience the following symptoms:

- General weakness
- Fatigue
- Loss of appetite
- Dizziness

Anemia can be brought on by recurrent infections, diseases affecting the entire body, certain drugs that destroy vitamin E and other essential nutrients, some insecticides, inadequate intake or impaired absorption of nutrients, or large losses of blood through heavy menstruation or peptic ulcers.

Anna Mae Gruca's case

The case of Anna Mae Gruca, of Indiana, Pennsylvania, a retired 75-year-old, is like many I see. She had multiple problems and a history of medical treatment that apparently contributed to her anemic state. She required a combination approach. The

> "I lived on Maalox and antibiotics."

beauty of alternative medicine is that we treat the whole body, not just a single symptom. The result is across the board improvements.

Anna Mae had spinal subluxations which set the stage for a hiatal hernia, an inflamed esophagus and stomach ulcers. She had arthritis and took medication for that, as well as drugs for sinus infections and repeated colds.

"I lived on Maalox and antibiotics," she told me.

In the spring of 1994, a series of medical tests, scopes and MRIs revealed that she had anemia and an inflamed esophagus. Her physician put her on a number of prescriptions, including Prilosec, Zantac, Gaviscon and Ferragon. She became ill and was hospitalized for a week. After release she felt light-headed and dizzy. Her anemia was not improving.

It was at this time that Anna Mae opted for the natural approach. She had almost given up when she came to see me. I felt that the loss of the "good bacteria" in her intestines from numerous antibiotic series had led to poor absorption of nutrients and was contributing to anemia. In addition, I suspected that the drugs for arthritis pain may have created the symptoms of hiatal hernia and ulcers. Moreover, the arthritis and ulcer drugs prevented iron and other nutrients from being absorbed.

Her problem could not be resolved by taking iron supplements alone. Along with dietary recommendations, I administered chiropractic soft-tissue manipulation to correct her hiatal hernia. Aloe vera gel, along with vitamin B-12, a multi-strain probiotic supplement and the British herbal therapy rhizinate (licorice extract), were used to repair the stomach lining and restore micro-organism balance.

The changes were dramatic. "I no longer have constant heartburn, spastic colon or anemia," she says, "and I take no more medication."

Anna Mae had also suffered from neuropathy in her legs and had given up dancing — a favored pastime. Through foot and hip manipulations we were able to help return her to the dance floor.

How we treat anemia

Q *"I have been chronically tired since my early twenties. Now I am 42 and the fatigue is getting worse. I really wipe out around my menstrual cycle. My gynecologist says it is because I am anemic and I have a lot of blood loss because of a heavy flow and clots. The doctor gave me iron sulfate but it made me nauseated. He told me to take it anyway. Aren't there herbs or other remedies that could help me?"*

A Although iron is the most common nutritional deficiency associated with anemia, there are many more palatable forms of it other than iron sulfate. You should also keep in mind that single vitamin and mineral deficiencies, in this case iron, are rare. Most people have multiple nutrient deficiencies that over time contribute to poor health and illness.

I frequently prescribe Hemoplex, a nutritional supplement complex featuring a different type of iron — ferrous peptonate — derived from spinach. The formula, which also includes folic acid, B-12, Vitamin C, and liver extract, is especially helpful in cases of excessive blood loss.

Ferritin, a unique nutritional prescription available in capsule form, is a natural iron-bound protein compound that simulates what your body manufactures and is well tolerated. I have found this supplement to work much better for anemia than ordinary iron compounds.

Deficiencies of vitamin B-12 and folic acid, another B complex factor, can also be involved in anemia. The form of vitamin B-12 I recommend is taken sublingually (under the tongue) with folic acid and provides an efficient and effective method of improving certain types of anemia..

Some words of advice here:

• If you take B-12 without folic acid for a long period of time you could develop a folic acid deficiency anemia — and vice versa

• Not all anemias involve iron deficiency. One should have a blood test (CBC and Ferritin) before using iron supplements. Iron is very beneficial if you need it but potentially harmful if you take too much. Excess has been shown to promote oxidation that can lead to cancer.

I often use applied kinesiology (AK) to quickly identify organ weaknesses associated with anemia.

Chiropractic manipulation of the thoracic spine (mid-back) to stimulate liver function, along with the glandular extracts of liver and spleen work remarkably well for this problem. I have helped many women whose anemia was either caused by, or aggravated by excessive menstrual bleeding, with manipulation of the lumbar spine (low back). This method will often enhance the nervous system—hormone connection and help relieve the pain, cramping, and excessive bleeding associated with menstrual problems.

Natural Remedies for Anemia

• **The Gallagher Wellness Program**
• **Chiropractic manipulation**
• **Hemoplex (chelated iron, vitamin B-12, liver extract)** *1 tablet daily*
• **Vitamin B-12 (sub-lingual)** .... *1-2 milligrams daily*
• **Ferritin** .... *1 capsule daily*
• **Livaglan (liver extract)** .... *2 capsules twice daily*
• **Spleen extract** .... *2 capsules twice daily*
Note: total iron intake should not exceed 30-60 milligrams daily unless indicated by a physician.

ANXIETY AND PANIC DISORDERS

About anxiety and panic

Anxiety is the most common psychological symptom of stress. According to the National Institute of Mental Health, some 24 million Americans suffer from an anxiety disorder at some point in their lives. At any given time, an estimated eight million people are believed to be afflicted. Less than a quarter of them obtain therapy, however. There are several reasons for this:

- Because of the stigma of having a mental disorder, some don't seek help.
- The problem is misdiagnosed
- Individuals have no medical insurance covering mental illness
- Treatment may be too expensive

All of us have experienced anxiety sometime in our lives. Perhaps before a stressful confrontation or test or speech. But for many people, anxiety is a constant companion. They are always anxious and fearful, beset by negative feelings of impending doom or rejection. Common symptoms include:

- Heart palpitations
- Lightheadedness
- Difficulty swallowing
- Excessive sweating
- Headaches
- Inability to take in enough air.

This experience can become so intense for some individuals that they lose all reason and reality. They develop what is called a panic attack. Psychiatrists regard panic attacks as a genuine mental disorder if it occurs at least four times a month or when one or more attacks are followed by at least a month of persistent fear of having another attack. Panic disorders affect more than a million Americans and two to three times as many women as men, says the National Institute of Mental Health.

A 1989 New England Journal of Medicine report indicated that people with panic disorders are 18 times more likely to have considered or attempted suicide than people with no mental illness. Twenty percent of people with panic disorders and 12 percent of those with occasional panic attacks reported having attempted suicide.

If left untreated, anxiety can be a strong contributor to many serious physical and mental conditions, including cardiovascular disease, gastrointestinal complaints, asthma, allergies, chronic low back pain, insomnia and depression.

Pharmaceutical drugs — something really to be anxious about!

For many years, psychiatrists emphasized pharmaceuticals to treat mental disorders. Anxiety is no different. In fact, more prescriptions are written for anxiety than for any other physical or mental condition. Medical statistics indicate that someone with anxiety can spend from $200 to $900 a year on drugs for anxiety. These costs multiply when anxiety leads to other disorders and the drugs create new problems.

Physicians typically confront anxiety disorders by prescribing tranquilizing drugs called benzodiazepines to block the arousal centers of the brain. Among them are Librium, Valium, Xanax, Restoril, and Halcion. Some 60 to 80 million prescriptions for tranquilizers are written annually despite their reputation for limited effectiveness, considerable side effects, and the liability for abuse.

In a highly-critical analysis of these drugs, the January 1993 issue of *Consumer Reports Magazine* said that "Xanax is just the latest in a long line of tranquilizers that have promised to deliver psychiatry's holy grail: relief from anxiety with no significant side effects. And like the pills that came before it, Xanax has fallen short." Xanax has turned out to be more addictive than Valium, causing rage and hostility, physical dependency and sedation, the magazine added.

Along with drugs, physicians may also probe childhood and/or relationship factors to uncover emotional clues. Often patients are told by their doctor that they have a "chemical imbalance." The prognosis of the anxiety/panic patient in the conventional medical maze is poor at best. Major underlying causes of the disorder are generally overlooked, leaving many folks wearing a "chemical (pharmaceutical) straight jacket" for the rest of their lives.

Janet Gavazzi's case

Janet, a 43-year-old accounting clerk from North Huntington, Pennsylvania, came to see me at the insistence of her

> **"I don't feel that anybody can help me."**

husband, a patient of mine. She said she had a "general anxiety disorder."

"I have become intolerant to loud noises and have had to leave certain places because of anxiety," she told me. "I was treated with Xanax (a tranquilizer) but continued to have anxiety, panic attacks and heart palpitations as well.

"As a result of the Xanax, my menstrual cycle stopped. The psychiatrists tried me on 10 different anti-depressant drugs but I had to discontinue them because of the side effects. Prior to seeing you, I was started on Pamelor, another anti-depressant, and I am also taking Ativan, a tranquilizer, because of my extreme nervousness. I have become completely disabled over the past year-and-a-half because of all this.

"I don't feel that anybody can help me," she said. "That's why I am here only very reluctantly."

Evaluation of Janet revealed a misalignment in the neck vertebrae as well as deficiencies in several minerals and the B complex vitamins. I started her on the appropriate natural prescriptions, that also included a low blood sugar diet.

She was very resistant to idea of chiropractic adjustments. It took all her husband's cajoling to convince her. But immediately Janet felt the difference.

"After beginning chiropractic adjustments I noticed I can sleep better and my worries have started to ease up," Janet said soon after starting the treatment program. "The effects last for about three or four days after each treatment. My mind also becomes clearer and I have more ambition. It is the only relief that I get."

After a few weeks of treatment, Janet was able to stop the tranquilizers. "In cooperation with my psychiatrist, I have now also cut the anti-depressant drug in half," she said. "I am looking forward to a complete recovery. I can see the potential for my problem to resolve naturally."

After 1 1/2 months of treatment, Janet's panic attacks ended. She was gradually weaned off the anti-depressant. Six months later there had been no recurrence. During a follow-up visit, she told me she was off all drugs. She was so happy she cried.

When she first came to see me, Janet's condition was so bad that she hardly ever left her house. Her turn-around was so dramatic that she even appeared on my television program and in front of the cameras happily told the story of her recovery.

Marcia Christ's case

Marcia Christ, an attractive 46-year-old high school educator from Clairton, Pennsylvania, was experiencing panic attacks.

"Initially, the attacks began upon entering stores and after subsequent attacks, it seemed as if

> **Recovery from panic attacks instead of hospitalization**

they were occurring in department stores," she told me. "I was reacting to something in that environment and would become <u>extremely</u> nervous and distraught. After trying deep breathing and relaxing methods, I would still continue to feel the panic and have to leave the store."

After testing Marcia, we found that she was reacting chemically to the odors in the environment such as perfumes. But there was much more to her case than "department store-itis."

Marcia had been diagnosed previously with Epstein-Barr Virus, also referred to by many as chronic fatigue syndrome. She had recurring sore throats and a long history of heavy antibiotics and conventional medical treatment which, over the course of decades, made her underlying condition more problematic. Her situation was worsening. She was unable to work for a year. She could hardly get out of bed because of the fatigue. Then came the panic attacks.

Had Marcia continued to be treated conventionally, she would have received the "panic/anxiety disorder" label, received anti-anxiety drugs, and maybe counseling about her relationship with her parents.

Instead, she came to Medical Wellness Associates. We found her lymphatic system was malfunctioning, preventing her body from eliminating toxins properly. She also had adrenal weakness. The stress gland of the body was out of sync. These underlying disorders had a corresponding mechanical problem in the nervous system. When we performed chiropractic adjustments we were able to correct Marcia's mechanical imbalances, so that her nervous system was now coordinated with her immune and hormonal systems. We also started her on a nutritional program with numerous vitamin supplements targeting the various areas of weakness in her body. Soon the attacks became less frequent.

"I became more confident," said Marcia, "and went back to the very environment that had caused such distress for me only a short time earlier. There was no problem. I have absolutely no doubt that I would have been hospitalized for these attacks, in particular, and would have fallen victim to medication for my nerves."

Living in constant fear

Q "*I live in a state of constant fear,*" the caller on a radio show told me. "*The psychiatrist I see calls it panic or anxiety attacks. My life has been on hold for five years because the attacks are unpre-*

dictable but happen every day. I get lightheaded and dizzy, my heart races and pounds, and I feel like everything is closing in on me. I try to talk to myself and I have joined a support group. It helps to talk about it, at the time, but I go right back to the problem. I tried the drugs but they knock me out. I have only been married one year, but I feel like my husband thinks it is something I should just 'snap out of.' I know there has to be some kind of treatment for me. What are my options?"

A There are indeed natural approaches for people like this woman, approaches that do not involve side effects and the medical treadmill. The Gallagher Wellness Program offers a safe and effective non-drug approach that evaluates nutritional, biochemical, allergic, and structural factors. Results of the evaluation are honed into an individualized program to bring the nervous system back into balance.

Conventional physicians usually ignore the eating and drinking habits of their patients. The fact is that alcohol, caffeine, dairy, and processed foods (high in sugar) can cause elevation of a chemical in the body called lactate. High lactate has been associated with anxiety. Several studies have in fact shown that anxiety and panic attacks can actually be triggered by injections of lactate found in milk products.

You don't have to inject offending foods to produce this kind of reaction. Routine consumption of allergenic foods, or exposure to certain chemicals, can act as triggering agents for many people.

Vitamin therapy can achieve many positive effects. We regard this as crucial for people with high anxiety, nightmares, insomnia, racing heart, dizziness and memory loss. A high-potency yeast-free B complex supplement, along with additional Niacinamide, are major players in improving anxiety/panic attacks.

Our nutritional recovery program also includes an amino acid you probably haven't heard about — GABA, short for gamma-aminobutyric acid. It naturally "calms down the brain," acting as a "drugless tranquilizer." I recommend it taken as 500 mg between meals or with fruit twice a day.

Along the same lines of natural tranquilizers are two herbal folk medicines: Kava Kava, long used during Polynesian religious rites for its ability to relax and soothe the mind, and Lemon Grass from Brazil. Both are beneficial and non-addictive.

Breathing exercises (see chapter 12) are often helpful for anxiety. Studies have shown that they can lower the lactate level in the brain. In addition, prayer and meditation have a synchronizing effect on the brain and should be an integral part of a recovery program for those with anxiety, panic, nervousness, and high emotional stress.

The chiropractic — anxiety connection

Chiropractic manipulation has an equilibrating effect on the nervous system. Frequent sites of spinal dysfunction in anxiety patients are the upper cervical spine (neck) and the upper thoracic (mid-back) area.

Cranial alignment may provide another avenue of treatment for panic and anxiety patients. Common findings in individuals with psychosomatic symptoms are cranial misalignment. This refers to the locking and tension that occurs at the divisions (suture sites) of the skull. Gentle pressure point adjustments performed by skilled chiropractic physicians can free the locked cranial structures. This may help to increase alertness, improve concentration, and decrease anxiety.

In chapter 13 I discussed the concept of how misalignments in the skull and spine can generate anxiety and panic attacks, among other conditions, as symptoms of a "hibernating" and malfunctioning brain.

Chiropractic research literature contains a number of interesting studies, including the following two:

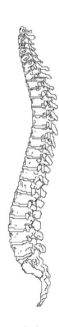

- A 42-year-old female suffered from anxiety attacks and agoraphobia (fear of leaving the house) following an automobile accident. She also experienced insomnia, dizziness, memory loss, difficulty in concentrating, and urinary bladder urgency. In addition, a previously well-controlled stomach ulcer had flared up. Chiropractic evaluation revealed major vertebral subluxation in the neck as well as the mid and lower back. After two months of chiropractic manipulation and counseling, the patient reported a sharp decrease in anxiety and low back pain, and an end to the agoraphobia, insomnia, bladder urgency, insomnia and dizziness. An additional four months of treatment resulted in complete relief from anxiety and ulcer symptoms (Journal of Chiropractic, September 1992).

- A 52-year-old female experienced frequent panic attacks. Over the years she had been prescribed antidepressants and tranquilizers. She had undergone counseling and relaxation training. All to no avail. Chiropractic evaluation showed a number of subluxations in her neck, and mid and lower spine. A series of adjustments were started. At the time this case was published in a chiropractic journal, she had been without a panic attack for some two months despite the fact that her medical doctor had cut her dosage of Xanax (a tranquilizer) in half (Journal of Chiropractic, December 1993).

Natural Remedies for Anxiety and Panic

- *The Gallagher Wellness Program*
- *Cervical (neck) manipulation*
- *Cranial manipulation*
- *Hypoglycemic diet (see chapter on hypoglycemia).*
    Avoid dairy, caffeine, and sugar
- *Identify food and chemical allergens*
- *GABA* .... 500 milligrams twice daily between meals
- *Niacinate (non-flush niacin)* .... 500 milligrams twice daily
- *B complex* .... 50 milligrams twice daily
- *Kava Kava,* .... 2 capsules as needed
- *Breathing exercises (see Chapter 12)*
- *Prayer and meditation*

ARTHRITIS

About arthritis

Wear and tear of the joints of the body leads to arthritis. Also known as Degenerative Joint Disease, it strikes more than 40 million Americans, especially those over age 45. The flexible bones in the spine, called vertebrae, are affected most frequently, but arthritis can also involve the shoulders, arms, hands, hips, knees, and feet.

Typical symptoms include:
- Soreness and pain
- Stiffness
- Discomfort relieved by movement
- Discomfort diminishing over the day and worsened by inactivity

Nora Bechtold's case

Nora Bechtold limped into my office.

"I have lost my ability to walk normally and exercise as a result of a tendonitis of the ankle that developed into a chronic arthritic condition," the 62-year-old Pittsburgh homemaker told me sadly.

> "The pain is so intolerable that my mind has become exhausted"

"I have gone to seven doctors. Podiatrists. Rheumatologists. And an orthopedic surgeon who wants to perform surgery to fuse the ankle. I don't want the surgery because there is no assurance I would walk again or be relieved of the pain. I am frightened by the possibility of complications.

"During all this time I have taken all types of tests, been given steroids, anti-inflammatory drugs, put into casts and also been sent to a physical therapist. No one could help me!

"I wanted to climb to the top of Mt. Washington (the highest point in Pittsburgh) and scream from the top of my lungs, 'ISN'T THERE ANYONE OUT THERE WHO CAN HELP ME? THERE MUST BE SOMEBODY!'"

Now Nora was in my office, showing me her foot. It was inflamed and swollen, resembling, as she put it, "an oversized club foot."

"The pain is so intolerable that my mind has become exhausted," she said. "I can no longer remember what was said to me two minutes before. I have even begun thinking of having the foot amputated and learning to walk with a prosthesis. The thought of this, or of being in a wheelchair for the rest of my life, is very painful for me."

I recommended a program that included hip and foot manipulation, special orthotic inserts for her shoes, and nutritional prescriptions. Gradually, we were able to restore the health of her foot.

"You told me that I had a 10-20 percent chance, or maybe 30 percent, of walking again," she reminded me during a recent visit. "Now, not only am I walking again but I can cover a mile in 15 minutes without any pain!"

Father Vernon's case

Father Vernon Holtz, a 65-year-old priest, psychologist and college professor from Latrobe, Pennsylvania, was facing two total knee replace-

> "Today, I walk with no cane"

ments after 10 years of pain and medication. Most of the cartilage was gone. He arrived at our clinic using a cane, limping noticeably, and in obvious discomfort. He could no longer tolerate any of the arthritic pain killers. As a teacher, he was having increasing difficulty standing in the classroom. He was looking for alternative solutions.

"After x-rays and an examination, Dr. Gallagher told me there was a possibility of restoring 30 to 60 percent of the original motion in the knee," Father Holtz recalls.

My recommendations included weekly chiropractic treatments, the detox diet, avoidance of certain foods, six months of electrical stimulation for the knee, myofascial therapy, nutritional supplements, and a rigorous exercise program for the knee mostly done at home.

"Today, I walk with no cane and my knees have been rehabilitated to nearly all of their original motion," says Father Holtz. "I have almost total reduction of the previous constant pain. And I am currently playing tennis! All this without taking any heavy medication. Occasionally I use Tylenol or chiropractic cream with capsaicin to control periodic flare-ups."

As a priest, Father Holtz was also interested in the spiritual influence on healing and made the following comment: "Beside the physical healing that has taken place, throughout the therapy discussions were held which pertained to the understanding of life, that is, the meaning of pain, the value of transcending pain and acknowledging a power greater than oneself which, if properly understood, could assist one in the healing process. Discussions were also held on how to 'center' and 'focus' one's energies in order to help heal the body through its own powers."

How we treat arthritis

Q *"I am 59-years-old but feel like 90. When I get up in the morning I hurt all over, especially my back, neck, shoulders and knees. I usually limp when I first get out of bed and I have a hard time getting out of a chair, or even the car. My family doctor gave me Motrin and sent me to an orthopedic surgeon. He did x-rays and a bone scan, and said I had osteoarthritis. He gave me a shot of cortisone in my knee and a new arthritis drug. He more or less told me to live with it. I can't live with it, and I keep losing ground. Isn't there something that can help me?"*

A I can't begin to guess how many times I have heard this kind of a story from arthritis sufferers. In more than 20 years of practice, it has probably been thousands of times.

Conventional medical treatment focuses on a "chemical assault" of the body to try and snuff out the pain temporarily. From aspirin and acetaminophen, to cortisone and non-steroidal anti-inflammatory drugs (such as Motrin, Advil, Nuprin, Naprosyn, and other ibuprofen compounds), pharmaceutical prescriptions are neither corrective nor preventive. Worse yet, they can be dangerous.

Current outcome studies have now demonstrated that up to 25 percent of those who take these drugs will develop ulcers within thirty days of regular use. Millions develop GI disturbances including irritable bowel and leaky gut syndrome. Shockingly, yet seriously under reported, is the death count which now numbers between 15-20,000 Americans each year for non-steroidal anti-inflammatory drugs. To further complicate matters these drugs have been proven to actually cause arthritis by damaging cartilage cells necessary for healthy joints.

A more logical approach is the kind of comprehensive wellness program we offer at our clinic. We have many weapons at our disposal against arthritis.

Diet

The typical American diet, high in animal foods, sugar and rancid fats, contributes to a complex biochemical process that promotes inflammation. Emphasizing more raw fruit and vegetables in your diet is a good first step. These foods are rich in enzymes and vitamins which help counteract the effects of arthritis.

Detoxification

Intestinal toxins, unleashed by unfriendly bacteria, yeast, and parasites, are now linked to arthritis, rheumatoid arthritis, cancer, allergies and a host of other illnesses. Colon detoxification, colonic hydrotherapy and improved digestion are musts (see chapters six and eight).

Medical research has found that toxins from the gut are often deposited in joints. Researchers aren't sure yet why this happens. They do know, however, that patients who have intestinal disorders such as inflammatory bowel disease experience joint inflammation, particularly in the major limb joints, and that the severity of the joint problem is often related to the severity of their intestinal disorder.

Eliminating Food Sensitivities

Food sensitivities may trigger joint pain among some arthritics. Nightshades (tomatoes, potatoes, eggplants, peppers and paprika) may also be problematic for some people. Gluten, a protein found in wheat, rye, oat and barley, can cause an inflammatory joint response in susceptible individuals (see chapter nine).

Herbals

In my experience, different people have different responses to herbs. One herb may work for one person and not the other. I usually start a person on one for six weeks and if there is no benefit I will recommend trying another herb.

Contemporary researchers and physicians are confirming 1,500-year-old recommendations on the anti-inflammatory, anti-arthritic and anti-pain applications of the gummy extract of the Boswellia serratta tree commonly found in India. Boswellia is being found to shrink inflamed tissue, improve blood supply, and promote repair of local blood vessels damaged by proliferating inflammation.

Capsaicin, the active component of cayenne pepper, can help with pain when applied topically. It has the ability to naturally block pain impulses.

Devil's claw, a native African herb and Yucca, a desert plant found in the Southwestern U.S., have long folk histories related to helping arthritic sufferers.

One long-favored herb is Hypericum (St. John's Wort). Used in the form of a cream it has analgesic properties when applied to the affected area. Taken as a capsule, it acts as a natural anti-depressant. This makes it notably beneficial for arthritis patients, many of whom experience a form of depression that actually magnifies the perception of pain.

Colchicine, derived from the saffron plant, can be used intravenously to decrease pain and inflammation in cases of arthritis, rheumatoid arthritis, gout, lupus, fibromyalgia and chronic pain.

Other Nutritionals

I often prescribe a multiple nutritional and herbal "anti-arthritic" compound that I found to be effective for many different types of arthritis.

Glucosamine sulfate has been proven to be 10 to 30 times more effective than many of the current risky prescription drugs. This natural substance repairs joints. Conventional drugs damage joints.

Black currant seed oil, primrose oil, flax seed oil, borage oil, and fish oils such as cod liver oil assist the body in the production of "natural anti-inflammatory substances."

L-phenylalanine is an amino acid that enhances learning, memory and alertness when taken supplementally. It is a major element in the production of collagen, the protein that holds the body's tissues together. A chemically-modified version, called DL-phenylalanine, or DLPA for short, has earned a widespread reputation as a pain killer.

When pain occurs, brain hormones called endorphins are produced. They have similar properties to morphine, a powerful analgesic drug. But lurking within your body are enzymes that tend to neutralize the endorphins. DLPA comes to the rescue by inhibiting the action of those enzymes, allowing endorphins a longer life span in which to counter pain naturally.

IV Treatments

For severe cases in our clinic, we use intravenous infusions of vitamin C, pantothenic acid, magnesium, and hydrochloric acid. Vitamin C and pantothenic acid have natural anti-inflammatory properties. These two vitamins are building blocks of our own natural cortisone. The mineral magnesium helps to reduce muscle spasms associated with arthritis.

Copper Braclets

The wearing of copper bracelets, often mocked by orthodox medicine, has been shown to decrease pain and swelling of arthritis. In a fascinating study reported more than 20 years ago, researchers divided 240 arthritic patients into three groups. One group of people wore copper bracelets for one month followed by wearing a similar looking, but non-copper bracelet, for another month. The second group wore the bracelets in reverse order. Group three wore no bracelets at all. An analysis of comments made by the participants showed that the copper bracelets produced an alleviating effect. Copper is actually absorbed from the bracelet into the skin and body. The mineral is known to complex with proteins in the body and produce an anti-inflammatory effect.

Sugar not so sweet for arthritis

Ron Lawrence, M.D., a Southern California neurologist specializing in pain problems, has made an interesting observation regarding sugar based on more than 30 years of practice.

Sugar, primarily white sugar, he says, can contribute to pain.

"I first learned this with arthritics," says the neurologist. "The more sugar in the diet, the more pain. You take people off sugar and the pain diminishes. I tell all my arthritics to cut out the sugar."

That means not only the sugar you put in your cereal, in your coffee or tea, but also the massive amounts hidden in soda pop, chocolate cake, chocolate chip cookies, and ice cream.

Lawrence says sugar interferes with calcium's role in electrochemical transmissions in the body, causing nerves to become "more irritable."

The chiropractic - arthritis connection

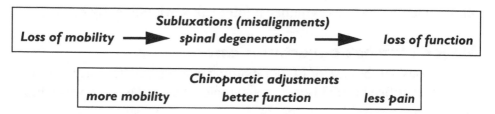

Based on my years of experience and a number of interesting studies, I believe that chiropractic manipulation may be the most important physical medicine treatment for the loss of motion and increase in pain and stiffness associated with osteoarthritis.

A common feature of arthritis is lack of mobility. Once a joint becomes immobile or locked, it will begin to degenerate. In fact, for your spinal disc to receive nutrition, each individual vertebral segment must be fully mobile. Subluxations of the vertebrae or other joints lead to loss of mobility of the joint. This hastens the degenerative progress. We have referred to this process as disc degeneration, cartilage erosion, calcium deposits, spur formations and arthritis. All are inevitable byproducts of loss of motion of joints. Chiropractic manipulation is a unique method of health care that will unlock immobile joints, increase mobility and decrease pain.

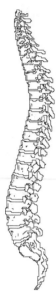

The following explanation helps to understand this process better:

Let's say that you are suffering from back, neck, shoulder, hand, or knee pain. You go to your family doctor who examines you and orders a series of X-rays of the affected parts. After viewing the X-rays and noting your age, the verdict inevitably will come down: "You have arthritis and you will have to learn to live with it."

So you say to your doctor, "I guess I am just getting older. Wear and tear, I suppose. Is there something I can do for the pain?"

"Something for pain" in mainstream medicine translates into an unlimited supply of arthritis drugs or surgery - a potential prescription for disaster.

The reality is that you have degeneration if you are over 45, and even before if your body has been through a lot of trauma. By trauma I mean a major event such as an injury or the gradual wearing away of tissue, bit by bit, over the years.

A distinguishing factor between people who have pain and those who don't is that people without pain have normal motion of the joints. That is the key - whether a joint can work normally or not.

Marjorie Strong's panarthritis case

Consider the case of Marjorie Strong, a woman in her early 60s, who came to my office in 1995 because of chronic arthritis. Over the years, her pain had progressively gone from back to knee to shoulder to elbow to wrist and to knee. She had panarthritis, that is, arthritis throughout her body. She had consulted a number of medical doctors over the years who prescribed a variety of anti-inflammatory drugs, but without any success.

Marjorie decided to try the chiropractic approach. I reviewed her X-rays and they clearly showed advanced degeneration of the joints and discs throughout her entire body. However, knowing that advanced arthritis like hers takes years to develop, I recommended chiropractic manipulation and lifestyle changes.

For the next three months she underwent a treatment program of chiropractic manipulation and dietary modification. At the end of that period, Marjorie was completely symptom free. She no longer suffered with the constant pain.

Her case is not unlike many hundreds of others that I have treated over the years. These are people who have been previously told that the cause of their pain is arthritis, disc degeneration, calcium deposits, spur formation, or disintegrating joints, but who have successfully responded to chiropractic manipulation and lifestyle modification.

How could it be that the pain was now gone but the arthritis, spurs and degeneration were still present? The answer to this one question holds the promise of relief for millions of arthritis sufferers. It seems to be some kind of a well-kept secret. I don't know who is keeping it. I'm not. I tell all my arthritis patients that degeneration is not the cause of their pain. Don't focus on it.

I treat people in their 70s and 80s with spines that are severely degenerated. If you look at their X-rays, you might think "why should I even bother." Yet these patients respond very favorably to chiropractic treatment that quickly restores improved or normal joint mobility. Simply stated, structure affects function. The pain is the byproduct of misalignment, which over the years promotes a loss of motion of the joints or vertebrae.

If degeneration were the sole cause of pain then everybody 50, 60, 70 or 80 years of age would be in agony. With loss of mobility, the discs, cartilage, joints, soft tissues, and affected organs cannot receive optimum nutrition. The blood supply decreases. The nerves become impaired or pinched. The nerve impulses are blocked. The joint surfaces undergo a premature wear and tear of degeneration. This is the process of arthritis. Arthritis is the effect. It is not the cause.

As an analogy, consider what happens when you break your arm. You put a cast on to immobilize the arm. When the cast is removed the arm has shrunk in size, the result of loss of movement and reduced blood supply.

You've heard of the saying, "use it or lose it." That applies to this situation. Normal movement of joints acts like a pump bringing the flow of sustenance to an extremity or body part.

Misalignments cause a loss of movement, be it within the flexible joints (vertebrae) of the spine or any other joints of the body, such as the hands, hips, knees, or shoulders. When the flow stops, you have problems. You have pain.

Drugs only stop the symptom of pain, they don't correct the underlying cause of the pain. Correction of the misalignment restores mobility of the joint, this in turn restores the flow of nutrients, vital energy and also opens the affected areas to endorphins, the body's own natural pain killers. Joint degeneration halts.

The healing effect comes from adjustments that recreate motion where there is loss of motion. After such treatments your X-rays will still show the degeneration but you will not have the pain or you will have much less. Don't buy into the medical model that "you are older and you have to learn to live with it."

Pass on this information to everyone you know with arthritis. Chiropractic should be the first treatment you ever receive from a physician for arthritic pain. Arthritis has many causes. An integrated wholistic approach using chiropractic manipulation, detoxification, natural anti-inflammatory nutrients, food allergy avoidance, exercise, and stress management promises a safer and more effective way to combat the problem.

Natural Remedies for Arthritis

- The Gallagher Wellness Program
- Chiropractic manipulation
- Extremity manipulation
- Stretching and conditioning exercises
- Boswellic acid .... 2 capsules 3 times daily
- DLPA .... 500 milligrams 4 times daily
- Omega 3+6 fatty acids .... 3 capsules twice daily
- Glucosamine sulfate .... 2 capsules 3 times daily
- Multiple herbal/vitamin anti-arthritic formula .... 2 capsules 3 times daily
- Chiropractic cream (cayenne) apply topically

ASTHMA

Sarah Hartzell, of Greensburg, Pennsylvania, was first brought to see me in 1989 when she was five. According to Joanne, her mother, the girl's young life had been dominated by the stress of severe asthma and allergies.

> "No more hospital trips in the middle of the night...no more hospitals at all."

"She has been hospitalized several times, each time worse than before," said Joanne. "She has received oxygen therapy, respiratory therapy, intravenous antibiotic therapy, along with bronchodilators, antihistamines, antibiotics and steroids. When not hospitalized she has frequently had to rely on medication as well as weekly allergy injections. The frequency and severity of her condition has become such that we invested in a nebulizer to use at home instead of running to the doctors everyday for inhalation therapy."

Sarah needed chiropractic treatment. Her primary problem was thoracic subluxation, that is misalignment of the vertebrae in the mid-back area, which caused her bronchial tubes to tighten, leading to chronic wheezing and asthma. Misalignments in her neck led to recurring sinus and throat infections. We also recommended a nutritional program and elimination of food allergens.

"What a difference the past eight years have made," says Joanne. "No more hospital trips in the middle of the night, no hospitals at all, no medications, no nebulizer, none of it, thanks to the gift of chiropractic and nutrition. She is allergy and asthma free.

"Six years ago we gave the nebulizer back to the pediatrician. For seven years Sarah hasn't required any pediatrician services. I am obviously grateful for this, I only wish I had known about this sooner."

I treat many Sarah Hartzells in my practice. Often, after six or eight adjustments, along with the removal of offending foods from their diet, these youngsters become asthma-free or have less frequency and severity of their symptoms. Sarah, as many of the others, continues to receive regular chiropractic wellness care.

It is worth mentioning that in some cases, individuals can — and do — revert back to their previous conditions unless they have regular follow-ups. If a weakness exists in the spine, the body can readily slip back into misalignment unless adjustments are given. However, I think you will agree that once-a-month preventive chiropractic plus nutritional care is far healthier and more cost-effective than daily drug care and frequent hospitalization.

Most people associate chiropractic with back pain. But as in Sarah's case, and in so many others, you can have misalignment in the spine without any back pain. Spinal problems also cause silent organ problems. Sarah had asthma. Other people have migraines, dizziness, ringing in the ear, or panic attacks. There can be a whole universe of symptoms, most of which conventional medical doctors don't relate to a structural problem, thus missing an essential element in helping a patient regain health.

About asthma

> "It has been suggested that the current prevalence of asthma can be likened to an epidemic which is out of control."
> – Nursing Times, 1992

Asthma is an inflammatory condition of the airways leading into the lungs. The airways become inflamed and spasm, causing excessive amounts of clogging mucous to build up, which in turn sets off a contraction of surrounding muscles. Asthmatic flare-ups can cause extreme difficulty breathing, and for increasing numbers of people the condition becomes as life-threatening as any killer disease.

The fact is that the incidence of asthma is increasing at a dramatic rate. Some 15 million Americans have the condition and 5,000 of them die each year, double the amount since 1978.

People usually think of asthma as a childhood thing, a condition that you will outgrow. Even many physicians believe so. It's not true. Symptoms may subside but asthma will often recur by the mid-20s. Today, asthmatics over the age of 50 are the highest at risk.

Conventional medicine recommends drugs that suppress symptoms, cause side effects, but never deal with the causes. Bronchodilating drugs (inhalers) are used to open the airways and anti-inflammatory drugs (oral pills and inhalers) are applied to counter the build-up of mucous.

The effectiveness and safety of these drugs is being increasingly questioned. One 1992 study concluded that regular use of bronchodilators may actually heighten the risk of death from asthma!

Airborne allergens are often involved in asthma, such things as pollen, animal dander, and dust. Food allergies and chemical sensitivities, usually overlooked, can be major culprits as well.

Refer to the allergy chapter. For more information, I suggest you purchase Doris Rapp's book, "Is This Your Child's World?" (Bantam

Books, 1996). It contains a wealth of practical options, many of which we offer in our clinic.

Marion Savasta's case

As I mentioned a moment ago, adults over 50 are the most at risk for asthma. Marion Savasta, of Irwin, Pennsylvania, now 80 years old, knows that only too well

> **80 years and going strong...no more lung problems**

from years of experience. When she came to see me in 1980 she had had a long history of chronic asthma that led to deteriorating lung function.

"Ever since I can remember," she said. "I have had a lung and bronchial condition. I always coughed and was prone to pneumonia two or three times a year and asthma. At one point as an adult, a lung specialist put me on antibiotics from September to April for five years until my body rejected it. Later, I went to another doctor who put me on four medications. I couldn't handle all this because of the side effects."

In Marion's case, I recommended chiropractic adjustments and a nutritional program that included the antioxidant vitamins A, C, and E. She has been following our program for all these years and has been able to avoid hospitalization. Only rarely has she needed to take medication. I feel our program has been able to add years to her life and life to her years.

"My health has greatly improved and for an 80-year-old I am quite active and enjoy living," she told me in a recent visit.

Thus at both ends of the life-span, in Sarah's case, and in Marion's, the natural approach offers patients a solid healing option without side effects.

How we treat asthma

Q *"My 14-year-old is asthmatic. He has been on Prednisone, inhalers, antibiotics and allergy shots since he was 8. I am very concerned about the drugs he is on, but I don't know of any options. What would be your approach?"*

A We find that asthmatic children and adults often have food sensitivities that can trigger bronchial spasms. Chief on this list are milk, eggs, wheat and citrus products.

Hydrochloric acid deficiency (stomach acid) is another consideration. It can impair digestion leading to food-sensitivity induced asthma.

For more than 20 years, I have prescribed Pneumo Forte, a combination of various botanicals that naturally relax the bronchial tube. This preparation, which includes anise, slippery elm, and wild cherry bark, is excellent for chronic cough, wheezing, and sore throat. It is also effective for recurring upper respiratory infections, bronchitis and emphysema.

Asthmatics are commonly deficient in vitamin B-12. Taking this vitamin as a supplement is often effective for asthma that has been caused by eating foods that are preserved with sulfates, such as dried fruits and wines.

The use of a liquid magnesium (18 percent solution) mixed into aloe vera juice provides a "double barrel" effect of relaxing the bronchial tube and enhancing the immune system.

The chiropractic — asthma connection

Chiropractic research has demonstrated that thoracic (mid-back) manipulation often helps to improve or resolve asthma, bronchitis and other respiratory problems involving difficulty in breathing (dyspnea). In one study reported in a 1995 issue of Chiropractic Pediatrics, Georgia chiropractors J.B. Peet, S. K. Marko, and W. Piekarczyk were able to

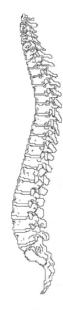

reduce or eliminate medication following chiropractic adjustments in seven out of eight youngsters with diagnoses of asthma. All individuals showed significant improvement.

In my clinical practice, I have seen chiropractic help countless patients over the years. Many were brought into the office with acute asthmatic attacks and frequently, with thoracic adjustments, we have been able to quickly alleviate their crisis.

Following adjustments, many patients say they can breathe deeply for the first time in months or years. This includes people with lung disease or even those with normal lungs. Why such quick relief? It's because all of our breathing muscles are attached to the spine. These muscles, as well as the lungs themselves, are either wholly or partially controlled by the nerves coming out of the spine. If you have pinched spinal nerves in that area of your spine due to a subluxation, the result can be that your normal breathing function becomes affected. Adjustments correct misalignments and help restore proper function to the mechanics of breathing.

Chiropractic is a prime weapons in our program against asthma. We also emphasize neutralization of environmental allergens, the avoidance of reactive foods, and reducing exposure to certain chemicals and cigarette smoke.

The successful combination of chiropractic along with elimination of environmental allergens was reported recently in the Chiropractic

Journal of Australia by Dean Lines, D.C., of the Royal Melbourne Institute of Technology, who described the cases of two children, age 2 and 5, and a mature adult, 30. At the time of writing the report, the patients were asthma-free anywhere from 6 months to 2 years.

Dr. Lines addressed the question of whether the environmental allergy approach alone would have worked. Possibly, but he noted that asthma patients often self-refer for an adjustment when an attack occurs. This, he says, is due to the immediate relief they experience.

The potential chiropractic contribution in this area goes well beyond cost-saving. For patients with lung disease, it represents a potential life-saver.

"With mounting evidence that current medical bronchodilator and inhaled steroid intervention may be contributing to the rising mortality, the conservative wholistic chiropractic approach...may provide for many sufferers a safer, more sustained and effective alternative," Dr. Lines stated.

Natural Remedies for Asthma

- *Gallagher Wellness Program*
- *Chiropractic thoracic manipulation*
- *Magnesium aspartate* .... 250-1000 milligrams daily
- *Vitamin B-12 (sub-lingual)* .... 1-2 milligrams daily
- *Primrose Oil* .... 2 capsules twice daily
- *Pneumo Forte* .... 2 capsules 3 times daily
- *Querciplex (Quercitin with vitamin C)* .... 2 capsules 3 times daily
- *Intravenous infusion of vitamin C, magnesium and HCL*
- *Pulsed diathermy (electromagnetic heat) applied to chest*

More tips for asthmatics:

• Studies indicate that asthmatics often have a minor type of chronic dehydration and by drinking more liquids can reduce the frequency of attacks. We recommend at least six eight-ounce glasses of water daily.

• Asthmatics respond better in cooler weather. It may be useful to lower the temperature in your home between 62 and 66 degrees. In Japan, children and adults take cold water baths to reduce asthmatic tendencies.

• Learn to breath with your diaphragm. Breathing correctly benefits asthmatics. For more on this subject, read Paul Sorvino's "How to Become a Former Asthmatic: Easy twice-a-day breathing exercises to prevent asthma, spasms, and reduce reliance on drugs" (Wm Morrow & Co., New York, 1985).

ATTENTION DEFICIT DISORDER
NOT JUST KIDS, BUT ADULTS, TOO

About ADD

• An inability to focus or concentrate.

That's the basic meaning of attention deficit disorder (ADD). Some 15 million Americans — both children and adults — are diagnosed with ADD and there are probably millions more who have not been diagnosed.

Among the individuals with ADD are people easily distracted, confused, poorly organized, and unable to function near the level of their natural potential. ADD affects four out of every 100 children in the U.S. The signs usually appear before the age of four but are not recognized until pre-school. By and large, symptoms persist throughout childhood. A quarter of affected youngsters show symptoms as teenagers and beyond into adulthood.

According to the experts, about 30 percent of these individuals are also hyperactive. In such cases, the condition is called ADHD — attention deficit hyperactivity disorder. Three times as many boys are affected than girls.

The medical names for these conditions have changed over the years. At first, baby boomers with the problem were called, simply enough, problem kids. Later, they were labeled hyperkinetic or hyperactive. Later still, children with minimal brain damage.

Research shows that almost all children and adults with ADD do not have any brain damage. Instead, there are varying degrees of brain chemistry imbalances that create a broad range of emotional, mental, and behavioral problems. including aggressiveness, temper tantrums, constant movement, destructiveness, abusiveness, inability to concentrate or to sit still, moodiness, nervousness, anxiety, fright, migraines, and distractibility.

No two ADD or ADHD patients are alike. They come from diverse backgrounds. Symptoms are influenced by personality, the environment and the specifics of biochemical imbalances. Even a child with a severe disorder will have some good days, be attentive, able to concentrate and stay on task. One of the most consistent features about ADD characteristics is, simply, inconsistency. On any given day, multiple ADD signs can be present.

Ritalin — Is it really helping?

The activity-modifying narcotic drug Ritalin, a mild form of amphetamine, has become the "quick fix" therapy of choice for ADD and ADHD. It, and other similar drugs, are being taken regularly by more than four million American children, double the number in 1993, with projections for as high as eight million by the year 2000.

"Do we have a miracle cure — or overmedicated kids?" asked Newsweek Magazine in a 1996 cover article.

Ritalin generates a calming effect in a large percentage of hyperactive and ADD children so they are able to concentrate and learn.

In many schools around the country, the use of Ritalin has reached epidemic scale. Prescriptions are doled out en masse daily because teachers send notes to parents requesting , and in some cases, even demanding it. The appeal of Ritalin is obvious for teachers overwhelmed by children who misbehave or don't learn. The appeal is similar for parents faced with difficult children.

In late 1995, ABC-TV's popular "20/20" news program investigated the Ritalin situation. Reporter Tom Jarrell concluded that "thousands of children nationwide are being rushed into taking Ritalin without proper evaluation. A note or call from a teacher and a brief doctor's office visit are often all that's needed for a prescription and though most experts say that Ritalin should never be given alone without also teaching children how to control their behavior, it often is."

During school hours, under the effect of the drug, the behavior of youngsters and ability to concentrate usually improves. After school, when the effects wear off, parents often say that children become more difficult to control. Some children are so numbed by the drug they lose their personalities and become zombie-like.

There are other problems with Ritalin. The Physicians' Desk Reference (PDR), the standard doctors' guide to the use of pharmaceutical drugs, lists 16 adverse reactions to Ritalin. Common side-effects include sleeplessness, irritability, nervousness, abdominal pain, and a slowing of normal growth activity due to lack of appetite. According to the PDR, the long-term effects of Ritalin in children have not been well established.

In addition, there are reports of a rising use of Ritalin for drug abuse because it is more readily available than street drugs. The Newsweek magazine article noted that Ritalin is attracting attention on the streets. "It's so common in some upscale precincts that a mini black market has emerged in a handful of playgrounds and campuses. 'Vitamin R' — one of its names — sells for $3 to $15 per pill, to be crushed and snorted for a cheap and relatively modest buzz," the magazine said.

The March 28, 1996 issue of USA Today carried the following item: "Drug Abuse Alert: Ciba-Geigy, the makers of Ritalin, a stimulant used to treat attention deficit disorder, this week is blanketing more than 200,000 pharmacists and doctors with pamphlets it hopes will prevent growing abuse of the drug. The Drug Enforcement Administration, which has charged the drug company downplays hazards and encourages overprescription for profit, views the movement 'with caution in view of the past,' says DEA's Gene Haislip. 'But I don't want to discourage anyone who wants to put out the good message.'"

According to the PDR, Ritalin is "not intended for use" in children with symptoms "secondary to environmental factors." The numbers of such children are significant, according to research cited in "Is This Your Child's World," (Bantam Books, 1996) by Doris Rapp, M.D., of Scottsdale, Arizona, a leading environmental illness expert. Some two-thirds of the millions of children diagnosed with ADHD have an environmental illness and/or a food allergy involved, she says.

Many physicians who practice what is called environmental medicine treat children with learning, emotional and behavioral problems whose problems are often related to allergies to food, pollen, molds, dust, mites, pets and chemicals.

"I wonder how many general practitioners, psychiatrists, pediatricians, neurologists, psychologists, teachers, or parents are aware that these allergies are all clearly environmental factors," says Rapp. "Any of them can cause some children to become hyperactive, inattentive, and impulsive. If environmental factors are not considered, many children can be needlessly placed on Ritalin."

Thomas Armstrong, Ph.D., a psychologist and author of "The Myth of the ADD Child" (Penguin Books, New York), which offers an insight on alternative and safe methods to help children, argues that indeed many factors can be involved that cause learning and behavioral problems. During a 1995 CNN interview, he cited such factors as allergies, stress, a chemical imbalance, and different learning styles.

Adam Clark's case

Leslie Clark, of Clarks Mill, Pennsylvania, brought her 12-year-old son Adam to my office in February 1996. She was desperate for help in sorting out

| From ADD |
| to all A's |

the learning problem of her son. Adam had been diagnosed ADD by one doctor and dyslexic by another.

The youngster's problem began at the age of nine, Mrs. Clark told me. Until that time he had been perfectly normal, she said.

"While in the second grade Adam got the flu and spiked a high temperature," she related. "He missed six weeks of school in 1990. He was put on Amoxicillin, an antibiotic, and sulfa drugs. When Adam recovered and returned to school, he was never the same child.

"All of a sudden he began having trouble reading and writing, even simple words. His writing looked like scribbling to all others. Only he could understand it. The school doctor told us he had ADD. We then took him to the Sylvan Learning Center in Ohio for academic testing. The diagnosis of ADD was confirmed. Later, a neurologist ordered an MRI and other tests, after which he diagnosed dyslexia and prescribed Ritalin."

Despite his difficulties, testing showed Adam to be an intelligent youngster — with a high IQ of about 130. He managed a B average in his schoolwork, accomplished through sheer willpower, by memorizing what was said in class. At home his parents would read him the lessons of the day, which Adam would also memorize. Instead of submitting written homework, he was given verbal exams in school.

This extraordinary effort was extremely stressful. By concentrating so hard, he developed severe headaches by the end of the day and would spontaneously begin to cry. In addition, the Ritalin was making him drowsy.

Since 1990, Adam's physical coordination had deteriorated. His hand/eye coordination also declined. He was unable to catch a baseball and play in Little League like his friends. This was very frustrating for him. He was physically inactive and spent much time in front of the television set watching what his mother said were "interesting programs" and trying hard to process the information.

Adam Clark was evaluated and found to have the "atlas syndrome," a misalignment of the first cervical vertebrae, and also cranial misalignment, specifically a rotation of the sphenoid bone in the skull. He was prescribed a series of 12 chiropractic adjustments. He was also placed on a dairy free, sugar free diet, but had a hard time with the program and couldn't stick to it. He was given nutritional supplements.

There was no change in his condition until after the third adjustment. After the treatment, the two returned to the family car for the drive back north. They lived near Erie, almost three hours to the north. As his mother was driving on highway 79, Adam began reading highway signs here and there.

Adam's mother never said a word until after the eighth treatment when she called me crying. Adam had read <u>all</u> the signs on highway 79. "It is amazing," she said. "He is reading the signs. And what's more, he started to read a book I had in the car."

"Let him try to read more books," I said.

The next day she called again to say he had read two books. He could never read a book before.

Following several more treatments, Adam was able to catch a ball and became reasonably coordinated in sports. Now, 1 1/2 years later, he reads books, writes better, and is getting straight A's in school. He no longer takes Ritalin. He is stable.

This case is very significant in my opinion. I believe there are millions of children in the U.S., unable to process information correctly, with ADD, ADHD, dyslexia and other problems, as a result of undiagnosed chiropractic, environmental and nutritional problems.

Young Adam was extremely bright, yet was frustrated because he could not make out words nor could anyone understand his writing. Chiropractic and cranial manipulation helped to correct a problem in the coordination between his brain and spinal cord so that information could be processed effectively once again.

Spinal misalignments can impair the proper function of the nervous system "wiring." In Adam's case there was both cranial and cervical stress. In the second grade, he became ill, in part due to spinal stress and nutritional factors. He went on antibiotics which suppressed his immune system and possibly caused a cerebral-like allergy. Ultimately, the boy developed a complex case of ADD because of spinal misalignments that prevented him from functioning normally.

How we treat ADD and ADHD

Most people view these disorders as mental or emotional conditions that need to be treated with chemicals. Unfortunately, natural therapies often are the treatments of last resort instead of the treatments of choice.

The problem with using drugs for ADD and ADHD is that they only mask symptoms, and do not address the causes. They should only be used on a short-term basis, if at all, while the causes of the problems are investigated and eliminated. The mainstream medical approach fails to do this. Ritalin and other drugs are not solutions.

There are many possible causes and varieties of learning disabilities associated with ADD/ADHD. As I have said before, each person is unique in many ways, including genetics, biochemical and structural individuality, trauma and disabilities.

Chiropractic alone is an extremely effective and often overlooked treatment for ADD and ADHD. In addition, food allergies, nutritional deficiencies, and toxic metals are frequently contributing factors. In our clinic we investigate for possible environmental and food sensitivities, drug side effects, diet and nutritional status, and for structural misalignments. This combined approach enables us to help many youngsters with learning and hyperactivity problems, as well as adults who have a difficult time concentrating (see the chapter on memory problems).

Environmental and food sensitivities:
(refer to chapter 11 and the allergy chapter)

Many individuals are sensitive to certain foods, inhaled chemicals, drugs, dust, mold, pollen or other substances. Reactions vary, but can include mood changes, hyperactivity, and problems concentrating.

Nutritional status:

We know that nutrition can impact the mood and behavior of individuals, even to a large degree.

Eating junk food, particularly refined, sugary carbohydrates, can send the blood sugar on a roller coaster ride. The brain is totally dependent on adequate blood sugar for its source of energy. When blood sugar levels dip, the result can be irritability, aggressiveness, hyperactivity, and an inability to focus.

A deficiency of certain B vitamins can lead to brain dysfunction and erratic thinking.

The chiropractic — ADD connection

> "Chiropractors correct abnormalities of the intellect as well as those of the body."
> — D.D. Palmer, founder of modern chiropractic

There is much evidence showing the potential benefits of manipulation for children with ADD and ADHD. Studies have confirmed clinical findings that chiropractic has a positive effect on anxiety, inability to concentrate, low mental stamina, hyperactivity, discipline problems, and even low grades and low IQ. After chiropractic care, energy, attitude and grades improve, attention span increases, discipline problems diminish, and neurological and other physical problems subside. Medication can often be discontinued.

Some of the many studies include these:

• In 1975, E.V. Walton, D.C., reported the benefits of chiropractic care on one group of 24 learning impaired students. Many of the youngsters showed dramatic results, including increase in IQ, improvement of behavior, increased grades, and better athletic ability. The children were on heavy doses of various medications after being diagnosed as hyperkinetic, non-verbal, passive, insomniac, and having poor gross and fine motor control. One group of children were treated medically with drug therapy while the second group received chiropractic care.

• Seven hyperactive children appeared to benefit from chiropractic adjustments and the researcher concluded that manipulation "has the potential to become an important nondrug intervention for children with hyperactivity."

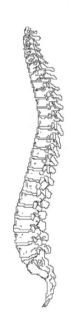

• A 10-year-old girl with ADD was taking 60 mg of Ritalin daily. She was diagnosed with severe scoliosis (curvature of the spine). After 10 adjustments, the mother reported a happier child, with greater immunity, and higher endurance. Within two months, the medication was stopped. The child's scoliosis reduced from 48 degrees to 12 degrees.

• A 12-year-old boy with ADD, asthma and seizures, was treated with chiropractic. After eight adjustments, his parents withdrew medication with the cooperation of the doctor. Positive personality changes were noted.

• A 10-year-old boy with a three-year history of hyperactivity, also suffered from ear infections, headaches, and allergic symptoms. Chiropractic examination determined multiple misalignments in his neck, back and skull. By the eleventh adjustment, his hyperactivity symptoms had abated. The other health problems had cleared up from earlier spinal adjustments. After 5 1/2 months, and being relatively symptom-free, he experienced two falls. His hyperactivity, headache and allergy symptoms returned. A single session of spinal and cranial manipulation resolved the recurrence.

• An 11-year-old institutionalized boy with ADHD had a history of behavioral disruptions, repeated ear infections, heavy metal intoxication, food allergies, environmental sensitivities, and multiple levels of biomechanical misalignments. The treatment program emphasized the need for care "in all aspects of the structural, chemical and mental triangle in children" with this disorder. As a result of the treatment, the youngster improved in his school work, attention span and temper, and recognizes he has control over his behavior. "There is hope he will be mainstreamed back into a regular public school setting soon," the report said.

• Following an automobile accident, a seven-year-old boy developed general agitation, memory loss, and inability to concentrate, along with loss of appetite, headaches, ear pain, difficulty in chewing, hearing loss, neck pain and bilateral leg pain. A medical doctor diagnosed ADD and Ritalin was prescribed. There was partial improvement. After four months, the boy's mother sought chiropractic care. A number of misalignments were found. Manipulation was performed three times weekly for 16 weeks and twice for one more week. The ADD symptoms cleared up as well as other symptoms. At 17 weeks, the Ritalin was stopped by the medical doctor. The mother discontinued chiropractic care after an insurance settlement was concluded. The boy's behavior symptoms gradually returned and he is back on Ritalin.

• In "No More Ritalin: Treating ADHD Without Drugs" (Kensington Publishing) osteopathic physician Mary Ann Block says that other osteopathic doctors have told her they have positively affected 50 percent of the children they see with the ADHD diagnosis just by using spinal manipulative therapy. Osteopaths are licensed to utilize medical drugs, surgery and spinal manipulation. "When a doctor considers the...nervous system in diagnosis and treatment, the patient is going to get a more wholistic approach to the treatment," she notes.

Natural Remedies for ADD/ADHD

* *The Gallagher Wellness Program*
* *Chiropractic manipulation*
* *Cranial manipulation*
* *Identify food, chemical and environmental sensitivities*
* *Check for toxic metals using hair analysis*
* *B complex* .... 25-100 milligrams daily
* *Pycnogenol* .... 2 capsules, twice daily
* *Chromium GTF* .... 2 capsules, twice daily
* *Trace minerals (calcium, magnesium,*
      manganese, vitamin D, vitamin B-6) ...... 2 capsules, twice daily.

BACK PAIN

About back pain

You have back pain. Perhaps leg pain as well.

You are not alone.

Elizabeth Taylor has suffered from recurring back pain for years. Ice hockey great Wayne Gretsky, like many athletes, has gone through his share of back misery. For the famous and not-so-famous alike, chronic lower back pain — and the leg pain that often accompanies it — is an all-too common and stressful reality:

• In the U.S., disability from back pain is growing at a rate 14 times faster than the population growth.

• The direct and indirect costs are at least $50 billion per year.

• Low back pain is the single most expensive health care problem and the most common cause of disability for persons under the age of 45.

• It's not just an adult problem. Half — that's right, one-half — of American children have low back pain by age 12!

• In the U.S., some seven million people are said to be temporarily out-of-work at any given time due to low back pain and 85 percent of people will be disabled by back pain at some point in their lives.

I myself have had my share of back problems. I first injured myself in sports as a teenager and later again as an adult in an automobile accident. As a result, my lower back has signs of degeneration. But I don't have back pain. Were it not for chiropractic and other natural treatments, I would be suffering like millions of others.

Just as I and my patients have done, you, too, can get substantial relief from back and leg pain — and perhaps eliminate it altogether — by following the recommendations in this chapter.

Conventional medicine often says the cause of your pain is arthritis, muscular tension and spasms, sprains of the ligaments that connect muscle to bone, or a disc herniation (also known as ruptured disc). Conventional treatment emphasizes drug and surgical solutions. Both are risky. Scientific research has clearly shown that chiropractic is the most effective, economical and safest treatment for sudden, acute and chronic back pain.

I'll talk about the chiropractic approach in a moment but first some facts on what back and leg pain are all about.

Back pain basics

Problems typically stem from two sources: the sacroiliac (hip) joints, and the five lumbar vertebrae in the small of the back.

Let's consider the sacroiliac first because that's where most back pain originates.

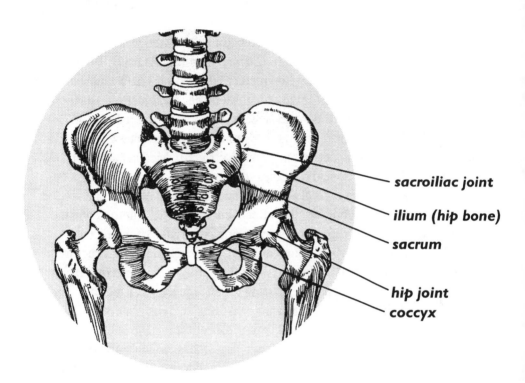

sacroiliac joint

ilium (hip bone)

sacrum

hip joint
coccyx

The sacroiliac problem

During the past two decades, research has demonstrated what chiropractors have known for 100 years — that the single greatest cause of back pain is sacroiliac misalignment. The sacroiliac joints, one on each side in the lower back region, are formed by the sacrum (the triangular bone at the base of the spine) and the two hip bones.

These large and powerful joints connect your upper and lower body. They have much to do with your well-being, or lack of it. All loads (forces and stresses) from the spine, trunk and upper body, and all forces from the legs, are transmitted through these pivotal joints.

The two most vulnerable groups for sacroiliac disorders are children and pregnant women. I have had thousands of children brought to my clinic over the years for chronic leg aches, often referred to as "growing pains" by pediatricians. Many times these pains will wake up a child in the middle of the night.

• One study found that 30 percent of elementary schoolchildren (ages 6 to 12) and 42 percent of older youngsters (ages 12-17) tested positive for sacroiliac dysfunction (Journal of Manipulative and Physiological Therapeutics, 1984).

• Sacroiliac joint problems have been implicated in 50 to 70 percent of adults with low back pain (British Medical Journal, 1979).

• In a study conducted by two medical doctors of 1,293 low back pain patients seen at a university hospital clinic, sacroiliac dysfunction was found to be the main problem in 23 percent of case (Clinical Orthopedics, 1987).

Until 1934 the sacroiliac joint was thought to be the source of most low back pain. In that year, disc herniation was discovered. Medical attention was diverted to the disc and surgical remedies for the next 40 years. Chiropractic continued to maintain a non-surgical mechanical treatment of back pain, in the form of manipulative therapy, but this effective method was smothered in the monopolistic and anti-chiropractic maneuverings of organized medicine.

Because the sacroiliac joints are pivotal to our physical structure, misalignments to one or both joints can and do trigger low and mid back pain, sciatica, disc disturbance, neck pain and headaches. Often they are involved as well in a variety of organic problems such as gynecological disorders, erectile dysfunction and bladder difficulties.

Toeing in and toeing out, limping, clumsiness, an inability to walk in the normal heel to toe fashion, are often connected to hip joint misalignments.

It is worthwhile to mention that the uterus is physically attached to the hip joints by ligaments. For this reason, chiropractic adjustments can reduce much of the suffering of pregnant women. I strongly believe that low back pain does not have to accompany pregnancy if a woman is managed chiropractically.

Years ago, I was the treating chiropractor for a number of patients who had chosen home deliveries. Chiropractic adjustments eliminated or reduced not just low back pain, but neck pain, leg cramps, nausea, and headaches associated with pregnancy. My patients also received adjustments and pressure point treatments during their labor, thereby facilitating an uncomplicated delivery. An obstetrician friend often remarked how chiropractic made the whole process easier.

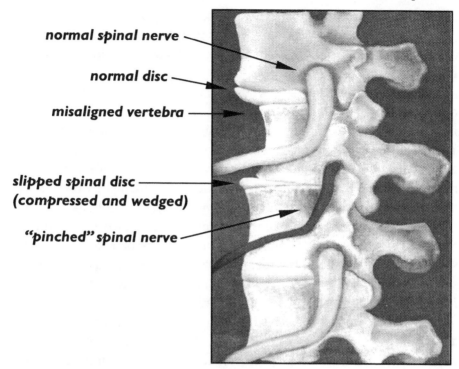

normal spinal nerve

normal disc

misaligned vertebra

slipped spinal disc
(compressed and wedged)

"pinched" spinal nerve

The lumbar problem

Between each of the spinal vertebrae is a disc that acts as a shock absorber. The disc is filled with a jelly-like substance, the consistency of an egg yoke, contained within a biconcave harder shell. When you twist, turn, run and jump, it is the discs that protect the vertebral bones from damage. And it is the joints of each vertebra that allow movement in each direction, so that we can twist, bend, and do a variety of movements without pain.

Spinal subluxations in the lower back can throw this marvelous mechanical arrangement in disarray, resulting in back pain and many other problems.

• Misalignments occur at any time in life, even as early as childbirth, from spinal stress or trauma. See chapter 13 for more details.

• Most of the time the lower back spinal misalignments involve the last two vertebrae. Technically, we say the L4 and L5 site, that is, the fourth and fifth lumbar vertebrae.

• When vertebral joints lose their flexibility and motion and become locked as a result of misalignment, pressure develops on the spinal nerves branching outward from the spine. This, in turn, creates an inflammatory, swelling reaction that causes back and leg pain.

• Painful lower back muscle spasms often develop as the result of pinched nerves not supplying the muscles with adequate electrical stimulation and oxygen.

• Subluxations and spinal stress can lead to disc tearing, also known as herniated, ruptured or slipped disc. This can cause the fluid inside a disc, or actual fragments of the disc, to protrude outside the structure of the disc. In most cases, doctors tell patients that their back pain is a disc problem. In reality, this is rarely true. And if it is a disc problem, surgery is rarely necessary. Chiropractic manipulation is effective for subluxations and disc herniation-related back problems.

• Calcium deposits (spurs) are often used as a justification for spinal surgery. But they are rarely the cause of back pain. Spurs develop as a result of spinal stress, trauma, nutritional and genetic factors, and especially wear and tear. Your body will attempt to "seal off" a damaged area by placing calcium in the region of injury.

• Spinal stenosis is a term referring to the narrowing of the spinal canal through which the spinal cord runs. This problem is sometimes congenital (at birth) or develops as a result of degeneration of the spine. It is much more common in those 60 years and older. Stenosis is rarely a cause of pain or a justification for surgery. Chiropractic manipulation and exercise work well to eliminate the pain associated with stenosis.

Types of back pain

• *Pain may come on suddenly and be either acute (sudden onset) or may become chronic over time, if uncorrected.*

• *It can be caused by the birthing process, difficult deliveries, C-section births, or the use of obstetrical forceps.*

• *Sudden pain can occur from trauma generated by a wrong move, such as during sports or exercise activity, or when lifting something heavy, or even working in the yard. Sports or automobile accident injuries are other common types of trauma.*

• *Pain may be a chronic condition due to years of bad posture, physical labor or degeneration.*

• *Pain may be triggered by long periods of inactivity or working in an abnormal position for an extended time.*

The chiropractic — low back pain connection

Worldwide recognition of the effectiveness of chiropractic treatment

Nearly a hundred years of clinical experience along with solid research show that chiropractic manipulation is a significant, safe and cost-effective healing method for back and leg pain. It restores normal motion to the vertebrae, which defuses the pressure and inflammation on the nerves, thus re-opening normal nutrient and nerve impulse flow in the affected area.

Chiropractic — and not medical doctors — should be the first line of management for low back pain, according to an independent study on health care effectiveness commissioned by the Province of Ontario (Canada) Ministry of Health. The comprehensive study, published in 1993, was conducted by Pran Manga, Ph.D., an economist and director of health administration at the University of Ottawa.

"The Manga Report" as it is called concluded that billions of dollars could be saved each year if chiropractors, instead of medical doctors, were the primary care physicians for workers suffering from low back pain.

Among the points made by the study were these:

• "...for the management of low back pain, chiropractic care is the most effective treatment, and it should be fully integrated into the government's health care system."

• "...injured workers...diagnosed with low back pain returned to work much sooner when treated by chiropractors" than by medical doctors."

• "Chiropractic manipulation is safer than medical management..."

• "The overwhelming body of evidence shows that chiropractic management of low back pain is more cost-effective than medical management, and that many medical therapies are of questionable validity or are clearly inadequate."

• "There would be highly significant cost savings if more management of low back pain was transferred from physicians to chiropractors. Users of chiropractic care have substantially lower health care costs, especially inpatient costs, than those who use medical care only."

Other findings support "the Manga Report:"

• In 1994, the U.S. Government's Agency for Health Care Policy and Research (AHCPR) and the Department of Health and Human Services recommended spinal manipulation as a first line treatment for acute back pain in adults. Acute back pain was defined as pain for less than three months. The recommendation also applied to patients with recurring pain.

The report, entitled "Acute Low Back Problems in Adults," said that costly imaging and other diagnostic tests should only be considered if a patient "continues to be limited by back symptoms for more than one month without improvement" under care.

- "Chiropractic treatment was more effective than hospital outpatient management, mainly for patients with chronic or severe back pain," stated T.W. Meade, an English medical doctor in a British Medical Journal published in 1990. His study, based on two years of monitoring 741 patients, was commissioned by the British Medical Research Council. Chiropractic patients did significantly better, the report said, with superior results maintained at one and two year follow-up.

- Guidelines published in 1996 by the Royal College of General Practitioners in England, in consultation with the British National Health Service, endorsed the importance of manipulation in the management of most back pain patients. Among the experts involved in establishing the guidelines (both in England and in the U.S.) was Scottish orthopedic surgeon Gordon Waddell, M.D., an internationally renowned expert who describes contemporary medical management of back pain as a "disaster."

- A 1988 study of 10,652 Florida workers' compensation cases by Steve Wolk, Ph.D., concluded that "a claimant with a back-related injury, when initially treated by a chiropractor versus a medical doctor, is less likely to become temporarily disabled, or, if disabled, remains disabled for a shorter period of time." The Wolk report, made for the Foundation for Chiropractic Education and Research said, "claimants treated by medical doctors were hospitalized at a much higher rate than claimants treated by chiropractors."

- A 1991 workers' compensation study in Utah and reported in the Journal of Occupational Medicine revealed that treatment costs for medical services were significantly higher than for chiropractic services. In addition, the number of work days lost under medical care was nearly 10 times higher than under chiropractic care.

- In a 1992 article in the Journal of Family Practice, "the number of days of disability for patients seen by family physicians was significantly higher (mean 39.7) than for patients managed by chiropractors (mean 10.8)."

- Of 1,996 low back pain cases studied in Australia, patients receiving chiropractic treatment averaged 6.26 compensation days compared to 25.56 days for medical patients (Chiropractic Journal of Australia, 1992).

The chiropractic — leg pain connection

The two <u>sciatic nerves</u> are the largest and longest nerves in the body. They branch out from the spinal column in the lower back, run through the pelvic area on each side and down each leg to the toes. The sciatic nerves supply your legs with the "electrical juice" to keep you moving.

<u>Sciatica</u> is the name of the painful condition that results when one of these nerves is pinched at the lower part of the back. This can result in low back pain, leg pain, knee pain, and foot pain. Additional symptoms include numbness, burning, cramping, hot or cold sensations, weakness, heaviness or feeling like your leg is giving out.

Research has shown that chiropractic can offer significant relief for sciatic pain sufferers. One study of 60 patients concluded that spinal care should, in fact, be the treatment of choice. (Journal of Manipulation and Physiological Therapeutics, 1982).

In an additional study that evaluated four different treatment methods — spinal care, traction, and two types of spinal injections — the patients who underwent spinal adjustments reported the greatest improvement (British Journal of Rheumatology, 1987).

In a more recent study, researchers at the Royal University Hospital in Saskatoon, Canada, reported improvements among the vast majority of 59 patients with leg pain from lumbar disc herniation who were treated with chiropractic manipulation. Most of the patients had been referred to a postgraduate chiropractic teaching clinic at the hospital by medical doctors.

The results, according to the study, included the following:

• 90 percent of patients improved,

• 75 percent of the cases were described as clinically successful, meaning they experienced at least 50 percent recovery and/or return to work, and a significant increase in range of spinal motion and leg function.

• No patient reported increased back or leg pain or other complications.

The authors of the study concluded that a course of non-operative treatment including chiropractic can be effective and safe for the treatment of back and radiating leg pain (Journal of Manipulation and Physiological Therapeutics, 1995).

Drugs and surgery — caveat emptor!

The above reports make it quite clear that chiropractic treatment should be the first treatment patients seek for back and sciatic pain.

Unfortunately, too many patients seek riskier routes first.

Often, on the recommendation of a physician, they will take painkillers. While this is a customary route, medication never gets to the cause of the pain, it just turns down the intensity. When the effect wears off, the pain returns. Moreover, pharmaceutical prescriptions, such as aspirin and non-steroidal anti-inflammatory drugs (NSAIDs) used for relieving pain, are associated with many side effects. As I pointed out in chapter three, the continuous use of these medications can have deadly side effects. NSAIDs, for instance, can adversely affect your stomach, kidneys and even contribute to joint destruction that will often worsen your back condition.

The other "usual" option offered by conventional medicine is surgery. Low back problems are the "third most common reason for surgical procedures," according to a U.S. Government study. There are an estimated 600,000-700,000 back surgeries performed every year in the U.S. — a figure 40 percent higher than any other country and more than five times the rate of England and Scotland, according to a 1994 report in the journal Spine. Daniel Cherkin, Ph.D., the report's author, stated that "back surgery rates (have) increased almost literally with the per capita supply of orthopedic and neurosurgeons in the country."

Recent data from the Department of Research and Scientific Affairs at the American Academy of Orthopedic Surgeons indicate that the total number of disc operations in 1994 was 317,000. An additional 163,000 spinal fusions were performed in the same year. These figures do not include surgeries for spurs, tumors, infections, fractures, or other conditions.

Spinal surgery is sometimes considered necessary in cases of severe bone and nerve destruction (due to a variety of causes, including infection or cancer). Disc fragmentation, a cause of leg pain, may occasionally require surgery. I have encountered a few cases like that over the years. The majority of patients, however, can be more effectively managed through conservative chiropractic treatment. In fact, a 1987 study in the journal Spine concluded that surgery is an effective means of dealing with low back pain in less than one percent of cases.

Unfortunately, some 87% of back surgery patients did not have the benefit of a prior chiropractic opinion. Afterward, they often wish they had.

If people were aware of the outcome statistics on back surgeries they would think twice about having operations. In a landmark review of published studies in 23 medical journals, G. F. Dommisse and R. P. Grahe, two medical doctors, found that 48 percent of patients suffer from recurrence of lower back pain, sciatica, or both, within one year of surgery. This particular review was monumental in scope, involving 7,391 cases and 71 surgeons, and appeared in a 1978 book appropriately entitled, "The Failure of Surgery for Lumbar Disc Disorders."

The reality of the situation is that patients often develop what is currently referred to as the Failed Low Back Surgery Syndrome (FLBSS). Yes, it happens so much that the phenomenon was given a name! And to make matters worse, if surgery is ineffective the first time, a second or third operation often will not help matters. Even successful operations can cause scar tissue, permanent spinal weakness, distortion and instability. Many patients of mine who have undergone back surgery can attest to that. See the cases of Bill Heinz and Kathleen Andrejko below.

In an analysis that appeared in the widely read professional book "Managing Low Back Pain" (Churchill Livingston, New York, 1992), researchers C.V. Burton and J. David Cassidy described conventional medical treatment as "the single greatest and most inefficient expenditure of health resources in our society today."

Beware: the disc treadmill

"You have a herniated disc and you'll need back surgery."

When you hear those words from a medical doctor, proceed cautiously.

My sincere advice is to have a chiropractic evaluation first, for all the reasons I have described above.

Chiropractic manipulation is effective for most back and leg pain, whether it is caused by a herniated disc or not.

A herniated disc is not the cause of back and leg pain in the majority of cases.

In the U.S., back pain sufferers usually go to a family doctor, who often refers them to an orthopedic surgeon. An MRI (Magnetic Resonance Imaging) study is prescribed. Often they are told they have a disc herniation and that is the cause of the back pain.

Don't fall into that trap.

MRI technology has contributed to and has been a source of justification for spinal surgeons to recommend back surgery. The really scary part is that MRIs, while helpful for determining fractures and tumors, are inaccurate for determining back pain from disc herniations.

Up to 60 percent of people between the ages of 50 and 60, who have no back pain, will show a disc herniation on MRI tests. The incidence of herniated or bulging discs increases with age. By age 75, the percentage of individuals found to have disc damage by MRI rises to something like 80 percent. Disc herniation, although typically cited as the reason for surgery, may even be a "normal" situation and not the cause of pain.

Chiropractic can generally deal effectively with herniated discs. Consider these studies:

• Of 517 patients with protruded lumbar discs, 76.8 percent reported satisfactory results after manipulation of the spine (Clinical Orthopedics Related to Research, February 1987).

• Twenty-one patients with diagnosed disc herniations experienced resolution of nerve root pain after chiropractic manipulation. A cat scan at least six months later showed the herniation reduced or disappeared in most patients.

Even though chiropractic is considered the most effective method for treating back pain, if you are unresponsive to treatment, it is advisable to obtain a second or third chiropractic opinion. There are a multitude of chiropractic techniques and schools of thought for correcting spinal conditions, including disc herniations.

Since chiropractic physicians are skilled at differential diagnosis, they may refer you to a medical doctor for an orthopedic or neurological opinion if your condition warrants that type of evaluation.

Bill Heinz's case — chronology of an ordeal

Remember Bill Heinz, the suffering salesman and ex-baseball player I mentioned at the beginning of the book? He had undergone two back surgeries, was dependent on painkillers, and was still in misery. Bill's case, unfortunately, represents the lot of many people. He asked that I tell his story in the hope that people will read it and not have to travel the same painful path.

1984

• As a freshman in college, he developed severe pain on the left side of his lower back. He underwent surgery for a herniated disc.

• After the operation, he contracted aseptic meningitis, meaning blood in the spinal fluid, and spent an additional two weeks in the hospital. Other than the complication, he regarded the surgery "a success."

1985

• For a year, he was pain free. In mid-1985, "a constant, dull, aching feeling" developed in his lower back, now on the right side. It was very painful at times, and he would have it for the next 10 years. Sitting was often uncomfortable because of the pain.

1987

• In 1987, he returned to the back surgeon complaining of the pain. The doctor explained that after disc surgery there is a settling of the vertebrae surrounding the disc that has been operated on. This often produces pain felt on the side opposite to where the surgery was performed. Shots of cortisone, called a facet block, were administered. "The shots were like a miracle cure," said Bill, but then, six months later, "the party was over. The pain returned. He received more shots. "Then, they wore off, and I would get more," he said.

1989-1994

• From 1989 through 1994, he didn't return for shots, although he had pain every day. "I guess I was getting used to it," he said.

• In April of 1994, he suddenly felt sharp pain on the right side. "It felt like someone stuck a knife in," he said. He had to quit playing baseball and take it easy. "I was taking all kinds of painkillers (Tylenol, Ultram, non-steroidal anti-inflammatory drugs, Vicodin, sometimes mixing them together) and nothing was helping," he said.

• Bill went to a pain clinic, took an MRI, and received another series of facet block shots. Relief was minimal. Pain was shooting down his right leg. He received an epidural steroid injection that helped substantially but wore off within a month. He repeated the shots twice in the next 10 months.

• The results of the MRI were negative. Two surgeons said Bill might have to live with the problem.

• A pain specialist performed a facet rhizotomy, an operation under local anesthesia where electrical currents are aimed at the nerves thought to be the source of pain. "The intention is to kill those nerves," said Bill. For several months afterward, he had "good days and bad days," but the pain gradually returned.

1995

• His doctors ordered another MRI. They now said the results indicated a herniated disc at the same vertebra level but on the opposite side of his operation 11 years before. "The pain was so bad and the leg numbness so great, that I was beginning to lose the control of my right foot," he said. "I could not wait to get operated on. I saw this as the light at the end of the tunnel." Surgery was performed in June of 1995. "This was my second disc surgery and I wasn't 30 years old yet," he said.

• Several weeks later, Bill was diagnosed with an infection in the area of the surgery. The risk of infection had been explained to him beforehand as a 2-4 percent chance. "I never thought it would happen to me," he said.

• Now Bill couldn't stand straight and almost fell down several times trying to walk. On July 4th he was taken by ambulance to the emergency room with muscle spasms that caused the worse pain he had ever experienced. He was given Toradol and Valium and discharged on high doses of Percocet, eight pills a day. "I spent the next two to three days in a daze, and can't recall anything except excruciating spasms several times per day," he said.

• Bill received another MRI. Then he underwent an aspiration procedure, meaning that a #18 gauge needle was injected into the disc space to drain out a sample of pus for culture.

• Bill was prescribed amoxicillin, an antibiotic, to eliminate the infection. People usually take 1,500 milligrams a day for 10 days to get rid of an ear or sinus infection. "I took 4,000 milligrams a day and I was on it for four months," he said. "I also took a lot of Motrin as well as other NSAIDs along with some Tylenol every now and then." He also was prescribed to wear a brace for his back.

• Bill began having trouble moving his bowels, a common problem associated with low back problems and the use of NSAIDs.

• A physical therapist helped him strengthen his back muscles. However, the old "nagging, aching stuck feeling" was returning on the right side. It became annoying enough to resume the NSAIDs, Ultram and Tylenol. In addition, pain had developed in the upper mid-back. The combined pain was beginning to "drive me crazy," he said.

• Then, he began bleeding from the rectum, a well-known side effect of NSAIDs. A colonoscopy test came out normal.

1996

It was at this time, in May of 1996, that Bill came to see me at the suggestion of his mother, a patient of mine.

"I went to Dr. Gallagher strictly for the pain I was having in my low right side," Bill said. "I also wanted to see about the pain in my upper mid-back. He told me what would be involved and gave me no promises, but he thought he could help.

"On May 16 I returned for my first treatment. I was still taking a lot of pain medication right up to and including May 16. The pain in my low right side was not crippling but it was extremely annoying and bothersome. The pain in my upper mid-back was very uncomfortable, but not debilitating.

"On May 17, the day after my first chiropractic adjustment with Dr. Gallagher, I did not take any pain medication. My right side low back pain was gone as well as the pain in my upper mid-back. I felt like a million bucks.

"I have returned to Dr. Gallagher's clinic on and off for eight months. In addition to the adjustments, I also have been working with their Cybex low back weight machines and been a routine recipient of deep muscle myotherapy treatments designed to break down scar tissue from all my surgeries. I am also on a nutritional supplement program designed to promote the healing process.

"As far as pain medication goes, I have had to use only an Advil or Tylenol for a rare headache, perhaps eight times in the last eight months. I have not taken anything for my back. The bleeding is gone. That's probably because I no longer take NSAIDs or from the improved alignment in my spine from the adjustments.

"The overall treatment plan is working. I still occasionally get the 'stuck' sensation in my lower right side, but it is not as severe as before. The amount of pain relief between once-a-week adjustments is growing with each treatment and I hope that soon I will be able to extend treatments to a monthly basis.

"I will never know if Dr. Gallagher would have kept me from having disc surgery. I know that things would certainly not have been as bad as they were. I will always have damaged spinal joints due to surgery, cortisone shots and the infection, but my joints have been saved in my opinion because of Dr. Gallagher's treatments."

The morale in this, and most other cases: Misalignment precedes pain

Bill's case is very poignant. I believe his misery could have been cut short immensely. He had a subluxation complex in his spine long before he started having back pain. <u>Misalignment precedes pain. It is the cause of the pain, not just in Bill's case, but in most cases</u>. However, he didn't have chiropractic treatments to resolve his spinal misalignments until after he had gone through the medical and surgical treadmill. The medication and surgeries never corrected the underlying problem. They created new ones. The adjustments we administered to Bill reversed his condition. He no longer has back pain and no longer lives on medication.

His case dramatically points out the need for early chiropractic evaluation, and certainly before anyone ever agrees to surgery. It also points out the need for chiropractic intervention for those who have undergone back surgery, whether the surgery is successful or not. Spinal care is necessary for everyone throughout life.

For the sake of your back, and your health, long-term drug therapy, cortisone injections, nerve blocks and surgery are drastic medical methods and should be considered only as treatments of last resort.

The two Kathleens

Ever make a false move and suddenly your back is out with a ruptured lumbar disc? It happened one night in 1996 to Kathleen Ponzetti, a 46-year-old emergency medical technician from Delmont, Pennsylvania, as she rolled over in bed in her sleep. A jolt of pain awakened her. Immediately the pain shot down her left leg and foot. She couldn't move without the pain increasing. Her left ankle felt like it was going to explode off of her leg. Soon there was no sensation in her lower abdomen and she experienced difficulty controlling her bladder and bowel. She couldn't sit. Her toes were numb and felt like rocks. She couldn't raise her feet.

In prior years Kathy had undergone a failed cervical disc surgery and was sent home with a bottle of pain pills. Her doctors told her they could do nothing more for her. Now, she opted for chiropractic treatment. She arrived by ambulance, flat out on a stretcher, in great distress.

Kathy had classic signs of herniation of the disc and spinal subluxation. I started administering daily lower spine manipulations and Leander distraction treatments, a specialized adjustment method for disc-related problems. She also received B-12 and B complex injections, muscle therapies, and natural anti-inflammatory supplements.

With this program we were able to make substantial progress rapidly:
First week:
After her fourth treatment, she was able to sit in the back seat of a car, and no longer had to be brought by ambulance. Her urinary function improved and bowel function restored, although painful. She was now able to get her foot on the floor, walk for a short distance and even stand for short periods.
Second week:
Standing longer with less pain. Increasing control of bladder and bowel function, although bowel movement still painful. Still pain at night.
Third week:
With some difficulty now able to dress and undress herself, except for shoes. She could stand and walk longer and could sit for a few minutes at a time in a hard chair. "It was so nice to eat a bit of something at the table, instead of lying on the floor trying to eat," she told me. Her toes starting to get feeling back. They didn't seem like heavy rocks anymore.
Fourth week:
Able to sit up in the car. Standing and walking time increasing. Bladder control back to normal. Bowel control improved and associated pain decreasing. Now able to get her shoes on.

Fifth week:

Able to drive to office for treatment. Improvement continues on all fronts.

Next three weeks:

Able to walk up to several miles a day, sit for more time, and felt substantial strength in legs. Feeling better overall.

Ninth week:

Passive therapy discontinued. Exercise rehabilitation started, along with spinal manipulation three times weekly.

Eleventh week:

She returned to work and soon afterward to the outdoor activities she loved to do.

Kathy's case was a classic herniated disc associated with loss of control of the lower extremities as well as the bladder and bowel. She would have definitely undergone a low back operation had she taken the medical route again...and if her mother had had her way, that's what would have happened.

Kathy's mother had accompanied her daughter in the ambulance to my clinic and followed as the paramedics carried her on a stretcher into a treatment room. There, she took me aside and said she wanted Kathy to go to the hospital instead. She had, understandably, a great deal of concern and fear for her daughter's well-being and thought that the only option was another operation. But Kathy had refused because of the complications she had experienced after her neck surgery.

Today, Kathy is functioning relatively normally. Her case again points out the importance of early chiropractic intervention so as to avoid the complicating conditions that often result from surgery.

Another patient of mine named Kathleen — Kathleen Andrejko, 54, of Swissvale, Pennsylvania — suffered incapacitating back pain for more than 10 years and then underwent two painful back operations. The surgeries didn't help her. She still had back pain plus numbness and weakness in her left leg.

Our program was able to rehabilitate her. She now has no back or leg pain. She was able to return to her favorite sport of bowling.

"You put me back on my feet again," she told us.

For those who have already had back surgery, stabilization through chiropractic is more challenging because of the scar tissue generated by the operations. Nevertheless, manipulations lessen residual pain and help improve the quality of life.

If chiropractic treatment is effective for patients with constant pain and impairment after back surgery, doesn't it make sense to use this method in order to avoid surgery in the first place?

How we treat back and leg pain

Sacroiliac and lumbar subluxation cannot be accurately determined through X-ray, CT scan, MRIs or any other conventional medical procedure. It requires the skill of a highly-trained chiropractic physician to evaluate each joint and correct each abnormality that is found.

We use a number of popular chiropractic techniques in our office for back and leg pain. Among them are:

• In cases of sacroiliac disorders, the Thompson Method allows for specific hip manipulations to be performed quickly and painlessly.

• The Leander Method, an advanced form of manipulation effective for disc herniations.

• Sacro-Occipital Technique (SOT), a method that helps balance the hip and low back in relationship to the head.

• Applied Kinesiology (AK), a major advancement in muscle balancing for spinal dysfunction.

There are many unique and innovative chiropractic techniques. If you do not respond to one particular method, consider a second or even third chiropractic opinion.

The frequency and duration of treatment are always an individual matter and depend on the condition, health and compliance of each patient.

Treatment of sudden pain

Most patients with sudden acute pain may require manipulation daily for one to two weeks, followed by a stepdown of two or three weekly treatments for another two to four weeks.

As your condition improves, the frequency decreases. Parallel to this is an increasing program of rehabilitative exercises.

Treatment of chronic pain

For patients with chronic (long-term) pain, a series of 15 to 25 adjustments over eight to ten weeks is often effective.

Results

Strong studies, both here and abroad, now show that patients with either acute or chronic back pain experienced excellent results under chiropractic care, and that the benefits of treatment last one to two years.

I would like to know what drug eliminates chronic back pain for that length of time.

I think it is very significant that chiropractic care provides up to two years of relief for chronic back pain sufferers. However, what makes more sense is to follow a chiropractic wellness program over the course of your life. That's the kind of proactive plan I myself follow. A regular once-a-month adjustment works for me, my family, and many patients. It helps maintain a healthy nervous system and prevent problems. Why let symptoms dictate your need for care. Don't you take vitamins and exercise for preventive reasons?

As I mentioned above, manipulation restores normal motion and alignment to the subluxated, misaligned or locked vertebrae and restores normal nerve and blood supply to the affected area. Once the series of adjustments is completed and pain relief is obtained, a follow-up program of active exercise rehabilitation is recommended. This is necessary to increase strength, flexibility and endurance, and help protect against recurrences. For more than 10 years, we have utilized a Cybex system in our clinic that combines unique computer measurements of muscle strength with state-of-the-art exercise programs.

The nutritional connection

The nutritional connection to back pain and sciatica is not nearly as strong as the chiropractic aspect. However, I have corrected some chronic back and sciatic nerve problems with vitamin B-12 and folic acid. Deficiencies of these nutrients can lead to nerve inflammation (neuritis or neuropathy).

Good nutrition for discs and joints, in any case, plays an important role in the restoration and maintenance of healthy tissue. Beneficial nutritional supplements we recommend to patients include Discazyme, which contains ingredients such as manganese, a key mineral for strengthening ligaments and disc fibers, and bromelain/papain, the anti-inflammatory enzymes found in pineapples and papayas. DEPA, another supplement, is an excellent source of omega-3 fatty acids which have a natural analgesic effect.

Herpes infections can sometimes simulate sciatica. In such cases, we will recommend the amino acid lysine, along with the mineral lithium arginate. Lysine and Lithium inhibit the herpes virus that can infect a nerve root.

The herbal medicine white willow bark and the homeopathic Ruta have natural pain modulating effects without causing damage to your stomach, a common consequence of using aspirin or NSAIDs.

Natural Remedies for Back Pain and Sciatica

- *Chiropractic manipulation*
- *Myotherapy (deep tissue massage)*
- *Cybex isokinetic rehabilitation exercise (following decrease of pain)*
- *Discazyme* .... 2 capsules, 3 times daily
- *DEPA (essential fatty acids)* .. 2 capsules, twice daily
- *Brom Pap* .... 2 tablets, 4 times daily between meals
- *Chiropractic cream (capsacin) apply topically*

BLADDER PROBLEMS

About urinary tract infections

Cystitis, or urinary tract infections (UTI) affect 25 million women each year. The condition is characterized by severe pain with urination, urgency to void and frequency of urination. Common contributing factors include E. coli bacterial infections, the use of birth control spermicide gels, a history of antibiotic therapy for upper respiratory infections, poor hygienic practices, spinal and mechanical dysfunction and dietary factors.

Individually or in combination these factors can lead to recurring infections and in some severe cases, to what is called "chronic interstitial cystitis."

Conventional medical treatment focuses on anti-bacterial drug therapy, including sulfa drugs and antibiotics, to kill the E.coli bacterium.

Sara Marusa's case

When she came to see me in 1994, Sara Marusa, a beautician in her fifties from Homer City, Pennsylvania, was feeling poorly and suffering from intensifying burning in the bladder. She had a history of recurring bladder and yeast infections and antibiotic treatments.

> "The burning was so bad that I felt like ending my life."

According to Sara, the first urologist she had seen many times had eventually told her to see a psychiatrist, that the pain was in her head. A second physician diagnosed her with interstitial cystitis but said he had no cure for her.

Sara was extremely uncomfortable from her condition, which now included itching and discharges. She had been to the emergency room four times in the previous four months.

"The burning was so bad I felt like ending my life," she told me. She couldn't stand the burning any longer. She also complained of low back and neck pain, blurred vision, right shoulder discomfort, tension headaches, depression, heartburn, bowel problems, a history of ulcers, sinus trouble and problems sleeping at night.

We put Sara on an intestinal cleansing diet. She drank purified water, took supplements and received chiropractic treatment for her back and neck.

"I started to feel better already on the third day," she reported.

"Today I am burn free. I am careful with my diet. If I start to eat junk food and go off my diet, the burning starts again. I go back on my diet and the burning stops. I do not eat bread, yeast products, wheat, or acidic foods."

Sara first came for chiropractic treatments twice a week for six weeks, then once a week, then twice a month, and now maintenance at one treatment a month.

"If people would have told me this was possible I would have laughed at them," she says. "I still get depressed but not as much as I used to and I can handle life's problems a lot better now. My life has been saved."

Adrienne Riethmiller's case

Adrienne, from Jeannette, Pennsylvania, is a patient in her 70s, who had been suffering with bladder infections off and on for more than 30 years. Doctors had prescribed antibiotics and other medication,

> **"My urologist said it was something I would have to live with."**

flushed her bladder and even stretched the bladder opening. For short periods of time she had relief, but as she grew older the infections came more often.

"I have tried to get off the medication," she told me at the time of her first visit to my clinic, "but after a week or so I would hurt so bad I had to go back on antibiotics. My urologist said it was something I would have to live with. It has been very discouraging. I haven't had much hope."

Adrienne had heard me on radio and decided to see me in September 1991.

"I am hurting so bad that I am ready to try anything," she said.

Adrienne tried our combined approach of nutrition and chiropractic. Her problem had been going on for many years and it took some time to resolve them. But resolve they did. In a matter of 12 weeks, Adrienne was free of bladder infections and antibiotics. The program also benefited her in other ways. Her cholesterol dropped from 242 to 176. She lost 20 pounds. A hiatal hernia condition cleared up.

"I used to wear socks to bed because of cold feet, but I no longer need them," she told me during a checkup. "It is amazing after going through chiropractic care in a period of time how you begin to notice the different things that aren't bothering you anymore."

Adrienne experienced what most of my patients do. That is, they come for a specific complaint, such as chronic bladder problems, and after a series of chiropractic adjustments and nutritional prescriptions, many other problems disappear.

Adrienne had thought about coming to see me a year or so before she finally made an appointment. She felt there wasn't any hope for her because she was taking many vitamins and following a healthy diet. As I told her, "you may have a set of keys but that doesn't always mean you have the right one to open a locked door."

How we treat bladder infections

Q *"I am 30 years old and I have constant bladder infections. I don't know what to do because as soon as I finish one set of antibiotics, I am back on them again. I am exhausted from frequency of urination at night. My marriage is suffering because intercourse seems to make it worse. Is there anything natural for me?"*

A In our clinic we use a variety of natural approaches, including nutritional supplements and chiropractic adjustments, and have very positive results. Raw cranberry juice is a great aid, long recognized as a folk medicine remedy. Indeed it has strong anti-bacterial benefits for individuals with urinary tract infections. It also has the unique ability to soothe and protect the bladder lining. We recommend one pint to a quart daily.

We also use Cran C Plex, a nutritional supplement that incorporates raw dehydrated cranberry extract with vitamin C and the botanical medicines Uva Ursi and couch grass. This product is helpful in inhibiting the growth of E. coli and combating even antibiotic-resistant infections.

The lining of the bladder responds favorably to vitamin A treatment. Vitamin C with bioflavonoids and zinc also add a helping hand through their ability to fortify the immune system. Vitamin C, when taken as 500-1000 milligrams every hour, is effective, and zinc, in the form of zinc picolinate, at 25 milligrams twice daily.

We also recommend a "natural herbal antibiotic" combination called DL Winter that contains echinacea, goldenseal and red clover.

You can make a big impact against bladder infections by flushing out your bladder with liquids. I suggest that patients drink two to three quarters of water daily, preferably distilled or mineral water.

For chronic bladder infections, one should consider the possibility of an estrogen deficiency. Although more common in menopausal women, recurring infections can be in part triggered by vaginal and urethral (bladder opening) dryness. Ostaderm V Cream, a natural plant form of estrogen and progesterone hormones, can be applied vaginally to help overcome menopausal symptoms and bladder infections due to vaginal dryness.

The chiropractic — bladder connection

Preliminary chiropractic research on bladder infections is promising. In my own practice, I have successfully treated many patients with both acute and chronic conditions. Chiropractic manipulation at the level of the lumbar spine often produces excellent results.

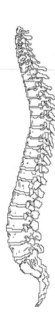

I strongly recommend a chiropractic evaluation. It is apparent that misalignments can —and do — trigger many different bladder problems, including acute and chronic urinary tract infections, bedwetting, incontinence, and urinary frequency and urgency. Manipulation eliminates spinal misalignments that may be interfering with normal nervous system control of the bladder as well as reproductive organs.

Although some cases of urinary tract infections may require medication, many are related to unsuspected spinal misalignments and nutritional factors.

Chronic interstitial cystitis, the more advanced condition, responds quite favorably to spinal manipulation along with nutritional supplementation and elimination of allergenic foods from the diet.

I have had several cases of patients whose chronic infections responded even dramatically to chiropractic manipulation. Anita Viviano, 57, was one. She suffered from considerable discomfort.

"Regardless of the frequency of bathroom visits, I was having pain and difficulty emptying the bladder," she told me. "It felt as if I was retaining about a pint of urine.

"As a consequence, I became feverish, nauseous, was unable to hold down food, developed cramping and diarrhea, along with a constant urge to urinate."

After examining Anita and hearing her problem, I determined she had a lumbar misalignment. I adjusted her low back at L5 — the last lumbar vertebra.

Anita explains what occurred:

"Dr. Gallagher had me lie down on my stomach and he proceeded to press quite firmly on a spot near my lower back. After this therapy was completed, I felt nothing whatsoever, except the urgency "to go," which I did as soon as I found the bathroom.

"To my surprise, I noticed immediately that I was completely emptying my bladder for the first time in a long time! I no longer had discomfort and bladder pressure. In fact, I felt great for the first time in nearly a week — no longer stressed out and nervous.

"I am convinced the trigger point therapy that Dr. Gallagher applied to my back allowed me to have almost instantaneous relief of a bladder infection. Unbelievable, but true."

The lower back vertebrae not only control the low back, legs and abdominal muscles, but also the bladder, colon and reproductive organs.

One case several years ago involved a woman in her 30s with chronic bladder infections so severe that she had been previously told by her doctors to take antibiotics preventively on a daily basis. When I saw her she had been on antibiotics for more than nine months. Despite the medication, she still had chronic infections.

Following two months of low back manipulation and dietary changes, the patient totally stabilized and never had to take antibiotics again.

I have treated several patients who developed bladder infections after intercourse. One patient, a newly married woman, had been unable to have intercourse other than a few times in her three years of marriage as a result. A series of lumbar and sacroiliac adjustments resolved this problem. She no longer had to take antibiotics or other drugs. I vividly remember the case because afterward, her husband visited my office to personally thank me for helping his wife and rescuing their sex life.

A three-year old boy was brought by his grandmother to our office several years ago because of a severe problem of urinary frequency. He was urinating up to 45 times a day!

The boy had originally been taken to a pediatrician. The physician had diagnosed a urinary tract infection and prescribed an antibiotic which failed to provide relief. The pediatrician then scheduled the child for surgery for what he described as a structural problem in the bladder. The family decided to try a natural approach.

Following eight low back pediatric manipulations, the child was urinating seven times a day. He has continued to be symptom free ever since.

Keep in mind that the bladder is an organ located in the lower abdomen. It is controlled by nerves extending out from the lower part of your back. If your sacroiliac joint or lower part of your back is misaligned, the consequences can include urinary frequency, urgency, incontinence and bladder infections.

Chiropractic research literature includes a number of reports describing the alleviation of bladder conditions, among other abdominal malfunctions, following spinal manipulation.

As I have said before: structure affects function.

The coughing/sneezing connection

A young mother, age 44, came to my office in 1995 complaining that whenever she coughed or sneezed, she would lose some urine. The situation was becoming very embarrassing for her. She consulted with her gynecologist, who could find nothing wrong. There was only the suggestion that perhaps her bladder was dropping and that she may need bladder surgery at some point.

I examined her and found a spinal misalignment. Following one lumbar manipulation, her problem was gone. She was able to cough, sneeze and even do aerobics without losing her urine.

I have treated similar cases involving coughing or sneezing and often the difficulty resolves with one or two manipulations.

Bedwetting

In 1992, the following item appeared in the popular "Dear Abby" syndicated newspaper feature:

"Dear Abby:

"I took my 15-year-old twin sons, both daily bedwetters, to a chiropractic and within a month both boys were completely cured. Regular medical doctors could not help.

—True Believer

"Dear True Believer:

"I believe you. I had several hundred letters bearing the same message concerning chiropractors." (San Francisco Chronicle, 3/5/92).

Enuresis (bedwetting) in children may be connected to misalignments in the lower part of the back. I have successfully treated many youngsters of all ages with lower back spinal manipulation.

One case involved an eight-year-old boy. The pediatrician had no answers over a period of several years, his mother said, other than to repeat, "Let's just wait and see if he grows out of it."

The mother told me she got tired of this reply, and concerned about the psychological effect the continued bedwetting might have, decided to seek the natural approach. Through chiropractic manipulation, we were able to resolve the problem within four months.

"He was finally dry through the night," his mother reported. "It was a God-send for my child and I am very happy for him."

This particular youngster had also suffered since infancy from bronchitis. He had been hospitalized many times for his severe lung condition, been on many medications, and was once even administered Last Rites. By following a comprehensive nutritional and chiropractic program, the boy overcame his bronchitis and today, at age 16, he is a healthy young man.

"No hospitalizations. No bronchitis. No medication," said his mother.

Over the years, chiropractic researchers have frequently reported on the benefits of manipulation for the problem of bedwetting. Among the recent reports is a 1994 study in which 31 children were given chiropractic treatments over a 10 week period. Of this group, 25 percent experienced a 50 percent or more reduction in wet night frequency.

In a 1991 report involving some 171 cases of persistent bed wetting at night, a series of eight chiropractic adjustments reduced the frequency from seven to four nights a week. At the end of the study, 25 percent of the children were classified as successfully treated.

Remember, mom and dad, chiropractic is for children, too.

Natural Remedies for Bladder Infections

- Chiropractic lumbar manipulation
- Drink 1-3 quarts daily of distilled or mineral water
- Cran C Plex (cranberry extract and vitamin C) ...... 2 capsules, 4 times daily
- Beta Carotene .... 200,000 I.U. daily
- Zinc Picolinate .... 25 milligrams twice daily
- DL Winter (a herbal combination of echinacea, goldenseal and red clover) .... 2 capsules, 4 times daily
- Ostaderm V Cream (phytoestrogen/progesterone for vaginal/urethral dryness) .... 1/4 tsp. transdermally if associated with menopause

CARPAL TUNNEL SYNDROME

About Carpal Tunnel

- *"I work as a hair stylist and I've noticed lately that while cutting hair, my hands start to go numb. I have even dropped the scissors a few times. What could be causing this?"*
- *"I work in the computer field. I am on the keyboard 6-8 hours a day. For relaxation, I have always played the piano. About 6 months ago, my hands started to fall asleep. I would shake them and then it would go away. Now it happens all the time. I am concerned because my job is at stake and I had to stop playing the piano. What is wrong and what can I do?"*

I hear questions such as these routinely from people who use their hands intensively in their work, individuals such as hair stylists, computer operators, secretaries, carpenters, musicians, meat cutters, truck drivers, assembly line workers, supermarket cashiers and construction workers. They are at risk for carpal tunnel syndrome (CTS).

This common condition occurs when the median nerve, which passes through a narrow bony passage in the wrist (the carpal tunnel), becomes compressed. Nine hard tendons also run through the tunnel. Any inflammation or swelling in the area can exert pressure on the nerve and trigger symptoms.

Typical symptoms can include:
- numbness, tingling and burning sensation in one or both hands,
- discomfort or pain, sometimes severe, in one or both hands,
- loss of grip strength and weakness of index, middle fingers and thumb,
- lack of feeling in hands,
- difficulty to execute fine hand skills.

Direct causes often involve continuous, forceful and repetitive hand and wrist motions that strain or damage muscles, tendons, ligaments and bones in the wrist. If not treated, the problem can develop into a permanent disability.

Most people have heard about carpal tunnel syndrome. Frequently you will see on television news an interview with a local physician describing the condition and the "cure," typically pain-killers, splints, ice, cortisone injections and surgery. CTS has, in fact, spawned a drug and surgical cottage industry that is dwarfing the "tonsillectomy campaign" of the 1950's.

Unfortunately, what you rarely hear about are the alternatives to medicine and surgery.

Joanne Hartzell's case

Joanne Hartzell, 49, a licensed practical nurse who operated a day care home in Greensburg, Pennsylvania, first visited our clinic in 1989 with carpal tunnel symptoms and a number of other problems, including migraines, and neck, back and leg pain.

> **"The surgery was the most painful procedure that I ever experienced..."**

"The medical community has no answer for the numbness and tingling in my arms and hands, my continuing pain, and extreme fatigue which interferes with my ability to function normally," she told me during her first appointment.

"I underwent many, many diagnostic tests. The doctors said the results were all normal. I was told I had arthritis in my back, given an unlimited prescription for Motrin and told that I needed to lose weight. That was it! The doctor had not answered anything about why I felt as I did or why I had numbness in my arms and hands.

"I then consulted an orthopedic surgeon. After more testing, he advised me that I had classic carpal tunnel syndrome in both wrists, but gave me no explanation for my back or neck pain. He recommended surgery on my right wrist, with surgery on the left to follow. The surgery was the most painful procedure that I ever experienced in my life, including multiple childbirths! The symptoms returned afterward.

"For my back, I was prescribed pain medication. The medication did nothing more than make me drowsy, not a good thing with small children of my own to care for, plus caring for others at my day care."

It was around this time that she came to see us. After taking a medical history and an examination, I determined that Joanne's numbness in the hands and arms were caused by misalignments in her neck and wrists. We initiated a treatment program that emphasized nutritional supplementation and chiropractic adjustments.

Later, Joanne told me she could not believe the changes that occurred.

"I began to have less pain and more energy," she said. "The numbness lessened and eventually disappeared. Since the very first day of treatment I haven't taken a pain pill — not prescription and not over the counter. I have learned to treat my migraine headaches, which are now rare, with chiropractic adjustments and Feverfew, an herb. Above all, I have learned how to care for the precious gift of health."

Ruth Hewston's case

Ruth Hewston, 60, also from Greensburg, decided not to go the surgery route at all. She had been diagnosed by her physician with CTS.

> "I no longer have the pain."

"I was having pain in the wrists whenever I overused my hands," she said.

She was told to wear wrist supports for six weeks before her insurance and HMO would let her have surgery.

"This is something I did not want," Ruth said. "When I asked if there was any therapy that I could take to help me, none was recommended."

Ruth happened to hear a radio program of mine during which I mentioned that carpal tunnel syndrome could often be helped with chiropractic neck adjustments. Hearing that, she made an appointment. After an examination and X-rays, we recommended a series of adjustments and a program of nutritional supplements.

Ruth no longer has the pain, nor any signs of carpal tunnel syndrome. The treatment also helped clear up a problem of chronic constipation.

How we treat carpal tunnel syndrome

For sure, there is an overuse and repetitive motion factor here — an occupational risk. Still, most cases of CTS have other contributing issues involved. Among them are the use of tartrazine dyes (yellow food dyes) in the food chain, psychiatric medications, oral contraceptives, menopause, cervical (neck) misalignment, pregnancy and nutritional deficiencies. Carpal tunnel is often found in patients with rheumatoid arthritis as well.

Years ago, John Ellis, M.D., a Texas physician, first found a striking connection between vitamin B-6 deficiency and CTS. A B-6 supplement is often helpful in alleviating this problem.

I always recommend B-6 along with other B complex vitamins. If one takes large doses of B-6 alone it is possible to create relative deficiencies in the other B vitamin factors that are not being taken. For this reason I recommend Coenzyme B Complex, a high-potency enzyme form of the B complex. For patients with a deficiency-type carpal tunnel problem, this treatment is often effective, however such deficiencies may take 8 to 12 weeks to resolve.

Boswelia serratta, an Ayurvedic herb also known as Indian Frankincense, is a traditional remedy against inflammation and is often helpful for this condition.

Plant and enzyme therapies are also useful. Turmeric, another natural remedy for inflammation, can be taken in capsule form several times daily. Brom/Pap, a natural anti-inflammatory extract from papayas and pineapples, is taken on an empty stomach between meals. This enzyme combination has a strong capacity to reduce pain, swelling and bruising.

Low thyroid function (hypothyroid), particularly in women, can contribute to carpal tunnel in both hands. The reason is not yet clear, but it is believed to be related to fluid retention. When we encounter low thyroid in patients with carpal tunnel, we usually recommend Thyrosine Complex. This is a natural thyroid extract with tyrosine, an amino acid, iodine, B-6, and other synergistic nutrients. The combination provides the raw materials to help activate a sluggish thyroid.

Refraining from foods with yellow dyes and monosodium glutamate (MSG) are helpful since they interfere with the uptake of vitamin B-6. Drugs such as tranquilizers and birth control pills can also interfere with absorption of vitamins, especially B-6, and may contribute to developing carpal tunnel.

Carpal tunnel will sometimes improve with the removal of allergenic foods.

The chiropractic — carpal tunnel connection

According to John Bourdillon, M.D., a medical expert who has written extensively on spinal manipulation, problems in the spine can be a major factor in the development of wrist swelling and carpal tunnel. In 1973, a study published in the medical journal Lancet showed that about 70

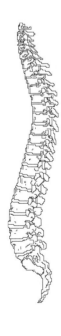

percent (81 out of 115) of patients with carpal tunnel had associated pinched nerves in the neck .

Keep in mind that your hands and fingers are controlled by nerves that originate in the spinal cord. The nerves supplying your arms branch out on each side from the spinal cord at the lower part of your neck and upper part of your back. They run across the shoulders and then down the arms, through the elbow, wrist and into your hands.

Subluxations of the cervical (neck) or thoracic (upper back) vertebrae or misalignments of the shoulders, elbows or wrists can lead to pinching or irritation of the nerves that control your hands. Individually, or collectively, these misalignments can cause carpal tunnel syndrome.

I have successfully treated hundreds of cases using spinal manipulation as well as wrist and hand manipulation.

One case involved a truck driver in his early 30s. He came to the office because of persistent numbness, tingling sensations, and loss of grip strength in both hands. These symptoms had developed gradually over a driving career of more than 10 years. He was now on disability and unable to work.

His family doctor prescribed anti-inflammatory drugs and wrist braces. They didn't help. An orthopedic surgeon recommended surgery, first on the left hand and then later on the right. Surgery was performed on the left hand. The procedure was a failure. Not only did this patient have continued numbness and tingling but additionally he now had a swollen left forearm and hand.

Following chiropractic evaluation, I found the source of the problem in his neck — quite removed from the wrist. I began a series of cervical manipulations. After five adjustments, the swelling and pain in the left hand decreased. Within two months, the numbness, tingling and loss of strength completely dissipated in both hands. He was able to return to his job and never had to have his right hand operated on.

Anyone with carpal tunnel should have a chiropractic evaluation for nerve stress before resorting to drugs and surgery.

Several years ago, I treated a professional golfer who had injured his wrist during the British Open. The injury forced him to withdraw from the tournament. A British orthopedic surgeon diagnosed torn ligaments and said that he would probably have to discontinue golf; he could not use his wrist or hold a golf club effectively.

I proceeded to examine his wrist and found misaligned, restricted wrist joints — the result of a single jolt from a bad shot when his clubhead struck into hard turf.

Following one chiropractic wrist manipulation, he was able to return to the golf course and play 18 holes the next day without problem. He quickly returned to the professional tour. Over the years I have treated many other golfers and tennis players with wrist problems.

Natural Remedies for Carpal Tunnel Syndrome

- *Gallagher Wellness Program*
- *Chiropractic cervical (neck) manipulation*
- *Wrist manipulation*
- *Vitamin B-6* .... 50-250 milligrams daily
- *Coenzyme B Complex* .... 1 tablet, 3 times daily
- *Turmeric* .... 2 capsules, 3 times daily
- *Thyrosine Complex (in cases of slight hypothyroidism)* 1 capsule, twice daily

CHEST PAIN
SURPRISE! IT MAY NOT BE YOUR HEART AT ALL!

About chest pain

There are two kinds of chest pain. The most familiar is the cardiovascular type, where blocked arteries and reduced oxygen to the heart muscle can produce a squeezing, painful pressure in the chest. Angina pectoris, as it is called, requires immediate medical attention. It can be life-threatening.

Few people know about the second type — a kind of musculo-skeletal angina. It is far more common, not life-threatening, but often debilitating and often mistaken for angina pectoris.

The difference between the two is this:

People with cardiovascular angina experience increasing tightness and pain in the chest with physical activity, emotional disturbance, and even intense elation. By resting and reducing stress, they can relieve the discomfort. Various types of medication are prescribed, such as nitroglycerine that temporarily dilates the arteries, to provide symptomatic relief.

With musculo-skeletal angina, the tightness and discomfort may be present constantly or brought on by certain movements or postures of the body. The cause is usually misalignments in the spine. Medication prescribed for cardiovascular angina doesn't help in this case, but is often prescribed anyway because the medical profession is unfamiliar with the spinal connection.

Patients with cardiovascular-type angina describe their chest pain in these terms:

- Heaviness
- Tightness
- Pressure
- Squeezing
- Centered under the breast bone

Individuals with a musculo-skeletal type will experience these kinds of variable signs:

- Any of the symptoms above
- Pain may be stabbing or radiating
- Pain may be reproduced by putting pressure on the sides of the ribs or by taking a deep breath or by turning over in bed
- Activities such as riding in a car over a bumpy surface, coughing

hard, raising your arm on the side you have the pain, bending forward, and pushing or pulling may increase the pain.

Because of the overlapping symptoms of these two conditions, it is critical for the physician to make a thorough evaluation to determine whether musculo-skeletal or insufficient blood supply to the heart is involved. In some cases, both conditions may exist. A differential diagnosis is accomplished through a medical history and physical examination in conjunction with EKG, X-rays, blood tests and other types of diagnostic procedures.

Mary Lindenberger's case

Mary Lindenberger is a 75-year-old health instructor from Latrobe, Pennsylvania who I have been helping for an arthritic condition for some 10 years. In 1995, she was rushed to the hospital with chest pain.

> **Angina medication "upset my whole system...I thought I was going to die."**

There, she had a heart catheterization and an echocardiogram.

"It was determined that I had the heart of a 30-year-old but the doctors said I had had a heart spasm caused by emotional stress and my thyroid medications," Mary told me. "They put me on Procardia and a nitroglycerine patch and lowered my thyroid medication. After a month or two I was so sick I thought I was going to die. These prescriptions have upset my whole system."

The doctors had found Mary's coronary arteries clear. But spasms, from emotional stress they believed, was causing narrowing of the arteries, and a resultant shortage of vital nutrition and oxygen to the heart. They wanted Mary to lower her activity level, wear a patch to keep her artery constantly dilated and take Procardia to slow her heart rate down.

Mary didn't want to accept this route. Had she done so she might have had all the signs and symptoms of angina and all the medications and their side effects. She wanted to find the cause of the problem.

She returned to our clinic for an opinion. I determined she had spinal misalignment in the mid-back and a hiatal hernia. Nutritional analyses showed she was short on a number of important nutrients, such as calcium, magnesium, co-enzyme Q10, and vitamin E. We starting her on a nutritional program, natural thyroid, and chiropractic adjustments. Before long, her chest pain symptoms were gone. Her medication was reduced and then eliminated. Today, she remains stable and medication-free. "My heart is doing fine," she says whenever she comes for an office visit.

There are too many cases like Mary's. In the system they are typically treated as "fixed" conditions and never eliminated, just "managed" at tolerable levels of symptoms through medication. We "unfixed" Mary's condition. That's what the natural approach is often able to do by searching for the cause of problems instead of just "managing" the problem.

The chiropractic — chest pain connection

Most people, when they experience pain in the region of the chest, mid-back, ribs and arms, become extremely anxious, fearing a heart problem. Particularly if the pain occurs on the left side.

In the chiropractic profession we know that often the heart is not involved, rather it is a musculo-skeletal problem related to mid-back or rib subluxations. Your chest muscles, ribs, heart, lungs and stomach are controlled directly and indirectly by your spinal nerves. Misalignment can cause musculo-skeletal angina that in many ways simulates cardiovascular angina, understandably creating great anxiety.

Consider these cases:

• A 45-year-old woman had a 15-year history of periodic chest pain and heart irregularity. She lived in a state of constant fear. She was told she had mitral valve prolapse and almost resigned herself to "learning to live" with the symptoms. Thoracic manipulation has stabilized her condition. She now receives periodic wellness adjustments.

• A 30-year-old mother experienced chest pain and heaviness, and a disturbing arrhythmia where her heart would skip beats. Previous electrocardiograms, stress tests, chest X-rays and cardiac exams were normal. She had been on and off medication to slow her heart rate. Her symptoms appeared whenever she would lean back into a chair or car seat. My assessment was that this slight pressure against her back was enough to aggravate an existing, but previously undiagnosed thoracic misalignment, and cause the angina-like symptoms. Eight chiropractic sessions resolved her problem.

• A 50-year-old man came to my office with repetitive chest pain. After exhaustive cardiac tests, he was pronounced "fit" but he was convinced that he had a heart problem because his symptoms of discomfort persisted. I found that he had three misaligned thoracic vertebrae and a misaligned rib. Following a series of chiropractic manipulations his symptoms disappeared. He returned three months later for a flare-up, which we resolved with a single manipulation.

From my experience, and conversations with other chiropractors, this type of disorder appears to be widespread.

M. Barker, D.O., an osteopathic physician reporting in a 1983 British medical journal that in a general medical practice there were less than two or three cases of "definite cardiac pain" a month, but "many more patients...with non-cardiac chest pains." The recognition of the mid-back misalignment, and its correction with manipulation, he went on to say, "reduces the patient's fears of underlying heart disease and can correct the cause of chest and back pain."

Harlen Johnson, D.C., a chiropractic researcher writing in a 1995 issue of the Journal of Chiropractic Technique, stated that "misalignments of the mid-back and ribs are an often overlooked cause of back, chest and arm pain. Many patients with this condition have had many costly tests and treated with little or no improvement. Spinal manipulation can provide effective treatment for this condition."

This reality is practically unrecognized in our contemporary medical system. Unfortunately, medical doctors and cardiologists have not been trained to look for this possible connection. As a result, there may be millions of Americans stuck on the treadmill. The overlooked use of manipulation, a powerful therapeutic tool for eliminating neck and chest pain without drugs as well as lowering blood pressure, is a tragic omission.

The fact is that any kind of physical, chemical or emotion stress can aggravate the misalignment and trigger alarms and dysfunction at weak spots in the nervous system.

In our clinic, once we resolve the problems of patients such as these, we encourage them to have wellness care, that is, come in for periodic check ups and "tune ups," if needed. Some individuals may have deep-seated weaknesses in their spine that will require occasional, or even regular, adjustments.

How we treat chest pain

In addition to chiropractic, other alternative aids we use include:

• Therapeutic massage and trigger point therapy should be considered directly over the chest wall in resistant cases.   Trigger point therapy , a type of pressure point treatment used by body workers, will often provide remarkable relief of chest pain and shortness of breath for those who experience musculo-skeletal angina.

Applied directly to tight muscles and soft tissue (fascia) of the chest wall and ribs, it releases deep spasms and rigid connective tissue often associated with this disorder.

• The therapeutic goals in cases of heart-disease related angina is to improve oxygen uptake by the heart muscle and improve energy metabolism. The three primary natural compounds critical to achieve this are carnitine, pantetheine, and co-enzyme Q10, or CoQ10 for short (see next page).

Several studies have shown that carnitine, an amino acid, alone allows the heart to utilize its limited oxygen supply more efficiently. Carnitine improves the contraction of the heart and reduces susceptibility to irregular heart beats. This translates into more exercise tolerance and better overall heart function.

Pantetheine, a derivative of vitamin B-5 (pantothenic acid), has the unique ability to lower cholesterol and triglycerides, another type of body fat, while raising HDL cholesterol (the so-called "good cholesterol"). This occurs, according to studies, without the side effects associated with cholesterol-lowering drugs.

Magnesium, calcium, potassium and even sodium represent critical mineral supplements that, when deficient, can lead to sudden heart attacks, hypertension, cardiac irregularity and swelling.

Hawthorn berry is a standard European cardiotonic (heart aid) herb rich in flavonoids that helps dilate peripheral and coronary blood vessels. This herb is also rich in procyanidins, natural chemicals found in plants that have sedative and antispasmodic effects. Interestingly, hawthorn is often used for restoring both high and low blood pressure, as well as in the treatment of irregular heart beats, spasms of the arteries (Raynaud's), and insomnia.

Herbal medicines including ginger, cayenne, ginkgo biloba and mistletoe exert powerful effects on the circulatory system that enhance circulation, lower cholesterol and naturally thin the blood.

A favorite nutritional supplement in our office is Neurosed, a combination of factors that includes the herb valerian root along with B vitamins that are known for their anti-stress and anti-spasmodic properties. For those whose chest pain is related to stress, this formula is often helpful.

Chelation therapy, an intravenous procedure performed by many practitioners of alternative medicine, has been documented to normalize 50 percent of cardiac arrhythmias, improve cerebrovascular arterial occlusion (blocked brain arteries), improve memory, concentration and vascular-related vision disorders. See chapter 11 for details on chelation therapy.

In our clinic we also utilize an oral supplement called Ora Key that generates chelation-type benefits. This formula combines many of the nutrients described here, such as CoQ10, ginkgo, magnesium, hawthorn, and niacin. Most of my patients receive oral as well as intravenous chelation therapy.

CoQ10 to the rescue of angina

CoQ10, a fat-soluble vitamin produced naturally in the body, deserves attention as a real "heart saver." Production, however, declines with age. In addition, our typical poor eating habits seriously impact our ability to make CoQ10. This set of circumstances can be deadly because CoQ10 is a major ingredient in cellular "bioenergetics," the chemical process that keeps you and your bodily machinery operating. It is absolutely essential for life. A shortage of CoQ10 can dramatically effect the efficiency of the heart muscle, where energy demand are extraordinarily high.

CoQ10 is also gaining recognition as one of the more powerful anti-oxidants, substances that combat the action of destructive molecular fragments in the body known as free radicals. Free radicals cause cellular damage leading to accelerated aging and degenerative diseases. Free radicals can be generated in quantities that overwhelm the body through such factors as stress, chemical contaminants, prescription drugs, radiation, processed foods, and toxic metals.

Cardiologist Peter Langsjoen, M.D., of Tyler, Texas, has participated in CoQ10 studies since the early 1980s and has logged more clinical usage of supplemental CoQ10 than any other physician in the country.

Langsjoen regards CoQ10 as "the backbone" of his practice. It won't unblock clogged arteries, he says, but it is a very useful addition at all stages of illness and patients definitely have less chest pain on CoQ. This is not because the arteries are being opened but rather because of better energy production in the areas that are poorly supplied.

"Patients just do so well with CoQ," he says. "For instance, we have a female patient in her 60s who previously had three bypass surgeries. Even after those surgeries, she was having chest pain many times a day and was absolutely bedridden. Just getting up and getting dressed she would have to take three or four nitroglycerines. She would get chest pain just sitting and watching TV. Four years ago we started her on CoQ10. Now she manages her own affairs and is quite active. She still has angina, but only from time to time. CoQ10 made a clear difference. This is somebody with extremely poor plumbing. Her arteries are a mess. Her grafts are a mess. There is nothing more to do surgically. You couldn't bypass her another time. I was amazed she even survived the third operation. It's a heart that's about as ischemic (lacking in oxygen) as you can get. We could never really improve someone in that shape without something like CoQ10. She takes 120 mg twice a day along with other anti-angina medications."

Natural Remedies for Angina

CARDIOVASCULAR ANGINA

Cardiovascular angina is a potentially-serious condition that requires medical supervision. For those whose chest pain is associated with arteriosclerosis (hardening of the coronary arteries) or an inefficient heart, congestive heart failure, irregular heart beats, or valvular problems, it is essential to seek the services of a physician.

* *The Gallagher Wellness Program*
* *Chiropractic manipulation*
* *Ora Key (hawthorn berry,*
      CoQ10, carnitine, niacin) .... 2 *capsules, 3 times daily*
                                       (may possibly produce a "niacin flush")
* *CoQ10 (sub-lingual)* .... 1 200 *milligram chewable tablet with meals*
* *Chelation therapy*
* *Intravenous magnesium therapy if indicated*

Note: refer to chapter on high blood pressure if condition involved
For information on the Dean Ornish method of reversing heart disease and chest pain, refer to chapter 4.

MUSCULO-SKELETAL ANGINA

* *The Gallagher Wellness Program*
* *Chiropractic thoracic manipulation*
* *Neurosed (valerian,*
      hops, B vitamins) .... 2 *capsules as needed for natural muscle relaxation*
* *Magnesium and calcium aspartate* .... 100 *milligrams, twice daily*
* *Trigger point therapy. Massage to chest muscles*

CHRONIC FATIGUE SYNDROME

About chronic fatigue

Chronic fatigue is a "catch all" term used for a general disorder that often includes:

- extreme fatigue
- recurrent sore throats
- low grade fevers
- swollen lymph glands
- headaches
- muscle and joint pain
- impaired sleep cycles
- emotional stress and/or depression
- irritable colon
- allergies
- loss of concentration
- low sex drive.

The condition is often referred to as adult mononucleosis-like syndrome, Epstein-Barr Virus Disorder, or "the Yuppie Syndrome."

Chronic fatigue syndrome is a label for a disorder of the nervous and immune systems that can have many contributing causes. Although the Epstein-Barr virus and other viruses may play a role, most nutritional doctors recognize that the body first becomes weakened in order for the germs and viruses to take root. We look for the causes of the weakness and attempt to correct them. If the patient is willing to work with us and with their own innate healing mechanisms, rather than simply taking drugs that mask symptoms and create new problems, we are usually able to reverse the problem.

Common causes of chronic fatigue:

- **A**ntibiotics
- **B**irth control pills
- **C**ortisone treatments
- **D**iets high in sugary foods.

For most people, conventional medical treatment represents a tragic detour away from the goal of real healing. It leads through a maze of repetitive antibiotics, anti-depressants, anti-inflammatory agents, sleeping pills, medical specialists and tests. Patients often gravitate to "support groups" and "learn to live with it."

Do these radio show callers sound like you?

- *"I am 42 years old and have been teaching school for 20 years. I have been on sick leave from my school district for 1 year. There are days I can barely get out of bed because of severe fatigue, sore throats, muscle and joint aches, sinus problems and headaches. I have been to 12 different specialists and have taken about every medical test and drug there is. One doctor said it might be Lyme's disease. Another said it was depression. The last one said it might be a virus. I am confused, run down and depressed. I'm sick and tired of being sick and tired."*

- *"For a number of years, my health was failing. I was feeling very sick, tired, and weak. Every time I went to a medical doctor, they only could 'guess' at most of the complaints I gave them. My diet consisted of red meat, potatoes, cold cereals, dairy, and lots of sugar; and my exercise was very limited."*

- *"I am suffering from chronic fatigue and am unable to be helped by the medical doctors. I become tired without exerting effort, gasping for breath after a short time teaching, falling asleep at the wheel of my car, and unable to hold my head up by the time the work day finishes."*

Sheila Kay Laney's case

The ordeal of Sheila Kay Laney, a Mechanicstown, Ohio, homemaker in her forties, began after the birth of her third son, Dillon, all

> **"I have no energy left...no strength"**

10 pounds, three ounces of him, in June 1989. The delivery was C-section.

Here is her story:

"It was during the three or four months afterward that I began to feel fatigued and achy. Previous to the Dillon's birth I was full of energy, a picture of health. I walked 6 to 12 miles every other day, lifted weights, was nutritionally aware, and in short I felt great. Now after this pregnancy I felt ill at ease, and not quite right.

"The feeling continued and increased. When Dillon was 18 months old, my hair began to fall out. I was gaining weight. I developed a rash on my face. My energy level was going down and down. My bones ached so badly that after I'd get my other two sons off to school and my husband out the door I would collapse. The pains in my legs were so horrible I would crawl around the house on my hands and knees, or curl up in a ball on the couch. I cried a lot, worried myself sick. My physician told me this was all post pregnancy problems due to my age, then 39.

"My problems worsened. When I would get up at night I could hardly walk. I had to take teeny tiny steps, as if my feet were bound. I began to feel like a balloon with a slow air leak. By now, my arms and hands ached, and my back, and I couldn't sleep. I was having bowel problems. Again I went to the doctor. This time I was lead to believe that I might have lupus.

"The loss of strength continued. My life was a shambles. A different doctor said he would test me for MS and recommended medication. It turned out to be Prozac, which when I was informed as to what it was, I stopped taking it.

"I felt lost, alone, empty. To function on a basic daily level took every ounce of energy I had. Now to this recipe add two teenage sons, an impatient husband, a 79-year old mom, who was widowed and a cancer patient, along with financial problems and medical bills, you have the perfect formula for insanity. I began to feel as if I were fighting to live.

"By the time Dillon was six, I was getting throat infections and antibiotics one after another. I'd given up on doctors but ended up in the emergency room on New Years Eve. I had to be rehydrated because I had been throwing up for three days. The ER doctor prescribed antibiotics mainlined into my body. I could feel a wave of nausea sweeping over me as the medicine went in me. I was given a shot for the nausea. I remember laying in the ER looking at the ceiling thinking how in the blazes did I get to this point, what is wrong with me? I'm so sick all the time, I've taken enough antibiotics to kill a horse ten times over and I just get worse every time. The tears were running in my ears. I wanted to go home. I thought, here I am, my face is broken out like I'm 12. I'm 70 pounds overweight. Every bone in my body hurts so badly. I rattle when I walk from all the Tylenol. I have no energy. No strength. I can't stand my husband to touch me. This hospital stuff is not working!! I left the hospital. I run up and down steps again. I'm smiling again. I'm singing while house cleaning again. I'm alive. I'm crying for happiness.

"It was after this episode that I happened to hear Dr. Gallagher's radio program while I was doing the dishes. People were calling in. Some sounded just like me. I stopped the dishes and listened. What I heard Dr. Gallagher say in reply to questions made sense to me. I was super-energized with something I hadn't had for years: HOPE. I called for an appointment. Then I called my best friend Lynn and said, 'Lynnie, I've found somebody who I think can help me. Get a map and find Jeannette, Pennsylvania. In two weeks we're going.'

"There are no words that can express my thanks to God for the miracle of letting me hear that program that day on the radio. Now approximately seven weeks later, I'm ALIVE. Dr. Gallagher evaluated my disease through hair analysis, blood test and x-rays and pinpointed my multiple problems."

How Sheila Kay's health plummeted

Sheila Kay Laney is a typical example of a person who appears to be doing all the right things to be healthy. She exercised, lifted weights, followed a nutritional program, but nevertheless wasn't prepared for the physical toll of a particularly hard childbirth.

Pregnancy creates significant stress in the body. It accelerates a person's nutritional requirements and puts mechanical pressure on the spine and pelvic joints. The combination is capable of generating chronic fatigue, depression, and immune dysfunction.

Sheila Kay had significant mechanical misalignments of her spine following pregnancy and childbirth that in turn adversely affected her nervous system. Additionally, we found that the upper part of her neck was also misaligned. She received a series of chiropractic manipulations to the lower part of her back and neck which played a major role in her recovery.

We also suspected that she was hypoglycemic, and had low blood sugar, which is often associated with after-delivery depression. She was placed on a low blood sugar diet of small frequent meals, higher in protein and lower in carbohydrate. She supplemented this with B vitamins, trace minerals and magnesium, and other factors to strengthen weakened organs. She also underwent a thorough detoxification program to clear her body of accumulated toxins.

As a result of this wholistic treatment plan, she soon regained her prior health status and once again became the same energetic person she used to be.

"I take my supplements faithfully," says Sheila. "Dr. Gallagher and his associates have educated me in nutrition, made me aware of my body functions and its miraculous abilities to heal itself. Hallelujah. A real doctor who really cares about people, and guess what, NO antibiotics.

"I could go on and on because I'm so excited to feel alive, feel good again, on my way to feeling GREAT again. I'm going to live to raise my son Dillon. I run up and down steps again. I'm smiling again. I'm singing while house cleaning again. I'm alive. I'm crying for happiness.

"Two days ago I got a wonderful gift. My 22-year old son Garrett came to visit and while hugging me he looked at me and said , 'you look so good Mom. The lights are back in your eyes.' My heart soared.

"Lynnie and I drive three hours one way to Dr. Gallagher's. But it's a trip of joy."

One teacher's story of "paralyzing fatigue"

A 48-year-old West Virginia teacher came to see me with what she called a "paralyzing fatigue" that had increased over the years in frequency, duration and intensity. She told me the following story:

> **"Eventually I realized that the drugs and the medical system complicated my situation."**

"Annual physicals resulted in clean bills of health with various physicians offering advice to lose weight and exercise to fight the fatigue and leg weakness. I tried diets but never succeeded in permanently shedding the 35 pounds gained during my first pregnancy many years before. One doctor suggested I try Prozac to give me an energy boost. I refused to take it.

"During the last three years my health seriously began to decline. I endured back, neck, knee and joint pain, gynecological problems, increasingly lower energy, and an irritability totally incongruous to my nature.

"I elected to have a complete hysterectomy in hopes of regaining my life and my soul. For months after the surgery, I endured a total body weakness, sensitivity and itching in the lumbar back, a prolonged bladder infection, a yellowing of my nails, numbness in my arms on waking, numbness of leg and foot after sitting, severe groin pain, a need for 12 hours of sleep at night, and naps during the day.

"My gynecologist continued to prescribe medication. I continued to feel ill after taking them. Eventually I realized that the drugs and the medical system complicated my situation."

The woman heard about our clinic from friends and with a strong determination to heal herself has made a dramatic recovery. She lost her post-pregnancy excess weight and enjoys renewed energy and vitality. She has faithfully followed a program of diet, exercise, conditioning and chiropractic manipulations.

"When I discipline myself to the regimen," she told me, "I can live cheerfully and calmly again without the thread of discontent and lack of energy. Living well requires discipline. Now I want to eat healthy foods. Gone are the fats and undesirables from my diet. Other health care providers dismissed my complaints as societal, unimportant or emotional. Here I have received knowledge and a concrete approach to health care that has inspired me."

This particular patient's condition had been dismissed as emotional which served to <u>add</u> an emotional burden to her already weakened physical state. Her problems included spinal misalignment, toxicity and nutritional deficiencies. Because medical doctors don't usually consider these factors, many patients live "half lives" of constant pain and debility.

How we treat chronic fatigue

Technological breakthroughs have allowed healthcare practitioners to carefully evaluate and more effectively treat chronic fatigue patients. Sophisticated blood antibody studies have made it possible to assess a person's chemistry to help determine unsuspected causes.

We can, for instance, find clues that enable us to learn if parasites, candida (yeast syndrome), chemical toxicity, food sensitivities, exhausted adrenal glands, or digestive and malabsorption problems are involved. In addition, we evaluate patients for "toxic metal syndrome," that is, the accumulation in the body of harmful levels of certain heavy metals such as lead, mercury, cadmium, aluminum, and nickel.

In my experience, most chronic fatigue patients have many of these factors as underlying causes. They are people with multi-factorial health problems, meaning there is neither one cause nor one cure.

Our strategy against chronic fatigue syndrome includes the entire Gallagher Wellness Program.

Initial phase

The initial phase of treatment emphasizes detoxification. Refer to chapter six for details. Detox is based on a timeless natural hygienic principle: "first and foremost allow the organism to discharge its toxins."

We recommend a ten-day detox diet, special supplements for cleaning out the body, lymphatic drainage, colon hydrotherapy, and herbal medicines that are particularly helpful for reducing sore throats, swollen lymph glands, and stimulating the immune system.

The herbals include Baptista, ADP (a time-released oregano supplement that acts as an anti-fungal agent), Burdock root and Yarrow.

Vitamin C with Vitamin P (bioflavonoids) is useful, along with Nutri Tox, to help clear heavy metals from the tissues. Brom Pap (papaya and pineapple enzymes), Nutri Zyme (comfrey and pepsin) and Colon Cleanse (ground psyllium and liquid bentonite) help remove mucous and toxic debris from the small and large intestines.

Chiropractic adjustments activate the immune system and are critical in both phases of treatment.

Recovery phase

During this phase of treatment we focus on strengthening and repairing the body.

We use glandular therapy that consists of extracts of spleen, thymus and lymph to help rejuvenate primary immune organs. Adrenoglan Chelate is a supplement containing adrenal glandular extract along with potassium and the amino acid tyrosine. I recommend it to patients whose stress has contributed to adrenal fatigue. Studies indicate an association between chronic fatigue syndrome and weak adrenals. The adrenals produce stress hormones. Excessive stress for prolonged periods can deplete these important endocrine glands and lead to a wide array of symptoms, including fatigue. (Refer to the chapter on stress and the adrenal glands)

In connection with the adrenals, an interesting report appeared in the New Zealand Medical Journal in 1995 describing the experience of a physician who used licorice in his recovery from chronic fatigue. That's right. I said licorice, the stuff of candy. There's also a medicinal side to licorice. It has been used traditionally by herbalists as an anti-inflammatory agent for allergies, ulcers and arthritis, and contains chemicals that act similar to cortisone, the important adrenal gland hormone. Whole licorice is said to be beneficial for cases of adrenal insufficiency.

In the journal article, the author said he had tried various therapies in vain to overcome chronic fatigue. After taking licorice, his physical and mental stamina returned "in a few days." He said he found licorice dissolved in milk at 2.5 grams per 500 milliliters particularly effective for him. His theory is that the licorice may potentiate adrenal hormone activity in patients with chronic fatigue syndrome and associated adrenal exhaustion.

High dosages of vitamin C, from 1,000 milligrams up to bowel tolerance, should be considered. When using vitamin C in large amounts, it is advisable to take it in divided doses throughout the day. If you take too much at once, you may develop temporary diarrhea. If that occurs, you simply stop for a while or cut back the amount you are taking. Many people find that a powder form of vitamin C, mixed with juice or water, is easier to take than swallowing tablets or capsules. If you use powder, we recommend the buffered (non-acidic) form of vitamin C known as sodium ascorbate.

If you are prone to sore throats use the vitamin C gargle (1/2 teaspoon of vitamin C powder in 4 oz. of water) as often as needed.

Hair analyses often reveal deficiencies in magnesium and chromium. Magnesium aspartate and GTF chromium are critical for recovery. Chronic fatigue is often associated with magnesium deficiency. Chromium helps to stabilize the blood sugar.

For those whose condition is associated with candidiasis (the yeast syndrome), a diet is recommended that eliminates yeast and dairy products and emphasizes protein and vegetables. Refer to the yeast chapter in the book. If yeast is involved we also use YPD (a combination supplement with anti-yeast factors that help boost the immune system), probiotics that replace beneficial bacterial in the intestines, grapefruit seed extract, and Pau D'Arco tea. Homeopathic preparations of candida albicans (30c) and penicillium notatium (8x) are often helpful.

For chronic fatigue patients with parasite disorders we utilize a herbal combination with Chinese wormwood and grapefruit seed extract called MFP herbal (take 2, 3 times daily) for 3 months and Biocidin (4 drops, twice daily). These herbals can naturally interrupt parasite cycles.

Chronic sufferers who have been treated with conventional treatments are often weary, anxious, fatigued, and depressed. Remember, though, that these feelings are usually the result of your state of health and not the cause. Although stress management techniques such as prayer and meditation are helpful, take care of your body first. You will be amazed how your mind will follow!

The chiropractic — chronic fatigue connection

Unfortunately, most patients and medical doctors don't have a clue that there is a chiropractic connection. The reality is this: the primary symptom of spinal subluxation is not back pain. It is loss of energy and function. Remember that your nervous system controls your immune system and your immune system ultimately controls your ability to fight infection. So if your spine is misaligned, your defenses become weakened and dis-ease is often the consequence.

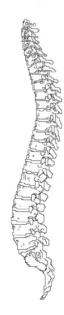

Consistent with chronic fatigue cases is an impairment of the nervous and immune systems. Chiropractic manipulation activates both systems and restores lost communication. It can be a vital link in recovery.

I have treated patients with histories of chronic fatigue varying from months to years, who have gone to multiple medical specialists and taken a wide variety of drugs, and who, following a brief period of chiropractic manipulation alone, experienced complete resolution of their symptom complex.

One patient suffered from chronic fatigue and insomnia for 20 years. She had consulted multiple specialists who told her to relax and "learn to live with it." Over the years she had been on tranquilizers, sleeping pills and anti-depressant drugs, none of which were effective for her condition. She ultimately stopped the drugs because of side effects and concern for addiction.

Following a series of chiropractic manipulations over one month, she was sleeping six to seven hours a night and her energy level soared.

I continually see patients in my practice who have been basically labeled as emotional or psychosomatic cases by their physicians because they "pass" the conventional medical tests. Yet they have real problems and the solution isn't the chemical straightjacket of medical drugs.

In chronic fatigue, we often find weaknesses of thymus, spleen and liver. Organ weaknesses can often be determined through Applied Kinesiology testing. Both the thymus gland, located in the upper portion of the chest behind the breastbone, and the spleen, located on the left side of the abdomen, are key organs in the production of important disease-fighting cells. The liver, of course, is the chemistry factory of the body.

A gymnastics teacher I started treating some years ago had a five-year history of chronic fatigue with recurring sore throats. She became debilitated to the point where she couldn't teach anymore. Her family doctor had told her she would eventually shed the problem. He treated her sore throats with antibiotics which, over time, made things worse.

When she came to see me, she not only had the debilitating fatigue, but also neck pain, headaches, chronic recurring infections, swollen lymph glands, and premenstrual syndrome. I started adjusting her neck. I gave her thymus extract as well as spleen extract after determining weakness in those two organs. The combination worked and totally reversed her condition.

Keep in mind the individuality factor. The combination that worked for this one woman may not work for the next person. This is why we have to treat the patient and not just the symptom or a label of chronic fatigue.

I remember a case of a young grandmother in her fifties suffering from chronic fatigue for more than two years. She swore up and down that her problem was due to pesticides. She lived on a farm where large amounts of pesticides had been used in the past. She had been to many doctors but they couldn't find the connection. They told her to "learn to live with it." She took more than 130 vitamins a day and still felt terrible.

We evaluated her body and found that she had a weak thymus, spleen, liver and lymph system, and multiple subluxations of the spine. We started adjusting her spine. In a matter of a few visits she said that she was able to think clearly again, that "the coating around her brain" was gone.

We also worked with her on detoxification in an attempt to rid her body of toxins I felt were contributing to her problem. Her situation, however, turned out to be almost exclusively structural. Following 15 chiropractic manipulations over a 60 day period, she no longer had any signs or symptoms of chronic fatigue, and was able to substantially cut down her intake of supplements to a more manageable and effective regimen.

I mention this case because often I encounter patients with histories of chronic fatigue syndrome, fibromyalgia, and other immune-related problems who insist their problems are related to pesticides, chemicals or that they work in a so-called "sick building" with poor ventilation. Although we recognize that chemical agents, food allergens and nutritional deficiencies are primary causes of some conditions, often patients have unresolved problems because of spinal misalignments.

Interestingly, the grandmother I just mentioned subsequently referred her grandson to the office. At age five, he suffered from projectile vomiting and hyperactivity. Following 30 days of chiropractic manipulation, the boy no longer vomited and no longer suffered from hyperactivity. Both the mother and grandmother were amazed at the benefits of chiropractic treatment.

Natural Remedies for Chronic Fatigue

Initial Phase (Detoxification Phase — First Two Weeks)
- Applied kinesiology for organ depletion evaluation
- Chiropractic spinal manipulation
- Myotherapy with lymphatic drainage
- Detoxification program
- Colonic hydrotherapy
- DL Winter (Goldenseal, echinacea, red clover) ..... 2 capsules, 3 times daily
- Raw juice, such as carrot and green juices
- Yarrow (standardized extract) .... 2 capsules, 3 times daily
- Nutri Tox .... 3 tablets before bed

Recovery Phase (After First Two Weeks)
- The Gallagher Wellness Program
- Spleenoglan (spleen extract) .... 3 capsules, 3 times daily
- Thymoglan (thymus extract) .... 3 capsules, 3 times daily
- Lymphoglan (lymph extract) .... 3 capsules, 3 times daily
- Adrenoglan Chelate .... 2 capsules, 3 times daily
- Licorice (standardized extract) .... 600 milligrams daily
- ADP (time-released oregano) .... 2 capsules, 3 times daily
- YPD (multi anti-yeast factors) .... 2 capsules, 3 times daily
- Vitamin C .... 1 gram to bowel tolerance daily
- Intravenous vitamin C and magnesium infusion

COLD SORES

About cold sores

Cold sores or fever blisters are eruptions that occur on and around the lips. They are associated with a type of herpes simplex virus called HSV-1.

Genital herpes are caused by a related virus, herpes simplex II, or HSV-II.

For most people, outbreaks on the skin are infrequent, but for some people they can become a continuous nightmare.

Most people harbor the virus within their body in a dormant stage. The virus can become active and cause breakouts as a result of emotional, environmental or dietary stress, excessive wind or sun, trauma (such as injury to the lips), the use of some pharmaceutical drugs, food allergies and nutritional deficiencies.

Conventional medical treatment focuses on interrupting the cycle of the virus with anti-viral drugs. These drugs may be effective but we are not sure about their long-term effects.

Many prescription drugs suppress the immune system and can interfere with the body's own natural defenses that control the herpes virus. Antibiotics, birth control pills, steroids, and chemotherapy agents are among the common drugs that may increase the risk of herpes infections.

How we treat cold sores and genital herpes

Q *"I am 56-years-old and forever "haunted by cold sores." I don't believe in drugs, so I have tried garlic, zinc and lots of herbs, but I am getting nowhere. I know there has to be a natural remedy for this. Are there alternatives for me?"*

A I have been asked this question many times. The answer is yes. There are natural alternatives that help. We use a variety of nutritional strategies to keep the virus in check by building up the immune system.

• Among the immune-boosting supplements, the amino acid lysine is particularly useful here. It helps inhibit viral growth.

• High doses of buffered (non-acidic) vitamin C, taken in powder form, is a natural substance that enhances the immune system as well as specifically counteracting viral activity.

- Zinc is an important mineral nutrient. It activates special infection-fighting cells in our body called lymphocytes. Topical application of zinc oxide can also be used effectively.

- Lithium, used topically and orally, is another helpful mineral. It has been found to inhibit herpes activity.

- Nutri E Derm has been a gold standard topical preparation used at our office for sores, cuts, burns, stretch marks, and many skin diseases. Composed of raw flax seed oil, lipids, and vitamin E, it exerts powerful on site antioxidant activity that helps to repair injured or damaged skin.

- Herpanacine, an effective oral herbal/vitamin combination, has provided great relief to many of our cold sore patients. The formula includes echinacea, a natural plant antibiotic and anti-viral factor, along with goldenseal and zinc.

- The homeopathic preparation Borax 5c is sometimes helpful for cold sores.

- We often recommend Ultradophilus, a probiotic supplement that helps to re-establish friendly bacteria in the mouth and intestinal tract. It is mixed into aloe vera juice. Many times people develop cold sores after taking antibiotics or medication which destroy the natural bacterial flora of the body.

- We suggest eating a diet that avoids foods containing another amino acid, arginine. Arginine foods include chocolate (sorry, chocolate lovers!), peanuts, nuts, seeds, and cereal grains. The herpes virus thrives on arginine.

- In addition, some people with cold sores are sensitive to acid foods. For them, avoiding citrus, tomatoes and perhaps vinegar is prudent.

The ice connection

Direct application of ice, at the immediate onset of a cold sore, may be effective in halting herpes eruptions. Apply the ice for two or three minutes several times a day if possible.

How we deal with stubborn genital herpes (HSV II)

Genital herpes requires significant dietary and lifestyle changes, including the elimination of sugar, caffeine and alcohol. These substances all tend to suppress the immune system and change the acid-alkaline balance in the body in a way that favors herpes activity.

We strongly recommend identifying and eliminating food allergies as well as reducing arginine-containing foods in the diet.

I have found that a combination of lysine, zinc picolinate and high dosages of vitamin A can be very effective at inhibiting this virus. The therapeutic use of vitamin A should only be undertaken with the guidance of a nutritionally-oriented health professional.

Wound gel, a specific topical compound extracted from the aloe vera plant, has medicinal properties we have found effective against genital herpes.

A word on stress

Excess stress of any kind can fatigue the immune system and open the door for viral infections, including herpes viruses.

Many women, for instance, will experience an outbreak of cold sores around the time of their period as a result of the physiological stress that is taking place.

Relaxation and stress-reduction techniques (see chapter 12) can be helpful in controlling herpes outbreaks.

Natural Remedies for cold sores

- **The Gallagher Wellness Program**
- **Low protein diet (diets high in animal protein raise the acidic level of the body)**
- **Eliminate arginine-containing foods**
- **Lysine** .... *1,000 milligrams 4 times daily when an eruption occurs, taken between meals.*
- **Vitamin C (buffered non-acidic powder)** ..... *2,000 to 10,000 milligrams daily (or up to bowel tolerance)*
- **Herpanacine**
  (lysine, echinacea combination) ...... *2 capsules, 4 times daily (in acute cases) or once daily (preventively)*
- **Lithium chelate** .... *50 to 250 micrograms daily*
- **Aloe vera juice plus probiotics (mix 1 oz. aloe with 1 teaspoon probiotics). Between meals, swish in mouth and swallow.**
- **Nutri E Derm, apply topically for HSV I**
- **Wound gel, apply topically for HSV II**

COLIC

Q *"My wife and I are finding it hard to cope. Our 6-month-old boy constantly screams and cries. My wife nurses him but he can't hold anything down. Our pediatrician suggested Karo Syrup and long car drives. Nothing is working and we are worn out. Any suggestions?"*

A The caller to one of my radio shows was exhausted and desperate. If we lived in Denmark, he probably would not have called. In that country, as in many other places in Europe, it is well-known that "colic," a common problem of infants, will resolve in most cases after a few pediatric chiropractic manipulations.

Colic is a painful, spasmotic condition that causes crying, irritability, digestive upsets, repetitive and projectile vomiting, and excess gas. Untreated colic often takes 12 to 16 weeks to resolve.

Medical treatments generally have limited success. Some medical doctors may recommend Karo (corn syrup), which is totally ineffective. Sometimes upper GI series and gastroscopic examinations are performed. In some cases, children are prescribed anti-ulcer drugs!

The chiropractic – colic connection

Many infants and children have spinal misalignments, as a result of vertebral stress at the time of birth. Although forceps, caesarian and difficult deliveries are the most common cause of infantile misalignments, even "normal" deliveries can be traumatic to the spine and skull, and especially the neck.

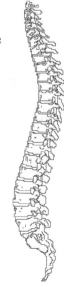

Such structural distortions can impair the normal nerve supply to the digestive tract and cause many problems, among them colic. If the stomach and intestines are affected, a child may experience upset, irritation, gas, constipation, and discomfort. If the tube leading down from the throat to the stomach — the esophagus — is affected, vomiting may occur.

Because of the frequency of pediatric misalignments and the positive results from manipulation that have been observed around the world, chiropractic evaluations should be recommended for all youngsters. In the case of colic, for instance, adjustments are often able to dramatically and <u>quickly</u> restore normal function and clear up symptoms.

Research in Denmark has demonstrated the powerful healing effect of chiropractic. In one study, 316 infants with moderate to severe colic received chiropractic care. The success rate was 94 percent within two weeks after an average of three treatments! A quarter of the children showed great improvement after just a single manipulation.

The median age of the infants was 5.7 weeks at the beginning of care. The most commonly adjusted site on the spine was the upper neck. The study involved 73 chiropractic physicians in 50 different clinics (Journal of Manipulative and Physiological Therapeutics, 1989).

Another international report described the benefits of manipulation on 600 babies with "suboccipital strain." There are seven cervical (neck) vertebrae. The uppermost is called the "atlas" and joins with the occiput (the back of the skull). The occiput-atlas joint complex frequently misaligns leading to colic, crying, a contraction of the neck muscles that produces an unnatural twisted position of the head (toricollis), fever, loss of appetite, swelling on one side of the face, and uneven development of the skull and hips. "Removal of suboccipital strain is the fastest and most effective way to treat the symptoms...one session is sufficient in most cases," wrote H. J. Biedermann, M.D. (Journal of Manual Medicine, 1992).

George Pluhar, D.C., and P.D. Schobert, D.C., two Michigan chiropractors, reported the case of a three-month-old girl with colic, disturbed sleep and poor appetite. Medication prescribed by the family's pediatrician eased symptoms temporarily for two weeks. Subsequently, a chiropractic evaluation determined subluxations in the neck and mid-back.

Following the first adjustment, the parents reported a reduction in colicky crying. The baby slept soundly for eight hours, and ate 32 ounces of formula, afterward. Until then the girl had been sleeping as little as two hours a day and would often consume less than five ounces of formula.

Of additional interest in this case history was the fact that the girl's father smoked in the house. The chiropractor advised him against exposing the child to second-hand smoke and cited published studies suggesting a connection between infantile colic and inhalation of tobacco smoke. The girl's misalignment may have been aggravated by the presence of tobacco smoke (Journal of Chiropractic Research and Clinical Investigation, 1991).

"This reflects the classical chiropractic tenet that chemical stressors (along with mechanical and emotional stressors) play a role" in the cause of spinal subluxation, said the Neurological Fitness Newsletter in a commentary on the study.

For many parents, the image of children receiving chiropractic treatment seems strange. Fear of the unknown and years of medical misinformation have prevented millions of children from experiencing better health through chiropractic care. Fortunately, this situation is changing.

I can assure you that the treatment is extremely gentle. Chiropractic physicians use light touch finger pressure to quickly and painlessly realign the vertebrae. We typically administer thoracic adjustments with a child lying comfortably face down on a parent's chest atop the treatment table. Adjustments to the neck are made while a parent comfortably holds the child.

How we treat colic

In our clinic we have successfully treated many infants. Generally, one or two treatments is all that it takes.

Let me share several examples with you:

• An eight-month-old boy, suffering with chronic colic and vomiting for two months, was brought in by his mother. The infant's pediatrician had been unable to help the condition. An evaluation determined a misalignment in the mid-back area. One single treatment resolved the problem.

• A three-month-old boy was constantly crying and frequently vomiting. The mother had taken the child to the pediatrician who suggested an upper GI series. The parents decided against the procedure and opted for chiropractic evaluation. I examined the spine and found misalignments in the area of the fourth thoracic vertebra in the mid-back. The child's symptoms vanished after manipulation.

• One fascinating case involved a one-year-old boy who constantly cried and was severely constipated. The only way the mother could calm him was by holding him against her chest. In turn, the boy would tuck his head under her chin and remain in that position while the mother patted him in the upper part of the back. The family pediatrician said the child would eventually outgrow it. However, the enduring problem was exhausting the entire family.

The mother had heard me on radio and decided to try the chiropractic approach, even though she lived 60 miles away. The child cried the whole way in the car. In my office, the mother put her child up against her chest. He tucked his head under her chin and quickly calmed down.

I decided to check the boy while he was in this position. I gently started to palpate his spine, starting with the lower part of the back and working my way up. There was no problem with the lower part of the back. When I reached the area between the shoulder blades, the site of the fourth, fifth and sixth thoracic vertebrae, the boy began to cry loudly. I had obviously arrived at the location of his spinal misalignment.

I had the mother lay on her back, with her son on top of her, and administered an adjustment. The child was thus treated twice a week for three weeks. At the end of six adjustments, the colic was resolved. The boy was able to sit in a car seat without crying. He no longer had to be continually held by the mother. He began moving his bowels two to three times daily.

• Over the years I have treated a small number of cases involving children who experience so-called projectile vomiting. In these situations, swallowed food is thrown up and out of the mouth with great force at distances of up to several feet. In my experience, this condition seems to be connected to spasms of the esophagus, a result of disturbed nerve impulses generated by misalignments in the neck or middle part of the back. In all cases, the problem was eliminated with a half-dozen or less adjustments.

Observations on nursing

I have treated many cases in which colic-like symptoms of breast-fed infants improve after the mother stops eating foods that have been identified as allergenic for her.

I have successfully treated infants who were unable to nurse because of subluxations in the spine. After adjustment, they were able to nurse again.

Many toddlers, on infant formulas, have chronic digestive disorders as a result of sensitivities to the ingredients in the products.

Natural Remedies for Colic

• **Pediatric chiropractic evaluation and appropriate manipulation**
• **Nux Vomica (30c) homeopathic** .... 2 pellets sublingually as needed
• **Establish breast feeding**
• **Check nursing mother for food sensitivities (dairy, wheat, corn, eggs, and beans are frequent culprits)**

DEPRESSION

About depression

The facts on depression are enough to make anyone depressed.

• More than 17 million Americans suffer from serious depression every year.

• Episodes of depression cost the country around $43 billion annually in lost productivity.

• Women are at higher risk than men for depression, although some researchers feel that depression is underdiagnosed in men. One in four women is likely to experience severe depression at some point in life, according to the American Psychological Association (APA).

The APA's Task Force on Women and Depression has found that women are not depressed primarily for biological reasons, but for a variety of social, psychological and biological causes. Among the risk factors cited are infertility, miscarriages, surgical menopause, sexual and physical abuse, poverty, alcohol, drug abuse and personalities that are passive, dependent, pessimistic or negative.

What the APA and other conventional groups fail to include in their risk factors are poor diet, food and chemical sensitivities, physical toxicity and spinal misalignments. I will talk about those later and show you how conventional medicine misses the boat.

Depression is characterized by feelings of persistent sadness, fear, unhappiness, pessimism, hopelessness, worthlessness and despair.

If not treated, serious depression can lead to suicidal thoughts and feelings, and physiological symptoms. Appetite may either decrease or increase. Depressed individuals may be insomniacs or have a need for excessive sleep.

If you own a pharmaceutical company, there is a very bright side to the depression epidemic. Drug companies make more than $3 billion a year in anti-depressant medication.

A word on Prozac

Prozac currently tops the chart of "best-selling" antidepressants.

According to the evidence, its popularity appears to be more the result of effective marketing than the effectiveness of the drug.

Prozac has a wretched record for stirring up serious side effects, INCLUDING depression. Among the other adverse reactions: convulsions, hallucinations, aggression, delirium, violent hostility, psychosis, and even death by suicide.

Peter Breggin, M.D., an outspoken critic of psychiatric medicine and author of "Talking Back to Prozac: What Doctors Aren't Telling You About Today's Most Controversial Drug" (St. Martin's Press, New York, 1994), says that both the research, approval process, and effects of Prozac are all questionable.

Breggin told New York medical investigative reporter Gary Null in an interview that "evidence from the FDA trials suggests this a very poor drug. Even a New York Times article...said that follow-up studies show Prozac as not very effective. But when you give something to people and tell them it's a miracle, they'll believe it. Also the drug does have stimulant effects. And while we no longer believe that stimulants should be given for depression, certainly people can feel like it's helping them."

Joanne Burke's case

Ten years ago, Joanne Burke, a hair stylist from Irwin, Pennsylvania, came to our clinic in despair. She said she was ready to jump off a bridge. She had had four babies and after the last was born she went into a post-partum depression.

> **Ready to jump off a bridge**

"Only I didn't come out of it," she said.

She had gone to several doctors for the depression, accompanying fatigue and severe anxiety. They put her on tranquilizers. A PMS clinic prescribed hormonal therapy. A psychologist helped some but didn't eliminate her highs and lows.

"Nothing was correcting my physical problems, which continued," she said.

Joanne had hypoglycemia (low blood sugar) and a yeast infection, the latter a result of antibiotic treatment over the years for bronchitis and sinus infections.

We started her on a wellness program which she followed strictly. It wasn't long before she started to improve.

"I am starting to feel so much better," she told me during a follow-up visit.

Soon she was feeling so much better that she began kidding me about treating her for burn-out because she had so much "new found energy," as she put it.

Joanne, now 48, comes in for monthly chiropractic adjustments.

Recently, she told me that she couldn't have survived in business without these treatments.

"And besides," she said happily, "for years I haven't had any colds, sinus infections or the yearly flu that I always used to get."

Joanne's case reflects the typical medical method of chasing symptoms with drugs and "talk therapy." I agree that medication and counseling play a role in some cases of depression, but based on my clinical experience I find that physical and chemical causes are often involved and usually overlooked.

The physical cause in Joanne's situation was "brain hibernation," the result of spinal misalignments. I talked about that in depth in chapter 13.

Her chemical imbalances related to low blood sugar and nutritional deficiencies.

Joanne didn't need psychiatric drugs. She is off that treadmill altogether. With our nutritional and chiropractic wellness program she is taking care of a full-time business and raising four children.

Nina Dancho's case

Nina, a 40-year-old accounting clerk from Greensburg, Pennsylvania, complained of debilitating migraines and depression.

> **Depressed no more**

"The stress in my life has taken a big toll on me," she said during her first appointment with me.

Nina had previously consulted with her medical doctor. He said she was stressed-out and gave her samples of Prozac along with a prescription when she ran out of the samples.

"I felt this was really not the plan of action I wanted to take," she said. "I felt that perhaps there was a better way to combat the stressful things in my life."

Around this time Nina met a patient of mine who had suffered emotional trauma from stressful life events. Our wholistic program had helped her. Nina decided to also try the natural approach.

Nina never had to begin a Prozac program because her main problem was not depression. The "stressful things" in her life had been severely aggravated by a long-term spinal subluxation along with nutritional deficiencies. Remember the "barrel concept" I talked about in chapter nine? Nina's barrel was overloaded and spilling over. That's why she had debilitating symptoms. Her body tried to cope by overproducing adrenal stress hormones, a constant burden that eventually led to chronic fatigue, dizziness, exhaustion, migraines and depression.

Nina no longer has any of these symptoms. Chiropractic adjustments and nutritional therapy have significantly reduced the level of physical stresses that had previously filled her "barrel." Now she has greater capacity and strength to deal with the stresses that come and go in her life.

"I have gained — and gleaned — so much," says Nina. "The treatments, and the knowledge I have learned, literally saved my life, I believe. The discovery of chiropractic and nutritional care has been the glue that has helped to hold me together, along with my faith in God. I have a much better understanding of my body and the way it works. I don't always follow the nutritional information as I should and when I don't I pay the price."

Nina's case is typical of many that I see. A person is told by a doctor or well-meaning friends that "your problems are emotional or psychological or stress-related." Nina still has stress in her life but no more depression or migraines.

How we treat depression

The medical establishment uniformly tends to overlook the nutritional and chiropractic connection to depression. To me this is a tragic oversight.

Depression is viewed broadly in alternative medicine as a multifactorial mind/body condition. Possible causes are many and we search for them instead of merely trying to smother the symptoms with a prescription of a strong, and often addictive, medication. Drugs, of course, may be able to jerk people out of their depression but they fail to help them deal with life or the causes of their condition.

The wholistic approach opens broad avenues for real recovery, not just a pharmaceutical respite. We explore causes such as low blood sugar, hypothyroidism, poor nutrition, chronic fatigue, allergies, spinal misalignments and psychosocial situations in life. All of these elements can impact the brain.

Cerebral allergies, for instance, are a type of allergy caused by food and chemical sensitivities that can trigger not only depression in vulnerable individuals but anxiety attacks, mood swings, insomnia, hyperactivity and even schizophrenia and psychosis.

When people are sensitive to dust or pollen, they may experience sneezing or swelling of nasal or bronchial tissue. Other people may experience a cerebral reaction, as if their brain "swells and sneezes."

The brain is an organ, and like any other organ, it responds to many different influences, some of which may cause it to malfunction. When that happens you get "brain related symptoms."

Virtually any nutrient deficiency can trigger depression. This was amply proven by investigations into the high incidence of schizophrenia during the 1940s among poor southern share croppers. This disorder, long considered a mental illness, is often characterized by the "3 Ds" — diarrhea, depression and dermatitis.

Agricultural studies pointed to the processing and removal of essential B vitamins from grain products. The B vitamins protect the body against the effects of stress and are critical for the health of the nervous system. This is why nutritional supplements that contain B vitamins are called the "stress B complex."

Supplements of niacin (B-3), vitamin B-6 and B-12, folic acid, magnesium, lithium and manganese are often helpful and are recommended depending on individual requirements.

One supplement you probably haven't heard of is S- adenosylmethionine or SAM for short. It is a natural chemical found in the body derived from the amino acid methionine and adenosine triphosphate, the basic energy compound that fuels cellular activity. This unique substance, originally discovered and studied in Italy in the 1950s, is responsible for the formation of many of the nervous system neurotransmitters. These are the chemicals that carry messages throughout the body. Michael Murray, N.D., writing in "The Encyclopedia of Nutritional Supplements" (Prima Publishing, 1996) reported that SAM supplementation has been proven effective for depression, fibromyalgia, migraines, liver disorders and osteoarthritis.

Blood tests to determine deficiencies or imbalances of amino acids have become widely available in recent years and are gaining repute as powerful indicators of mental and physical illnesses. Inadequate levels can contribute to depression. These substances are the building blocks of protein and are used, among many other functions in the body, as important chemicals in the conduction of brain activity. Amino acid supplementation is playing a greater role in health — helping people sleep and feel better, overcome anxiety, substance abuse and depression. Such key amino acids as tyrosine, glutamine, GABA, and phenylalanine can be effective at restoring healthy activity in the brain and nervous system.

Epidemiological studies in the U.S. and elsewhere suggest that decreased consumption of certain fatty acids (omega 3) correlate with increasing rates of depression. Such deficiencies may contribute to depressive symptoms in alcoholism, multiple sclerosis and post partum depression.

There are a number of herbs that are helpful for depression. Among them are Ginkgo biloba extract, a favored European treatment for tinnitus (ear ringing) and attention deficit disorder (ADD), that exerts natural anti-depressant activity. It improves blood flow to the brain.

In one study with 40 depressed patients, a daily dose of 240 milligrams of Ginkgo cut the symptoms of depressions in half after four weeks, and half again after eight weeks. The Ginkgo was added to the patients' regular program of medication.

The herb St. John's Wort (hypericum perforatum) has been used for centuries in the treatment of psychiatric disorders. In modern times, its anti-depressant effects have undergone thorough scientific scrutiny. To date, 25 controlled studies, involving more than 1,750 patients, have been conducted. In those studies, St. John's Wort extract has been compared against placebo or standard medical drugs such as amitriptyline, imipramine, or maprotiline. The usual dosage of the herb in these studies ranged from 300 to 900 milligrams a day over 2 to 3 weeks.

In general, St. John's Wort was just as effective in elevating mood states as imipramine and maprotiline for cases of mild-to-moderate depression.

Alan Gaby, M.D., an expert on alternative medicine commenting on St. John's Wort, notes that "although prescription drugs are usually effective in the treatment of depression, these drugs commonly cause side effects. St. John's Wort, on the other hand, hardly every causes significant adverse reactions."

Pharmaceutical preparations from this herb are approved in Germany as safe and effective in treating mild to moderate cases of depression. According to Mark Blumenthal, executive director of the American Botanical Council, St. John's Wort has become so popular in Germany that one leading brand alone is being prescribed by doctors at a rate of 7 to 1 over Prozac.

Prozup — not Prozac — is a nutritional supplement we often prescribe for patients with depression related to nutritional deficiencies. This formula contains St. John's Wort and Ginkgo biloba, along with zinc and an array of B complex vitamins including B-6, B-12, inositol, folic acid, and a non-flushing type of niacin called hexaniacinate. A number of our patients report favorable responses.

Toxic metal syndrome — that is, a harmful buildup in the body of certain metals such as aluminum, cadmium, lead and mercury — is often associated with depression, anxiety, panic, mood disorders, obsessive compulsions and many behavior and addictive disorders. We utilize specialized laboratory tests in our clinic, especially hair analyses and chelation challenges, to help us identify toxic metal involvement.

A chelation challenge involves a chelation treatment (see the section on chelation therapy in chapter 11) followed by collecting a 24-hour urine sample. The intention is to test for toxic metals. Toxic metals such as lead and aluminum are frequently stored in brain and organ tissue. Mere blood tests alone are inadequate to determine accurate levels. Urine testing, after toxins have been pushed out of the tissues by chelation, offers a better picture of an individual's toxic load.

The seasonal connection

Q *"I am 68 years old and I have been depressed on and off for the past 20 years. I always feel blue especially in the winter, or if I'm under stress. The psychiatrists say I have a "chemical imbalance." I have tried Elavil, Zoloft, Prozac and even Lithium. Counseling helps for a while but I just seem to slip back. It just seems there has to be a reason for this. Do you think nutrition or vitamins might help me?"*

A For patients whose depression is associated with seasonal changes and what is known as seasonal affective disorder (SAD), we employ 20 to 30 minute treatments of Medic Light, a unit that simulates light from the sun at high noon. It is worth pointing out that light waves are absorbed through our eyes and are converted by the pineal gland in the brain into the anti-depressant neurotransmitters serotonin and melatonin.

In this modern age, many of us spend much of our time indoors. For those of us who live in northern latitudes, we spend even more time inside during winter months. As a result of this situation, light-sensitive individuals can and do develop SAD, a condition characterized by depression, anxiety, mood swings, fatigue, sleep disturbances, cravings for carbohydrates, and weight gain.

An early morning walk for 45 minutes <u>outdoors</u> offers an effective natural antidote. If a walk isn't possible, we recommend the use of the Medic Light. This treatment, in conjunction with the rest of our wellness program, provides a remarkable non-pharmaceutical approach to relieving the seasonal blues.

The chiropractic — depression connection

Among the factors overlooked by mainstream medicine, and indeed much of alternative medicine as well, is a powerful connection between chiropractic and mental function. I have discussed this at length in chapter 13.

In brief, misalignments in the skull and the cervical (neck) spine can indirectly affect mood in two primary ways:

• Impairment of blood flow into the brain.

• Interference with the brain's normal electrochemical network as a result of "pinched nerves."

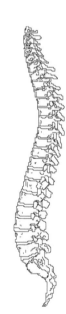

Either one, or both, of these scenarios can lead to what chiropractors call "brain hibernation," that is, certain areas of the brain do not receive normal nerve stimulation or blood supply. This results in decreased brain functioning.

Allen G. J. Terrett, D.C., of the Royal Melbourne Institute of Technology in Australia, has written extensively on the "brain hibernation" theory and linked it to many cases of depression, anxiety, memory problems, attention span and concentration difficulties, irritability and fatigue.

Frank Gorman, M.D., an Australian physician interested in spinal manipulation, has reported that a wide range of psychological disorders respond to chiropractic care. He believes that many people are disabled by "mental illness which has a simple physical cause," namely misalignments.

Clinical experience throughout the world, including my own, has demonstrated that chiropractic manipulations often help patients with these problems.

Over the years, I have had extensive exposure to patients who have been previously given a diagnosis of depression. I believe this is simply a convenient category in which to place patients.

Since chiropractic recognizes that the mind and body are one, please consider that you may be depressed because you have unresolved spinal misalignments leading to pain and impairment. I often see marked improvement in patients' mental outlook following a series of chiropractic treatments. Migraines dissipate. Insomnia improves. Anxiety lessens. Energy increases. We are often able to reduce medication or wean patients off of drugs altogether.

Moreover, chiropractic management, by improving the mind—body relationship, allows patients and psychologists alike to better understand what is truly emotional or mental.

Natural Remedies for Depression

- *Chiropractic and cranial manipulation*
- *Applied kinesiology (AK) to screen for allergies*
- *Vitamin B-12 sublingual* ....*1,000 to 5,000 micrograms daily*
- *Prozup* .... *2 capsules, 3 times daily*
- *Free-form amino acids* .... *2 capsules, 3 times daily*
- *Orthomolecular nutritional supplement dosages for resistant cases as determined by individual needs under supervision*
- *Medic Lite treatments if SAD present*
- *Chelation therapy (removes toxic metals)*

About diabetes

Diabetes affects 10 million Americans and is a leading cause of death behind heart disease and cancer. It has become the most common of the serious metabolic diseases. This disorder greatly increases your risk of heart disease, stroke, kidney disease, and loss of nerve function (neuropathies).

Diabetes is divided into two categories. Type 1 describes insulin-dependent diabetes, and usually strikes children and adolescents. It is caused by the destruction of tissue in the pancreas that produces insulin, the hormone that allows blood sugar to be transported into cells and burned for energy. Type 1 diabetics produce little or no insulin and must rely on insulin injections the rest of their lives.

Type 1 diabetes was long considered to be a genetic disorder but now it is believed to involve autoimmune responses, meaning that the body's own defense system turns on the body itself. This is believed due to such factors as toxic chemical overloads, viruses, free radicals, and food allergies.

Recently, researchers discovered that allergy to milk may be a frequent cause. Many youngsters are allergic to milk and because youngsters are encouraged to drink large quantities of it there is considerable potential for health problems. In some, reactions are triggered within the immune system that lead to insulin cell "burnout."

Ninety percent of diabetics are of the type II category, also known as non-insulin dependent or adult onset diabetes. Here, the pancreas produces sufficient insulin but cells throughout the body are resistant to it. This results in an elevation of both blood sugar and insulin. Telltale diabetic signs such as fatigue, excessive thirst, sugar in the urine may follow, as well as obesity and high blood pressure.

Diabetes dramatically raises the risk for devastating illnesses. As an example, a diabetic is 250 times more likely to suffer from heart disease and 25 times more from blindness.

Conventional medical treatment for both types of diabetes is primarily pharmaceutical along with standard American Diabetic Association exchange diets.

In the experience of nutritionally-oriented health practitioners, much of the problem of diabetes relates to poor eating habits, overweight, chromium and other nutrient deficiencies, lack of adequate exercise, and food allergies that cause a rise in blood sugar.

There is no question that Type I diabetics require insulin, but without appropriate lifestyle and nutritional strategies, these individuals face increasing insulin demand and serious complications.

Type II diabetics are commonly treated with oral agents (Diabinese, Micronase, and Tolinase). But drug therapy is not very effective beyond three months and long-term side effects abound. The standard ADA diet, a food exchange diet, although useful at one time is now regarded to have significant flaws, including excessive fat and deficient fiber content.

Carol Umbel's case

Carol Umbel, a 53-year-old homemaker from New Stanton, Pennsylvania, came to see me in 1992. She was unable to walk without a cane and had great difficulty rising from a chair.

> **"I had been told to expect to get worse and lose my ability to walk."**

"I had been on a downward spiral of deterioration from diabetic neuropathy," she said. "For about nine years I had seen traditional medical doctors and had received traditional treatment. I had been told to expect to get worse and ultimately lose all ability to walk. There was no treatment. All that could be done was to treat the pain."

Through diet, exercise, chiropractic adjustments, electrical muscle stimulation, and supplements of vitamins, minerals and herbs, we were able to help Carol's situation considerably.

"After only a few months of treatment, I was able to put the cane away," Carol says today. "Although I am not entirely cured, my condition has improved, and is currently staying at this improved state. My medical doctor is surprised at my physical ability and is genuinely impressed with my progress.

"When my son got married, I danced at his wedding. I never thought that would be possible."

When I first examined Carol I found subluxation of the sacroiliac joint. This misalignment was at the core of her problems. The sacroiliac joint is the foundation of the spine. If the joint is misaligned, it causes a person to shift weight to one side of the body which in turn can lead to balance problems, sciatic nerve pain, numbness and tingling sensations, neuropathy and other disorders.

Following one month of chiropractic manipulations, Carol was able to put her cane aside and walk securely without it. She also received wrist and hand manipulation and cervical spine manipulation which helped with neuropathy in her upper extremities.

After beginning treatment with us, Carol returned to the diabetic endocrinologist with whom she consulted at a local Pittsburgh hospital. Previously, she said, she would have to push herself up out of the chair with her cane and then limp over to the examination room. The medical specialist was amazed that following the consultation she was able to readily rise from the chair and proceed without the cane to the examination room.

He wanted to know what she had been doing.

"I have been receiving chiropractic manipulation, along with nutritional and vitamin therapy," she said.

The doctor asked her for my name and has since referred a number of diabetic patients with neuropathy.

How James Todd averted insulin

James Todd, 45, a Pittsburgh electrical engineer, was a diabetic who came to our clinic complaining of chronic fatigue, insomnia, intense neck, back and abdominal pain, and

> **"I have lost 15 pounds and I have more energy."**

daily headaches. When I first examined him he was legally blind from advanced cataracts and unable to work.

James' blood test results were consistent with diabetes. He had a high blood sugar count of 164 and a high glycohemoglobin level, a specialized test used to measure ongoing diabetes. He had liver disease, elevated cholesterol and triglycerides, multiple spinal misalignments, and deficiencies of calcium, magnesium, and zinc, based on hair analysis.

We initiated a program of chiropractic manipulation, detoxification, and nutritional supplements to improve liver function and lower blood sugar. Among our recommendations were Gymnema sylvestre, a well-known ayurvedic herb known to normalize blood sugar, and two important minerals for diabetics — vanadyl sulfate and chromium GTF.

For his eye condition, I referred him to an ophthalmologist for cataract surgery. When he went there, the eye doctor's nurse informed James he would have to see a diabetic specialist and begin insulin immediately before having surgery.

James politely refused and told the nurse he would take care of it on his own. He was keenly interested in natural remedies for lowering blood sugar and didn't want to start a long-term insulin program.

The nurse emphatically told him he should see an M.D. to get his sugar under control or there would be no surgery.

After one month of chiropractic and nutritional treatment, James returned to the ophthalmologist's office. His glucose level had dropped from 164 to 99, a normal reading. His glycohemoglobin test had also dropped into a normal range. The nurse duly noted the changes and commented that "it is miraculous that your blood sugar is normal." She wanted to know how and why he was no longer diabetic. According to James, when he explained to her that he received chiropractic adjustments, diet therapy and vitamins, the nurse was speechless.

James now felt confidant about surgery and underwent the operation without problem. On a follow-up visit to our clinic after his surgery, he expressed his satisfaction over the outcome and his overall improved condition. At this point, his blood sugar had dropped again — down to 95.

"I have lost 15 pounds and I have more energy," he said. "I don't have to take insulin or any medication."

Here is a case showing how effectively conventional and alternative medicine can work together. Surgery removed his cataracts and diet and nutritional prescriptions have brought his diabetes under control. James Todd is now free of headaches, pain, and insomnia. He understands that to prevent recurrences of his problems he has to take an active role on behalf of his own health. The susceptibility for diabetes is still there. He knows he needs to exercise and follow a healthy diet and nutritional program. We treat him once a month for preventive care and he is doing just fine.

Tammy Leister's case

Tammy Leister, 29, an administrative assistant from Somerset, Pennsylvania, had been taking insulin ever since being diagnosed with type I diabetes at the age of five. Despite the insulin, and carefully watching her diet, he blood glucose levels never truly stabilized. She was taking two shots of insulin per day and the doses were on the increase when she visited our clinic.

"I hope to improve my chances of avoiding future diabetic complications."

"I hope to improve my chances of avoiding future diabetic complications," she told me.

After initial tests, we recommended the 10-day detoxification diet and a program of nutritional supplements. We also prescribed weekly adjustments. A chiropractic evaluation determined a misalignment pattern in her neck. She suffered, in fact, from severe neck pain she described as "an electrical shock going up into my head."

Within one week, Tammy's insulin requirements had reversed.

Within a matter of months, Tammy was basically giving herself only one injection daily. She would take a second shot on the rare occasion that her glucose level rose above a certain point. In addition, her glycohemoglobin level began to decrease significantly, indicative of an improvement in her diabetic condition.

Tammy, like many of my diabetic patients, experience a rapid reduction of their blood sugar level with specific diet and vitamin therapy. Manipulation helped resolve her constant neck pain. Normally, such pain might be dismissed as an incidental finding associated with diabetes. But diabetics are subject to the same misalignments as are non-diabetics. The pain had nothing to do with her diabetic condition.

Tammy wanted prevention and that's exactly what she got. "Natural treatments may not be for everyone," she told me, "but they are another tool for me to utilize in order to live as long as possible, complication free!"

How We Treat Diabetes

Q *"My father is 56 and has been diabetic and taking insulin his whole life. He had many complications, including a heart attack, back pain, kidney problems, cataracts and difficulty walking. I am 30 years old, overweight with high blood pressure and my dad said I am headed for diabetes and a heart attack. He said to lose weight and exercise but I don't know where to begin. What do you recommend?"*

A Our strategy against diabetics and others with impaired glucose metabolism (hypoglycemics) targets the causes that unfortunately are often ignored in the medical system.

Perhaps the most effective dietary plan that we incorporate for diabetics is the modified high fiber content diet (MHCF). This plan emphasizes raw fruits, vegetables, whole grains, legumes and about 20 percent of the diet as proteins. It is effective for decreasing insulin requirements, lowering weight and improving levels of cholesterol and triglycerides, a form of fat found in the blood.

Additionally, we perform food sensitivity testing to identify reactions to food, which can destabilize blood sugar. Once offending foods are pinpointed, we help patients to eliminate those items from their menus by finding safe substitutes or showing them how to rotate the foods at intervals which will not cause problems.

Intravenous chelation therapy, which we administer in our clinic, should be strongly considered for diabetics (see chapter 11). This painless procedure is used by many wholistic practitioners to improve circulation and prevent stroke and heart attacks. It represents a major therapeutic weapon in the treatment of diabetes.

A number of nutritional supplements are known to contribute important healing benefits:

• Chromium GTF (polynicotinate), is known as the glucose tolerance factor. It is a special chromium-niacin complex that converts chromium into a biologically-active insulin co-factor. It will often lower insulin requirements, decrease body fat and retard arterial plaque (hardening of the arteries).

Most people think of chromium as the shiny metal parts on car bodies. Indeed, chromium has long been used in metal plating. However, in 1959 it was discovered that this mineral stimulates insulin activity. Insulin must first combine with chromium in order to effectively open the tissues to glucose and the production of energy. Experiments show that insulin is virtually powerless without adequate chromium to create energy.

Richard Anderson, Ph.D., the chief scientist for trace minerals at the U.S. Department of Agriculture's Human Nutrition Research Center in Maryland, believes that the vast majority of the adult population may be getting less than the recommended daily allowance (RDA) of 50-200 micrograms of chromium. The problem in part is processed food. Considerable losses of trace minerals, including chromium, are one of the many undesirable features of highly processed and refined food commonplace in the American diet. Up to 80 percent of chromium is removed from food as a result of milling and processing. Moreover, Anderson points out, diets that are high in refined sugars actually stimulate an extraordinary excretion of chromium. Thus low dietary intake along with increases in excretion due to diet and exercise carry the risk of health problems.

In a recent experiment, Anderson divided 180 type II diabetics into groups receiving a placebo or different intakes of chromium picolinate, a popular form of supplemental chromium. One group took 100 micrograms twice daily. Another group, took 500 micrograms twice daily. All subjects continued with their previous medications. After two months, Anderson found that the group taking the higher level of chromium had significant reductions of blood sugar (fasting glucose). After four months, this group also was found to have substantially lowered levels of cholesterol and positive changes in their blood hemoglobin, which transports oxygen. Anderson concluded that the higher dosage of chromium yielded more benefits for diabetics than at the 200 microgram level.

⊙ Magnesium is routinely found to be low in blood and hair analyses of diabetics. Inadequate magnesium is associated with glucose intolerance and diabetic complications, including retinopathy (blindness) and coronary artery disease. In addition, a deficiency worsens the body's reactions to stress.

Magnesium, Coenzyme B Complex and sublingual vitamin B-12 provide important nutritional support against eye damage and neuropathies (nerve damage) such as pain in the hands and feet. Since diabetics frequently have difficulty with conversion of vitamins for proper utilization, I prefer the coenzyme form rather than ordinary B complex vitamins. I found this especially important in difficult cases of neuropathy, retinopathy, and carpal tunnel syndrome.

• Vanadium is a mineral most of you haven't heard about. It has the ability to mimic the effects of insulin or increase its efficiency, thus reducing both glucose and insulin levels. People with both types of diabetes have had positive responses to vanadium. Among insulin-dependent diabetics, it appears to improve glucose management. Among adult onset diabetics, it both lowers glucose levels in the blood and improves tolerance to glucose.

• For individuals with failing eyesight due to retinopathy we recommend Opthalplex Plus, which contains raw eye concentrates, Vitamin A, zinc, eye bright herb, primrose oil, and European bilberry.

• Diabetics have an increased need for many nutrients, and particularly antioxidants. Here's why: Glucose appears to be prone to harmful oxidative processes that generate free radicals, the "molecular terrorists" that damage cells in our bodies, accelerating aging and disease. Experts believe free radicals are involved in more than 80 percent of degenerative diseases, including diabetes (see chapter 11 for details on free-radicals).

Free-radicals can attack DNA, enzymes, proteins, and cell membranes, producing a chain reaction of destruction; such membrane damage in the cells that line our blood vessels can lead to hardening and thickening of the arteries and eventually to heart attacks and strokes.

Antioxidants including vitamin E, selenium, and vitamin C, are essential to protect the blood vessels from free radical damage and heart disease.

A 1995 study at the University of Texas found that high doses of vitamin E may lower the common risk of atherosclerosis, or hardening of the arteries, among diabetics.

"This is exciting because it may be a new way to prevent heart disease in diabetics," said Ishwarlal Jialal, M.D., Ph.D., the study's lead author. "It is the first study to include men and women with both type I and type II diabetes who have a wide range of glucose control."

Numerous previous studies have shown that vitamin E's antioxidant properties can reduce susceptibility to heart disease in nondiabetic patients by curbing the oxidation of low-density lipoprotein (LDL), the so-called "bad cholesterol." It is known that oxidized or free-radical damaged cholesterol presents a larger risk factor for cardiovascular disease than cholesterol itself. Diabetic patients are more prone to premature atherosclerosis. They are known to have a lower concentration of antioxidants and a tendency to oxidize more "bad cholesterol." Moreover, high levels of glucose in the body appear to promote free radical activity.

In the Texas study, 28 diabetics were assigned randomly to receive either a placebo or 1,200 International Units (IU) of vitamin E for 8 weeks. Compared to the placebo group, the supplemented group had significant reductions in oxidation.

An earlier study by Jialal, but not involving diabetics, indicated that a daily dose of at least 400 IU is necessary to decrease oxidation of LDL cholesterol. The recommended daily allowance (RDA) of vitamin E is 8 to 10 IU!

Vitamin C, along with bioflavonoids, help improve the strength of blood vessel and capillary tissue. Diabetics are known to have fragile blood vessel tissue.

• Impotence, a frequent complication of diabetes, often responds to vitamin E and Glandplex M, a glandular vitamin and herbal male formula. The herb Ginkgo biloba (two capsules twice daily) has been found in studies to help tinnitus (ringing in the ears) and promote increased blood flow to the head, hands, heart, feet and penis. It has a remarkable effect on impotence.

• Brewers yeast, popularized by naturopaths and early nutrition researchers such as Adelle Davis and Linda Clark, is truly a miracle food of nature. Although bitter to taste, two to four tablespoons per day offer a cornucopia of B vitamins, chromium, protein, and complex carbohydrates. The combination helps improve the course of diabetes and lower insulin requirements.

• Niacinamide, a form of niacin (vitamin B-3), has been shown in European studies to restore the so-called pancreatic beta cells — the insulin-producing cells — that are damaged in Type 1 diabetes. The supplement can also slow down or stop destruction in newly diagnosed cases.

• Botanical and ayurvedic medicine have much to offer in the treatment of diabetes. Aloe vera juice, which taken orally in purified form, acts on a variety of intestinal complaints and has been used as a folk medicine for centuries in the Middle East. Aloe is known to have a blood sugar lowering property.

Onion, garlic, chives and leeks contain liberal amounts of allicin, selenium and flavonoids which strengthen blood vessels and help make insulin more readily available. The ayurvedic herb Gymnema sylvestre, literally used for thousands of years in India, has been validated by modern research to decrease insulin requirement and lower blood sugar among diabetics. Interestingly, in healthy individuals it does not lower the blood sugar.

The importance of exercise

Diabetics need regular aerobic forms of exercise. See chapter ten.

Exercise conditions the heart and blood vessels, lowers body fat and weight, and increases cellular sensitivity and uptake of insulin and nutrients.

The chiropractic — diabetes connection

Chiropractic manipulation, which has known antihypertensive and immune enhancing effects, should be a vital component in any diabetic management or recovery program.

Since 20 percent of insulin-dependent diabetics develop neuropathy (nerve damage such as numbness and tingling), chiropractic care can improve and in some cases alleviate this disorder. My experience is that indeed many of our diabetic patients, whether they are insulin-dependent

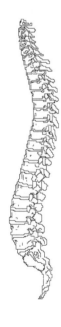

or non insulin-dependent, have neuropathy or nerve damage and benefit from chiropractic treatment.

A 1994 article in the Journal of Manipulative and Physiological Therapeutics described the case of an 80-year-old man with diabetes mellitus who complained of low back pain, poor balance and burning in the lower extremities. A treatment program with chiropractic manipulation of the hips and feet was begun.

While driving home after the first visit, the patient reported "a rush of warmth" in his feet. The restoration of warmth was permanent. Improvement continued over four months of chiropractic care.

In my experience, foot manipulation often helps to restore circulation and relieve nerve pressure in the foot.

Two cases of diabetic retinopathy, or damage to the retina, have been reversed in my clinic following chiropractic manipulation and nutritional therapy.

We have also treated and resolved a number of patients with diabetes-associated carpal tunnel syndrome, using wrist and hand manipulation and chiropractic cervical adjustments. These were individuals who had been considering hand surgery.

Many individuals consider themselves hopeless cases once they are diagnosed with diabetes and its associated arterial and neuropathic conditions. But there is hope, as Carol Umbel, James Todd, and Tammy Leister learned, through chiropractic, nutrition and other wholistic methods.

How sweet we are!

The average American consumes more than 125-130 pounds of refined sugar a year. That means, if you're average, 7,280 teaspoons, or 2/3 of a cup a day. Now compare that to what your grandparents ate: maybe 7 pounds in a given year.

The more sugar and sugary products you eat, the more you rob your body of important nutrients that are needed to metabolize it. The deeper into nutritional debt you go. Such deficits are involved in many common disease processes, among them hypoglycemia (low blood sugar) and diabetes.

Natural forms of sugar are present in fruits and vegetables, along with vitamins, minerals and other nutrients. This natural form of sugar is utilized by the body for energy, and the nutrients that accompany it are used in its metabolism.

But commercial sugar, refined from sugar cane or sugar beets, is another story altogether. The natural nutrient content is stripped away in the processing. That's why when you eat it, your body has to use its own reserves of nutrients to metabolize it.

Refined sugar has another downside. It is rapidly absorbed into the bloodstream, causing wild swings in the blood sugar level that can trigger a wide variety of physical and emotional symptoms, ranging from fatigue to severe depression.

Refined sugar is not just what you put in your coffee or ice tea. It serves as a sweetening ingredient in many processed foods. Some foods have different types of sugars. Cakes, candies, coughdrops, syrup, doughnuts, jellies, ice cream, cereals, and ketchup are loaded with sugar.

About a quarter of all sugar is consumed in soft drinks. Each 12 ounce can of soda contains 9 teaspoons of sugar! Americans drink over 250 cans of soda a year.

Now something new is coming. The dairy industry wants to boost sales so it has developed fruit-flavored milk, with as much sugar in it as soda pop!

There is a saying that we dig our own graves with our teeth. Native cultures that consume a traditional diet of fruits and vegetables are virtually free of diabetes. When they start eating refined food, diabetes is sure to follow. Our own Native Americans, with a terribly high incidence of diabetes, are prime examples of how disastrous the Western diet can be.

Natural Remedies for Diabetes

- **The Gallagher Wellness Program**
- **Chiropractic spinal manipulation**
- **Applied kinesiology to identify organic weaknesses**
- **Panglan (pancreas concentrate)** .... *2 capsules, 3 times daily*
- **Livaglan** .... *2 capsules, 3 times daily*
- **Coenzyme B Complex** .... *50 milligrams, twice daily*
- **Chromium GTF** .... *250 microgram capsules, 2 twice daily*
- **Anti Oxidant Complex** .... *2 capsules, twice daily*
- **Magnesium aspartate** .... *250 milligram capsules, 2 twice daily*
- **Ayur Gymnema (standardized extract)** .... *2 capsules, 3 times daily*
- **Vanadyl sulfate** .... *50 to 100 micrograms daily*
- **Glandplex M** .... *2 capsules, twice daily (for impotence)*
- **Aerobic exercise daily**
- **Chelation therapy**

DIGESTIVE
AND INTESTINAL DISORDERS

See also:
- **chapter 6 (detoxification)**
- **chapter 7 (the "biotype diet")**
- **chapter 8 (optimizing your digestion — including section on constipation)**
- **chapter 9 (food sensitivity identification)**
- **chapter 11 (nutritional rehabilitation)**
- **chapter on heartburn and hiatal hernia**
- **chapter on yeast infections**

Q *"I always either have constipation or diarrhea. One doctor said I had spastic colitis and another said it was nervous indigestion. They tried me on tranquilizers but I got side effects and quit. Is there a food or vitamin I could take?"*

A Patients are frequently confused by conflicting diagnoses of intestinal and digestive disorders, many of which have similar symptoms. But one thing is for sure, that whatever the precise condition, tranquilizers aren't the solution. There are indeed a whole gamut of natural prescriptions that can resolve these problems by eliminating their causes, not by tranquilizing the anxiety they cause.

Glossary of digestive and intestinal disorder terms

Irritable bowel syndrome (IBS)
Irritable bowel syndrome is the most common gastrointestinal condition reported to general practitioners. Thirty to 50 percent of all patients referred to gastrointestinal (GI) specialists suffer from this condition.

IBS is the name that physicians give to cover a group of symptoms (a syndrome) affecting the intestinal tract. Symptoms usually include abdominal pain, bloating, diarrhea or constipation.

IBS basically means that the intestines do not work in a normal orderly manner and that other diseases have been ruled out.

Other names for this condition are irritable colon, spastic colon and "nervous stomach." It is estimated that approximately 22 million Americans may be affected by IBS.

The symptoms of irritable bowel:

• Pain — Occurs usually in the lower left side of the abdomen. Also felt as heartburn or indigestion.

• Bloating and gas distention — Worse after eating. These symptoms are caused by spasms of the muscle fibers in the wall of the large intestine (colon), which compress normal or excess amounts of intestinal gas. Passage of gas or bowel movement may sometimes provide relief.

• Constipation — Lack of fiber (vegetables, fruits and whole grains in diet) and sufficient water causes an unhealthy slowdown of waste products through the intestines. This largely self-inflicted discomfort is a byproduct of modern day eating and lifestyle. It affects some four million people on a regular basis in this country. Americans alone spend $1.4 million daily on laxatives. Improper elimination may be the cause of headaches, low energy, low back pain, abdominal pain and bloating.

• Diarrhea — Stool passes through the bowels too rapidly for a variety of reasons, including intestinal infections and lack of beneficial bacterial flora in the gut.

• Mucous in stool — Normally some mucous is present. In IBS, it may increase and coat part or all of stool. This condition rarely involves blood in the stool.

• Heartburn — Stomach acid or contents migrate upward into the esophagus (see chapter on heartburn).

Crohn's Disease and Ulcerative colitis (IBD)

These two conditions comprise the two major categories of inflammatory bowel disease (IBD) and includes a group of chronic disorders that cause inflammation or ulceration in the small and large intestines. Other names used to describe IBD conditions include colitis, enteritis, ileitis, and proctitis.

The most common symptoms are abdominal pain, often in the lower right area of the abdomen (IBS pain is usually felt in the lower left), diarrhea and poor absorption of nutrients.

• Crohn's Disease — an inflammatory condition extending into the deep layers of the intestinal wall. Usually involves the small intestine, and particularly the lower part (the ileum). Some cases involve both the small and large intestine, the mouth, stomach, esophagus, and anus.

• Ulcerative colitis — an inflammatory and ulcerative condition of the inner lining of the colon and rectum.

There are a number of theories about the causes of IBD. They include infectious agents, a genetic predisposition, dietary factors, abnormal immune function, psychosomatic reasons, and trauma.

Standard medical texts fail to place proper blame on the Western diet loaded with fat and sugar and deficient in fiber and important nutrients. In cultures where whole foods and natural diets are eaten, IBD is practically non-existent.

Food allergies are known to create disorder and malabsorption of nutrients in the intestinal tract. Diets that eliminate such offending foods, followed by correction of nutritional deficiencies, can be most effective in the treatment of IBD. Structuring a diet rich in foods containing fiber is another critical measure in counteracting IBD.

Ulcers

Ulcers are sores or lesions that develop in the lining of the stomach or duodenum (the first part of the small intestine). Doctors will often use the term peptic ulcer to describe an ulcer in the stomach or duodenum. The most common symptom is a gnawing or burning pain in the abdomen between the breastbone and the navel. Pain usually is felt between meals and in the early morning, and can last for a few minutes to a few hours. Bleeding ulcers can cause weakness and fatigue.

Presently, about 20 million Americans are thought to develop ulcers during their lifetime. More than 40,000 individuals undergo surgery each year due to persistent symptoms, and about 6,000 die of ulcer-related complications.

Duodenal ulcers are most likely to develop between the ages of 30 and 50, and occur more frequently in men. Stomach ulcers tend to develop over the age of 60 and more frequently in women.

Lifestyle factors such as stress and diet were long believed to be the major cause of ulcers. Later, researchers found that an imbalance of digestive fluids (hydrochloric acid and pepsin, an enzyme) could also create ulcer problems. Most recently, scientists have incriminated a bacterium with a spiral shape and the colorful name of helicobacter pylori. Researchers now agree that this micro-organism, which penetrates the mucous lining of the stomach and upper small intestine, and causes infection and inflammation, plays the most significant role in the development of ulcers.

Antibiotics are now being widely prescribed to effectively deal with ulcers. However, while they may resolve one problem, they create new ones. They upset the beneficial bacteria population in the gut, which can lead to many digestive and other disturbances. The bottom line may be that we are resolving one condition and creating new ones. I personally treat many people who have been damaged from antibiotic treatment for ulcers.

Among the lifestyle factors are these:

• Smoking increases the risk of developing an initial ulcer and recurrent ulcers.

• No direct link between alcohol and ulcers has been found, but ulcers are more common to individuals with cirrhosis of the liver, a disorder associated with heavy drinking. Alcohol increases the production of hydrochloric acid in the stomach, which in turn increases the transit time of food through the digestive tract.

• Caffeine stimulates acid production in the stomach and can aggravate the pain of an existing ulcer.

• Emotional stress is no longer believed to cause ulcers, however pain from existing ulcers is often increased by such stress. Physical stress increases the chances of developing stomach ulcers.

• Non-steroidal anti-inflammatory drugs (NSAIDs), both the over-the-counter and prescription types that are used against fevers, arthritic conditions, headaches and pain, increase the risk of ulcers by making the stomach more vulnerable to damage from hydrochloric acid and pepsin. These drugs interfere with blood flow, cell repair, and the natural defenses of the stomach.

• Antacids used to treat heartburn temporarily neutralize stomach acid. The problem with that approach is that once your brain senses stomach acid has been neutralized it naturally tells your stomach to produce more acid. This phenomenon is known as "acid rebound." Repetitive use can lead to stomach ulcers.

Since most antacids contain aluminum, a toxic mineral, repetitive use of these drugs can contribute to neurological problems, possibly even to the development of Alzheimer's disease.

Excess consumption of antacids contributes to a deterioration in the physical integrity of the intestinal wall, similar to alcohol, nicotine and NSAIDs. These substances can create holes in the lining and a condition know as "the leaky gut syndrome." In this situation, large and incompletely digested molecules readily leak through the intestinal wall and into the bloodstream. There, they are attacked by the immune system as foreign matter. Their presence in the bloodstream can unleash a wide array of symptoms, including fatigue and allergic reactions.

- Anti-ulcer drugs block stomach acid secretion. But when they are discontinued, 90 percent of patients experience a recurrence of their original ulcer symptoms. They also cause impotence in 20 percent of male patients and depression among many others. Unfortunately, prodded by the endless advertising messages on television, most Americans rush to prescription and over-the-counter drugs to suppress their symptoms

Dianne's Crohn's Disease case (continued from chapter one)

Remember, Dianne Burkhart, the medical researcher from Pittsburgh with Crohn's Disease and ulcerative colitis who I mentioned in the first chapter? She had been on Asacol, Azulfidine, Flagyl, numerous antibiotics, Prilosec, Cortenema,

> **"...I felt like a prisoner of my bathroom."**

cortisone suppositories, Prednisone and Solumedrol. They had caused her moodiness, depression, insatiable appetite, excessive weight gain, hair growth, blood clots, peeling skin, and severe bloating.

Following a long course of antibiotics in 1994, she experienced a severe flare-up and was hospitalized. The doctors told her she would need immediate surgery for removal of the colon. In the hospital for three weeks, on intravenous steroids and pondering surgery, Dianne happened to hear a radio show during which I discussed digestive wellness. She phoned my office from her hospital bed. "What I heard made sense," she told me when I returned her call. "I need nutritional support."

Dianne said she was willing to put her conventional medicine bias aside and give alternative options a try before having surgery. She then had her physician wean her off the steroids so she could check out of the hospital.

When Dianne came to my clinic, I did a chiropractic evaluation and determined she had sacroiliac and lumbar misalignments. A hair analysis showed deficiencies of several minerals. She was also allergic to several foods, particularly dairy.

We started her on a comprehensive program that included chiropractic adjustments, nutritional supplements with aloe vera juice and powdered soluble fiber drinks, and dietary changes that eliminated the junk food she normally ate and the specific foods she was sensitive to.

In time, her energy started to increase. Discomforting symptoms lessened. Under the supervision of her gastroenterologist, she was able to substantially reduce her use of medication and eventually eliminate it altogether.

"I can't believe the difference," she told me within a few weeks. "I am feeling significantly better. My body is really responding to the sensible diet, supplements, and chiropractic adjustments," she told me.

Dianne had become increasingly interested in natural medicine. Around this time she happened to hear a radio show with Donald Carrow, M.D., an alternative practitioner. She called him to discuss her case. Carrow made a few suggestions, including using more glutamine. Within a month, her stools firmed up considerably.

Within six months of starting treatment, Dianne's colon was normal. Today, she is another person.

"I am delighted to say that I no longer have any rectal bleeding or cramping," she says. "My bowel movements are twice a day and firm. There is no pain. Before I felt like a prisoner of my bathroom. It had become increasingly difficult for me to go to work or even leave my home. In my desperation I had cried my eyes out and poured my soul out to the Lord. I am no longer a prisoner of my bathroom. I am so thankful to God, who I feel must have been speaking to me in my heart and told me to hold off with the surgery. I suffered 14 agonizing years with bowel disease going the traditional medical route. In under two years of natural care, I am completely symptom free. And I still have my colon."

Interestingly, during a follow-up colonoscopy by her GI specialist, the doctor told Dianne that it appeared as if she had grown "a new colon."

Patricia Lafko's case

To say the least, 1992 wasn't a good year for Patricia Lafko, 56. The homemaker from Mount Pleasant, Pennsylvania, was suffering from chronic constipation, being treated for irritable bowel with anti-inflammatory drugs, and, in September, underwent a painful hysterectomy.

> **No longer bothered by chronic diarrhea and constipation**

Three months after the operation, she experienced severe abdominal cramps, nausea, vomiting and diarrhea and was rushed to the emergency room. Her internist told her that the probable cause of this episode was a virus.

Patricia returned home but disquieting symptoms continued. She felt feverish, weak, and experienced a sore throat and laryngitis. She was not able to obtain relief or an explanation from her physicians.

"By May of the following year, I found myself with bouts of nausea, vomiting and diarrhea to the point that it was necessary to be hospitalized again," she told me later. "Tests at that time showed an absence of the bacteria which are necessary for the proper functioning of the digestive system.

"After returning home from the hospital, I found myself not being able to eat much in volume or variety. Visiting the gastroenterologist again, I was told to take Flagyl, which was supposed to help the problem. To my disappointment after the prescription was finished, I still had constant problems with indigestion.

"Around Christmas, I felt much worse and started to have many joint pains along with all the previous symptoms. During that period of time, I also needed dental work which required antibiotic therapy. To my amazement, one of my dental trips sent me home very ill which led me to make an appointment with a specialist for a sinus infection.

"I told my gastroenterologist that my health seemed to be deteriorating. At that point he referred me to an allergy specialist. My visit to the specialist showed that I had an abnormal number of food allergies, sensitivities and environmental problems. He prescribed a very limiting diet which was very hard to follow and by the end of one month I had lost too much weight."

It was around this time that Patricia made an appointment at our clinic at the suggestion of one of her physicians. It was June 1994.

After quite extensive testing, we found a range of problems, including candidiasis (yeast infection), bacterial infections, muscle deterioration, chemical sensitivities and spinal misalignments.

On a comprehensive program of nutritional supplements, diet changes, colonics, chiropractic adjustments, and exercise therapy, Patricia started to turn around. She has made considerable improvement.

"There were a few setbacks along the way that discouraged me, but I talked to other patients who had been made totally well with this type of health care," she says. "That helped. I overcame and today my life is full of health and happiness. I take care of my family and home. I am no longer bothered by chronic diarrhea and constipation. I have lots of energy and don't need a nap. When I am doing physical work, play or exercise, I don't have the pain of bursitis and arthritis that I had in the past. I am now able to eat, enjoy and digest foods that I couldn't go near before. And one benefit that I hadn't noticed until others pointed it out to me is that my skin is looking much younger and healthier than before."

Debbie De Sellems' case

Deborah De Sellems, a 48-year-old dental receptionist from Uniontown, Pennsylvania, told me this story when she came to see me about six years ago:

> **"After just three days, the pain was completely gone."**

"I have suffered for three years with severe pain and bloating after eating. I have migraine headaches, and irregular bowel movements usually once every two weeks. I am constantly tired.

"During this time I have taken prescriptions of Zantac and Reglan for ulcers. I have had many medical tests: upper and lower GI, small bowel series, barium enemas, colonoscopy, sigmoidoscopy, and numerous blood analyses. Results were all negative and I was diagnosed with irritable bowel syndrome, not ulcers.

"At that point I was given a new medication every week for five weeks, but nothing helped the pain. I just gave up."

A friend recommended Deborah to visit my clinic. After not receiving meaningful help from other physicians, she was reluctant but made the appointment anyway. We suggested colonic irrigation, chiropractic adjustments and a complete change in diet.

"After just three days, the pain was completely gone," Deborah reported. "I soon lost 10 pounds and eventually dropped 25 pounds. I went from a size 14 to 8. Today, I feel fantastic and pain-free. I wish I had known nine years ago to remove sugar from my diet. I could have saved myself years of pain."

An additional side benefit for Debbie was the remarkable regrowth of her very thin hair following several months of nutritional and vitamin therapy.

How we treat intestinal disorders

As far as the colon is concerned, and going in and out of spasm, I often prescribe an enteric-coated form of peppermint oil known to relax the intestinal tract. The term enteric-coating refers to specially-treated products able to withstand the acidic environment of the stomach and exert their properties in the alkaline intestine.

Acidophilus, and better yet, a multi-strain probiotic bacteria (dairy free) supplement available in health food stores, should be considered to "re-inoculate" the colon with healthy bacteria. This is especially important for those individuals who have had antibiotics or other drugs that affect the health and bacterial balance of the colon.

High fiber, low fat diets that eliminate food sensitivities are often crucial.

Chamomile tea, often given by Italian mothers to treat colic, offers a natural sedative effect for irritable colon patients.

Two standard intestinal detoxification methods we frequently recommend are colon hydrotherapy and Colon Cleanse, especially in resistant cases where parasites or candida (yeast) infections are involved.

Glutamine/FOS is a unique nutritional supplement that we frequently recommend to patients for irritable bowel syndrome, ulcers, colitis, Crohn's disease, diverticulitis and many other difficult colon disorders. Glutamine is an amino acid that repairs inflamed gut lining as well as helping conditions such as low blood sugar, fatigue, sugar craving and alcoholism. I generally recommend a tablespoon of this supplement two times daily between meals in one ounce of aloe vera gel. Aloe also helps to reduce inflammation.

For individuals who have continuing GI complaints despite taking acidophilus or eating yogurt, keep in mind that "friendly bacteria" cannot become activated without FOS. FOS stands for fructo-oligosaccharides, a type of sugar which acts as food for the beneficial bacteria and enhances their proliferation.

The combination of aloe, glutamine, and FOS is a "colon cocktail" that most patients find very effective.

Castor oil, known biblically as "palma christi" (the palm of Christ), has remarkable therapeutic qualities when applied as a warm topical pack over the colon or any other part of the body.

Diathermy, a form of deep electromagnetic heat, provides great benefit to patients by direct application over the intestines.

Visceral manipulation, a type of chiropractic pressure point treatment used at the ileocecal valve (a site near your appendix) is often successful in relieving irritable bowel symptoms. I will talk about that later in the chapter.

How we treat ulcers

Q *"I have been diagnosed with stomach ulcers. I have been on Zantac and Pepsid for the past three years. When I try to wean myself off the drugs, I get heartburn, nausea and chest pain. My doctor says I'll probably have to live with it. Isn't there some thing I could do?"*

A Our approach includes a high fiber diet, which can decrease stomach acid and aid cellular repair. We also suggest that patients drink aloe vera gel mixed with papaya juice between meals. Aloe, as I have indicated, repairs the lining of the gut, and helps soothe the pain of ulcers without the acid rebound associated with antacids. Drink 2-4 oz. between meals. Aloe Vera, as well as calcium carbonate, are natural antacids.

We also recommend a nutritional supplement containing deglycyrrhizinated licorice (extracted from licorice root) and vitamin U, nutritional factors which promote the repair and regrowth of the digestive tract lining.

Natural ingredients in raw vegetable juices have healing effects for ulcers. The best are carrot, celery, parsley and especially cabbage juice (up to 1 pint daily). Cabbage juice is rich in vitamin U, the anti-ulcer factor.

Beta carotene is a natural wound healer. So, too, are vitamin B-6, zinc picolinate, and buffered vitamin C.

Glutamine FOS, which I mentioned above, is also a helpful natural remedy for ulcers.

Botanical medicines including marshmallow, dandelion and chamomile can be used as tinctures, teas and drinks to safely and effectively repair the stomach lining.

Cases of ulcer associated with helicobacter pylori will benefit from elemental bismuth (120 milligrams four times daily). Liquid forms of bismuth taken several times a day, mixed into aloe vera or raw carrot juice, help to inhibit the growth of helicobacter. According to Michael Murray, N.D., writing in "Natural Prescriptions to Over-The-Counter & Prescription Drugs," the mineral bismuth acts as a natural antacid.

The chiropractic connection

Most people — doctors or patients alike — are unaware that spinal stress may be related to visceral disorders, that is, digestive problems. But I have many patients whose conditions have totally resolved after manipulation, including colitis.

From my experience, it appears that misalignments are often connected to non-specific abdominal pain and other symptoms. By that I mean people with complaints that are seemingly related to ovary, uterine, gallbladder, or intestinal tract disorders may in fact have problems related to their spine. This includes pain, severe abdominal bloating, digestive upsets, nausea, heartburn, fluctuations between constipation and diarrhea, and chronic diarrhea. Often times these patients seem to be normal by conventional medical testing measurements. They have gone through cat scans, upper GIs, lower GIs, colonoscopy, gynecology evaluations and internal medicine evaluations.

I have had hundreds of cases of patients receiving chiropractic manipulation for non-specific abdominal pain and other symptoms. I have seen resolution of their problem in a short period of time through chiropractic treatment alone.

Remember, your digestive system does not work independently. Just as your immune, reproductive and glandular systems are controlled by your nervous system, so, too, is your digestion.

Spinal misalignments create nerve interference that can trigger a variety of abdominal complaints, including but not limited to ulcers, gastritis, hiatal hernia, reflux, constipation, diarrhea, irritable bowel syndrome, ulcerative colitis, and hemorrhoids.

Another extremely common problem I have found, especially among children, is chronic stomach or abdominal pains related to misalignments.

Spinal misalignments represent a potentially major physical cause of digestive and abdominal disorders. Yet the spine is always overlooked by conventional doctors and by patients at large who have been programmed into the medical model of taking a drug if something hurts or doesn't work right in the body. What most doctors and patients perceive as psychosomatic or stress-related gastric disorders are often related to physical, mechanical interference in the nervous system that can be readily improved or corrected with chiropractic treatment as a single modality of as part of a wholistic health program.

Don't omit the spinal connection — and the potential benefits of chiropractic manipulation — when considering treatment of stubborn digestive and intestinal disorders. This may just be the missing link between you and good health.

Since 1921, the relationship between spinal misalignment and colon dysfunction has been documented in medical literature.

A Scandinavian study published in 1990 demonstrated a significant connection between individuals with digestive ailments and spinal subluxations impacting the nerves that lead to the abdomen.

Andrei Pikalov, M.D., Ph.D., a researcher at the Cleveland Chiropractic College in Kansas City, along with V. V. Kharin, M.D., Ph.D., of the Medical Research Institute of the Russian Ministry of Internal Affairs, conducted a pilot study at the Moscow Central Hospital in 1993 in which they compared chiropractic with conventional ulcer medication.

In the study, 11 adult men and women, aged 18 to 44, and all with endoscopically-confirmed diagnosis of ulcer disease, underwent chiropractic treatment. They received spinal manipulative therapy treatment from 5 to 22 days with a range of 3 to 14 procedures.

A comparison control group of 24 similarly diagnosed individuals received conventional medication.

The chiropractic group experienced pain relief and full healing of the ulcer after 1-9 (average 3.8) days. The control group took 10 days longer on an average.

The Russian study demonstrated that manipulation of the thoracic (mid-back) spine may offer excellent healing potential for ulcer sufferers. Rather than blocking normal stomach acid production, manipulation stimulates the regrowth of damaged mucosal lining tissue by restoration of the nerve supply. When the mid-back is misaligned (with or without the presence of pain) the nervous system can be disturbed. This can cause, among other effects, an excess secretion of stomach acid.

The results of the Russian study suggested that manipulation could have a positive impact on the disease process and reduce symptoms "with greater success than traditional medical care," the researchers said. "It appears likely that a substantial (about 40 percent) reduction of the treatment period required for full clinical remission is possible in cases of noncomplicated duodenal ulcer. This pilot study indicates a very promising direction for research in the conservative care of duodenal ulcer."

Moreover, they added, an advantage of chiropractic treatment is that patients "do not need medication" which typically are known to cause side effects including headaches, tiredness, dizziness, diarrhea, constipation, and nausea.

Visceral manipulation, a type of chiropractic pressure point treatment, used at the ileocecal valve (ICV), is often successful in relieving irritable bowel symptoms.

For those unfamiliar with the ICV, this is where the last section of your small intestine (the ileum), the site of nutrient absorption, is connected to your large intestine, where waste products are removed.

Infections, food allergies, subluxations of the low back, drugs, alcohol, tobacco, caffeine products, and especially antibiotics can destabilize the intestinal tract and lead to an inflammation of the ICV.

In this condition, called the ICV syndrome, the valve dilates so that the toxic materials that would normally be eliminated from your large intestine can actually move back into the small intestine. Auto intoxication, or self poisoning, can result. Some of the symptoms associated with ICV include intestinal disturbances, headaches, pain in the back, abdomen, hips and legs, and general feelings of fatigue and lassitude.

Chiropractic visceral manipulation helps to re-establish the normal functioning of the ICV.

Mike, 40, came to my office because of a history of ulcerative colitis. He had been treated in the conventional medical way with steroids and Azulfidine. Although the drugs would temporarily control the symptoms, he would develop symptoms in times of stress or change of seasons.

A chiropractic examination was positive for lumbar subluxation. Remember that the intestinal tract is a muscle and misalignment of the lower spine can cause nerve irritation resulting in the intestinal wall going into spasm. Following a series of 10 chiropractic manipulations, Mike's ulcerative colitis completely resolved and he no longer required any medication.

Chiropractic spinal manipulation of the lumbar vertebrae, at the lower part of the back, can have a marked improvement on a wide variety of intestinal and digestive disturbances.

Several years ago, Joyce, one of my patients, brought her 5-year-old son to my office because of constipation that had been going on for 10 days. Joyce, who was well versed in natural healing, had tried a wide variety of things including bran, prune juice and increasing the boy's fiber and water content in the diet, but to no avail. After reviewing the boy's history, I proceeded to do a spinal examination of the lower part of his back. The examination was positive for lumbar subluxation, misalignment of the first two vertebrae of the lower part of his back. He then received a type of chiropractic manipulation we call a lumbar roll.

Four hours afterward, Joyce called my office and asked to speak to me. When I picked up the phone, I heard an ecstatic mother say that following the manipulation the youngster had hardly left the toilet. He never again had a problem with constipation.

Another case of constipation involving a five-year-old was reported by Kirk Eriksen, D.C., in a 1994 issue of the Chiropractic Research Journal. In this particular instance, the patient was a girl with severe, chronic constipation. A "dramatic change" in her bowel functioning resulted from correction of misalignments in her neck.

Natural Remedies for Intestinal and Digestive Disorders

- *Chiropractic evaluation and lumbar manipulation*
- *Visceral manipulation*
- *Pulsed diathermy (abdomen)*
- *Castor oil packs apply to abdomen for 45 minutes*
- *Colon hydrotherapy*
- *Allerzyme (pancreatic enzymes, 10x)* .... 2 tablets, 3 times daily
- *Probiotic bacteria* .... 2 capsules, twice between meals
- *Peppermint oil (enteric-coated)* .... 2 capsules, 3 times daily
- *Aloe vera juice* .... 1 oz. between meals, twice daily
- *Glutamine /FOS* .... 1 teaspoon, twice daily

Natural Remedies for Ulcers

- *Chiropractic thoracic manipulation*
- *Avoid caffeine, alcohol, dairy, citrus, nicotine, sugar, strong spices*
- *Deglycyrrhizinated licorice* .... chew 2 tablets, 20 minutes before meals
- *Gastromet (Vitamin U — anti ulcer supplement)* .... 2 capsules, 3 times daily
- *Zinc Picolinate* .... 25 milligrams twice daily
- *Beta Carotene* .... 200,000 IU daily for 6-8 weeks
- *Buffered Vitamin C powder* 1/4 teaspoon 4 times daily or up to bowel tolerance
- *Vitamin E* .... 1,000-2,000 IU for 90 days, then cut to 400 IU
- *Bismuth* .... 120 milligrams, 4 times daily before meals
  and bedtime for 8 weeks, if associated with helicobacter pylori bacteria

See also: chapter on tinnitus

Peggy Barry's case

Margaret (Peggy) Barry is a 52-year-old teacher from West Homestead, Pennsylvania. For years she had been suffering from intense migraine headaches, dizziness and a balance problem. The problems were getting worse.

> **Her doctors believed her sense of balance was destroyed, but chiropractic manipulation restored it**

She had seen several doctors for her headaches, undergone EKG testing, and received prescriptions for painkillers.

"When one medication didn't help, the doctors always suggested trying another," she told me on her first appointment. "But nothing providing lasting relief."

For her vertigo, the doctors believed an inner ear infection had destroyed her sense of balance. She had taken a leave of absence from teaching because of the dizziness and the difficulty in driving to school. Her balance deteriorated to where she began stumbling. Her internist sent her to an ear, nose and throat specialist who, in turn, recommended an MRI and evaluation by a clinic that specialized in balance and ear problems.

After the results were in, the specialist overseeing her case told her he had both good news and bad news for her. The good news was that she wasn't crazy and imagining her difficulty, that she definitely had balance problems. The bad news was that they had no clue as to what was causing it.

The consensus of the experts was a recommendation for special training to learn to control her balance through her vision. It didn't help. After the program ended, she was told there was nothing more that could be done for her and she would have to learn to live with the problem.

It was around this time that Peggy's sister heard one of my radio broadcasts and her attention was drawn to a caller suffering from severe headaches. Peggy still had her headaches as well as her unresolved balance problem. On that particular show I commented that chiropractic and nutrition could often help migraines. Peggy's sister told her about what I had said and encouraged her to make an appointment. But Peggy was reluctant to deal with another doctor. Understandably, she was discouraged. But the sister made the appointment for her anyway and actually drove her to my office.

On her first visit, Peggy told me about her headaches but didn't say a word about the balance problem because, as she confided later, she didn't believe anything could be done about it. That's what the specialists told her.

When I examined her, she had pronounced pain in the area of the upper neck, just below the skull. The problem was a serious misalignment of the atlas and axis vertebrae, the two uppermost vertebrae of the spine. Because of this, the vestibular (balance) center in her brain was being bombarded with abnormal nerve signals. I then initiated a series of chiropractic adjustments to correct the misalignment.

Peggy was amazed at the results.

"After just three manipulations, my headaches seemed to disappear," she reported. "As an added bonus, my sense of balance began to improve tremendously." It was at this point she told me about the balance problem. It was so bad, she said, that just looking at the moving windshield wiper in her car during a rainstorm was enough to make her ill with vertigo.

I wasn't surprised. Peggy was paying the price for subluxations in her neck. Such physical distortions can and do cause both headaches and balance problems.

Peggy is no longer disabled from vertigo. Nor does she suffer from constant headaches.

Like many patients caught in the conventional medical web, Peggy was inaccurately told she had a permanent problem with no cure. It is true there was no drug or surgical cure but there was a chiropractic cure. Unlike drugs that generate serious side effects, adjustments generate "serious side benefits." Here is another example of why I believe much of our medical terminology, diagnoses and jargon needs to be replaced with a simple term: spinal subluxation. In the contemporary medical system, the widespread presence of simple structural misalignments are not being recognized. Because of this, countless millions of people are suffering unecessarily.

How we treat dizziness/vertigo

Q *"I have been dizzy for six months. It has gotten so bad that I am afraid to drive a car or go anywhere. My family doctor told me it was an inner ear problem and a neurologist diagnosed 'dysequilibrium' (poor balance). I take vitamins and eat a good diet but nothing seems to help me. Could you suggest a remedy for me?"*

A Vertigo, the sensation that you or the world is spinning, is a common form of dysequilibrium. Medical drugs in most cases are not only ineffective against vertigo, but often contribute to the problem. Among the most frequently prescribed are antihistamines, such as Antivert, which are designed to reduce fluids and swelling thought to be associated with vertigo. Side effects include fatigue, drowsiness, dry mouth, and impaired ability to operate machinery.

In some cases, patients with this problem even undergo brain surgery.

Chiropractic treatment is extremely effective for these conditions. See the chiropractic connection below.

I have found that many patients with a loss of balance associated with fatigue benefit in particular from Adrenoglan Chelate, a glandular supplement containing adrenal extract. It is important to keep in mind that the adrenal glands are major producers of stress hormones. Chronic stress is often associated with these problems and when the adrenals are overworked for long periods of time they can become depleted. One of the many consequences of this is decreased blood flow to the brain, leading to dizziness and light-headedness. (see chapter on stress and the adrenal glands).

Ginger capsules are also high on my natural remedy list. Ginger is one of the most widely used roots in the world for both culinary and medicinal purposes. It is a wonderful remedy for motion sickness and the nausea of pregnancy. A study published in the medical journal Lancet in 1982 documented another beneficial role — for vertigo. The research showed that ginger neutralizes intestinal toxins and acids that, if otherwise left unchecked, have the ability to interfere with the brain's balance and nausea centers.

Vitamin B-6, (the anti carpal tunnel vitamin), may improve cases of vertigo that are caused by allergies. Food allergy testing through applied kinesiology, as well as anti-body testing (IgG4), can be useful in determining causes of balance difficulties that may be associated with reactions to food. Food sensitivities can cause cerebral allergies which may in turn trigger vertigo.

The homeopathic remedy cocculus 6X provides good symptomatic relief for mild cases.

Over the years I have successfully treated several patients who suffered dizziness as a result of aluminum and lead toxicity. The toxicity was determined by hair analysis, a simple diagnostic method used by many alternative medicine practitioners. High levels of so-called toxic metals are known to create neurological disturbances, vertigo among them.

Patients with Meniere's syndrome (hearing loss, dizziness, ringing in the ears, and neck pain) respond remarkably well to a comprehensive program that includes chiropractic and cranial manipulation, myofascial release, colonic hydrotherapy and nutritional care (please refer to the tinnitus chapter).

Mary Lou Jones' case

Mary Lou Jones, 52, is a retired teacher in Greensburg, Pennsylvania. She was suffering from vertigo, along with neck and lower back pain, extreme fatigue, and yearly bronchitis, when she first visited us in 1988.

"These symptoms have been going on for many years," she told me. "I considered ending my teaching career because of the pain. My medical doctor decided the pain was due to the stress of my job. He recommended I try muscle relaxants for my neck and back. I was on these for several months with little relief.

"He also recommended I see a neurologist for the vertigo. I went through many tests to determine if there was anything neurologically wrong with me. The tests were all negative. I returned to my family doctor and informed him I was still in a lot of pain. He told me we would try a stronger medication. When I went to the pharmacist for a refill of my prescription, I was informed my medication was Valium. That was the last straw."

Mary Lou made an appointment at our clinic. I recommended

> **"When I went to the pharmacist for a refill of my prescription, I was informed my medication was Valium. That was the last straw."**

chiropractic and nutritional care. She received a series of chiropractic upper cervical manipulations to correct spinal misalignments. This markedly helped her dizziness and vertigo. She received thoracic (mid-back) manipulations to help against the recurring bronchitis.

We also discovered that she had hypoglycemia (low blood sugar). We put her on a blood sugar stabilizing diet along with nutritional supplements, including B complex vitamins and adrenal extract.

The natural approach has worked well for Mary Lou. "I am feeling much better," she said shortly after her treatment started. That was nine years ago.

For years now, Mary Lou has been receiving "wellness care" — a maintenance program designed to keep a patient's health at an optimum level once major symptoms are resolved. During a recent checkup, she told me she hasn't experienced vertigo or bronchitis since she started chiropractic and nutritional care.

"The neck and back pain have also been helped with manipulation," she said recently. "My energy level has improved. And I haven't had to take any medication in all these years."

When Mary Lou first started treatment under my care, she was so sick and exhausted that she wanted to retire prematurely from the vocation she loved — teaching elementary school children. She was so dizzy that she couldn't do any work above eye level without feeling as if she was going to fall. She was so tired that when she came home from school she would have to go straight to bed. She would drag herself out of bed to eat and then go right back again. She also had chronic fibrocystic breast disease, and she took antibiotics for severe bronchitis every winter.

With wholistic health care, Mary Lou taught for another nine years before retiring in 1996 — healthy and functional. No vertigo, neck pain, exhaustion, breast disease, or yearly bronchitis.

The chiropractic — vertigo connection

"A cervical (neck) factor may be present in all forms of vertigo and dizziness...(and) in no field is manipulation more effective than in the treatment of disturbances of equilibrium," states Czechoslovak neurologist Karel Lewit, M.D., a leading European medical expert on spinal manipulation.

David Chapman-Smith, editor of "The Chiropractic Report," commented in a 1991 issue of the journal that "with vertigo, the brain

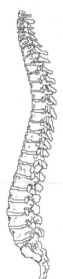

has a false perception of balance and motion because of flawed information from the nervous system."

The most common causes of such flawed information are:

• Cervical misalignments, affecting the nervous system directly. Such misalignments create abnormal stress in the neck. A situation develops known as "cervical vertigo," where continuous abnormal nerve signals from the spinal joints, muscles, and ligaments bombard the specialized centers in the brain responsible for balance — the vestibular nuclei, by name — as well as the inner ear.

• Cervical misalignments leading to vertebral artery compression or irritation. This causes reduced blood flow and oxygen in the arteries that supply the specialized brain centers.

• Muscle trigger points or spasms

• Injured spinal ligaments

A landmark study reported in 1988 by D. Fitz-Ritson, D.C. involved 112 patients with a confirmed diagnoses of "cervical vertigo." A total of 112 patients received chiropractic manipulation, along with stretching, nutrition, trigger point therapy and lifestyle management. After 18 treatments, 101 (92.2 percent) were symptom-free. The 11 patients who did not respond were all chronic cases — seen 21 to 43 months after their symptoms began. Their lack of response strongly suggests that individuals with vertigo should not delay chiropractic evaluation.

Pierre Cote, D.C., along with Don Fitz-Ritson, D.C., at the Canadian Memorial Chiropractic College in Toronto, reported three cases of vertigo resolved by neck adjustments.

The first case involved a 65-year-old male who had suffered for two decades from vertigo and neck stiffness. Whenever he extended his neck he experienced a "side-to-side movement of the room." Chiropractic evaluation revealed misalignments in the upper neck vertebrae. Eight adjustments over a three-week period resolved the vertigo. When checked again 18 months later, the condition had not returned.

Case # 2 was a 62-year-old male with a 10-year history of vertigo and associated neck, head and upper back pain and occasional nausea. Bending his head downward or up and back caused him to become "woozy." Misalignments were also determined in the upper neck. Chiropractic manipulation and soft tissue massage were recommended. After the first adjustment, the patient said the vertigo was eliminated.

Some neck pain persisted. After six years of follow ups, the vertigo was found to recur about once a year at which time the patient would undergo a single neck adjustment.

The third case involved a 30-year-old female patient who developed headaches, neck pain and dizziness after an automobile accident. Misalignments were determined in the neck, upper back, and the temporomandibular joint (jaw). Adjustments were administered along with soft tissue work on the jaw. After one month of treatments, the woman was free of dizziness and headaches, but still had some residual neck pain. After three years, she had had only one episode of vertigo, which was readily resolved with a single adjustment (Journal of the Canadian Chiropractic Association, 1991).

The findings I have just described reflect my own experience with several thousand vertigo/dysequilibrium patients over the years. Their problems are often related to the "atlas syndrome," a misalignment of the first vertebra of the neck.

Sometimes I will also find misalignments in the cranium and jaw joint. Cranial and temporomandibular joint (TMJ) adjustments often resolve these difficulties.

"Like being drunk"

Joseph, a patient in his mid 40s, came to my office in 1995 describing himself as a person who felt drunk on and off all day, even though he consumed no alcohol. He stated that the problem began a little over a year before when he began having sensations of being off balance, feeling lightheaded and dizzy.

"It's like I'm drunk," he said, "or like being on a ship out at sea and being rocked back and forth."

He had undergone several neurological examinations, CT scans, brain scans, and had consulted numerous ear, nose and throat specialists. He was told that his problem was vertigo or dysequilibrium, and that it was something that he would have to learn to live with.

I determined he had misalignments in the neck and TMJ. I administered a series of upper cervical spine manipulations and TMJ realignment. The latter is a type of treatment using acupressure to realign the structures of the jaw.

The patient began improving within two weeks and resolved totally in 90 days.

In the case of Joseph, and many other patients, there was no neck pain to indicate a cervical spine or neck-related problem. Remember what I said in chapter 13 about misalignments that cause no pain but adversely affect the healthy functioning of your body. Most alignments work that way. No pain. Just silently creating problems without you ever knowing what the cause is. That's why I call such misalignments "silent robbers of health." They can cause vertigo, visual and hearing problems, mental confusion, fatigue, and a wide array of health problems.

Chiropractic physicians address the underlying mechanical and lifestyle factors contributing to the causes of these often disabling problems. Few M.D.s have the manual training and skills to find and treat such dysfunction or movement restriction in the joints and muscles (subluxations).

Structure affects function. Don't forget it! And don't forget to have regular chiropractic checkups. If you have your teeth checked regularly, why not your spine? Your teeth won't disable you, but a misaligned spine can and does! Don't wait for pain to occur. Do it for the sake of your nervous system, which, after all, controls your whole body.

Natural Remedies for Dizziness and Vertigo

- *Chiropractic cervical manipulation*
- *Chiropractic TMJ manipulation*
- *Vitamin B-6* .... *25-100 milligrams daily*
- *Vitamin B-12 Sub-lingual* .... *1,000 to 5000 micrograms daily*
- *Ginger (standardized extract)* .... *2 capsules, 3 times daily*
- *Adrenoglan Chelate* .... *2 capsules, 4 times daily*
- *Cocculus (6X)* .... *2 pellets under the tongue as needed*
- *Ginkgo biloba (standardized extract)* .... *40 milligrams, 3 times daily*
- *Chelation therapy, if associated with circulatory problems*

EAR INFECTIONS

Q *"My children are ages 3 and 5. They are always sick with either ear infections, tonsillitis, congestion or runny noses. The pedia trician has loaded them up with antibiotics but the infections come right back. He said they both need ear tubes. I'm frightened. Isn't there something natural?"*

A Over the years I have heard variations of this question hundreds of times from concerned parents. In fact, most children brought to our office have a long history of antibiotic "abuse." Many of them have undergone ear tube surgeries.

What I see in my clinic is the tip of a health and treatment epidemic. Up to 40 percent of children under the age of six are affected by chronic ear infections or otitis media, as it is known medically. It is the leading health problem treated by pediatricians, accounting for more than 50 percent of office visits. How it is treated is also a major problem.

There are a number of basic reasons for ear infections:

• Up to two years of age, the immune system hasn't fully developed. Infants are more vulnerable to infections.

• Trouble occurs in the Eustachian tube, a tiny passage connecting the ear and throat. This tube regulates gas pressure in the middle ear, where the delicate organs of hearing are located, and protects them from nose and throat secretions and bacteria. It is the channel through which fluid is cleared from the middle ear. However, colds and allergies often push micro-organisms and contaminants into the tube, where conditions are ripe for infections to develop. The parade of symptoms that results often includes inflammation, swelling, pain, fever, crankiness, loss of appetite, and tugging at the ear.

• Risk factors associated with ear infections include early introduction of cow's milk or grain into the diet, food allergies, exposure to cigarette smoke, frequent changes in atmospheric pressure and nutritional deficiencies.

• As you will see later in this chapter, there is also a strong, but totally overlooked, connection between spinal stress and ear infections. Most people don't realize it. Certainly medical doctors aren't aware. Nor, for that matter, are many wholistic physicians. Research has shown that chiropractic manipulation may be extremely helpful in overcoming both acute and chronic cases of infections for children, and even adults. During more than two decades in my own clinical practice, I have seen literally hundreds of improved or altogether resolved cases following manipulation. I will talk more about that in a moment.

Antibiotics – The "cure" that's worse than the disease?

Conventional medical treatment often doesn't get to the cause of ear infections — and according to scientific evidence may even make matters worse.

Primary treatment consists of antibiotics. Pediatricians and family physicians prescribe half a billion dollars worth of antibiotics each year for ear infections alone. See my comments about antibiotic use in chapter three.

There is widespread concern in the medical community about over-prescribing antibiotics for this condition. And yet, many doctors say, parents demand it and will go elsewhere if they do not receive a prescription.

The facts on antibiotics are these:

• Most infections clear up on their own. Research shows that 80 percent of children with acute ear infections become free of symptoms in two to three days without treatment.

• Studies suggest that antibiotics do not shorten the course of respiratory infections, nor do they prevent complications, reduce pathogens in the nose, throat and Eustachian tubes, or exert any benefits.

• The perennial overuse of antibiotics has spawned antibiotic-resistant strains of bacteria that cause, among other things, ear infections.

• Outcome studies have clearly shown that every time a child is given an antibiotic at the start of an ear infection, there is a three to six times increased risk of developing another infection.

• "If you immediately interfere with antibiotics," says Erdem Cantekin, Ph.D., professor of otolaryngology at the University of Pittsburgh, "then children's immune systems don't have the ability to recognize these common micro-organisms and do not develop the necessary natural defense mechanisms. Antibiotics beget antibiotics, and eventually these children end up in surgery."

• Frequent use of antibiotics can foster food allergies, sensitivities, recurring infections, irritable colon, rheumatoid disease, depression, and chronic fatigue syndrome.

• As I mentioned in chapter three, antibiotics destroy the beneficial bacteria in the intestines, nose and throat that counteract the growth of harmful bacteria and yeast in the body. Without the protective colonies of bacteria, we become vulnerable to many health problems and infections.

Ear tube surgery

Ear tube surgeries are commonly prescribed when rounds of antibiotics fail to curb repeated infections. More than 1 million children have ear operations each year, at a cost of $2 billion. The surgical procedure involves inserting tiny tubes into the eardrum in an effort to drain blocked fluid in the middle ear.

"Fifty percent of these children get a second set of tubes, because, three to six months later, the tubes drop out, and the fluid comes back," says University of Pittsburgh's Cantekin.

According to Stephen Berman, M.D., professor of pediatrics and director of health policy at the University of Colorado in Denver, "there are times when tubes are important." But, he adds, "we're doing too much surgery. About 65 percent of tympanostomy tube surgery is not consistent with the (U.S. Government's) Agency for Health Care Policy and Research guidelines."

Surgeries are also known to increases the rate of ear infections while subjecting a child to potential anesthetic complications and permanent loss of some degree of hearing. In one 1976 study, researchers cited psychological trauma, anesthetic risks, secondary infection and eardrum scarring as the paramount complications. As possible long-term effects they mentioned the development of more serious ear disease and/or permanent hearing impairment.

The evidence surely indicates that antibiotics, and obviously surgery, should not be treatments of first choice in most cases. Because they have become so, this disorder is a nightmare example of unregulated and unscientific conventional medicine.

During my entire professional career, I have never had a single case where a child needed ear tube surgery after natural treatment. Rarely has a child even had to take an antibiotic afterward. The natural approach also works <u>successfully</u> for children who previously have been treated <u>unsuccessfully</u> with antibiotics and multiple tube surgeries.

Brennon Meadow's case

Nine-year-old Brennon Meadows, of Scottdale, Pennsylvania, began treatment in our clinic in 1994. He suffered from chronic ear infections, starting at six months of age.

> **Antibiotics...and tubes...and facing hearing loss**

He was under the care of his pediatrician who kept recommending antibiotics, which would help for a time. But the infections would return one or two months later.

At age 1, tubes were recommended by a specialist.

Brennon's mother told me the following: "The tubes were to stay in the ear canal for approximately one year. But the infections would come back. From age one to four years, my son had tubes inserted four times.

"The last time he had tubes inserted, he had his adenoids removed. The doctors also felt he had an ear disease that affected his ear drum due to scar tissue from the constant ear infections, and from surgery. They thought they would have to reconstruct the ear drum. He would also have hearing loss due to the disease, they said. Throughout that time he was placed on maintenance dosages of antibiotics at bed time.

"Somehow I knew that the antibiotics had to be bad for my son but our pediatrician kept reassuring me that they were fine and that they could not hurt him. Finding out years later what damage antibiotics can create, such as candida, I was a very desperate mother.

"When your child is in so much pain and there is nothing you can do you feel so helpless as a mother because you could not make the pain go away. He would finally get some relief when his ear drum would rupture and he would have fluid-like pus draining from his ear."

I saw Brennon after he had had five years of conventional treatment. We started him on chiropractic care and a nutritional program. We recommended avoidance of all dairy.

Brennon is now earache free simply through supplements, staying off dairy, and occasional chiropractic care.

Many years ago, Robert Mendelsohn, M.D., a pioneer of alternative medicine, said that there isn't a single ear infection case that requires antibiotics and/or ear tubes. Originally, I thought he was off-base. But my experience in treating hundreds of kids and even adults confirms the validity of his statement. Just think about Brennon Meadows. Not only was his ear tube surgery unnecessary, but doctors were ready to perform "reconstructive ear surgery" on the boy. Where are we going with this kind of medical madness?

The dairy connection

Charles Attwood, M.D., a well-known pediatrician and author of "Dr. Attwood's Low-Fat Prescription for Kids" (Penguin Books, New York, 1995), echoes the opinion of many nutritionally-oriented health professionals who feel that allergy to dairy is a major cause of ear and other childhood infections.

"Dairy protein is highly allergenic," says Attwood. "I have personally observed the damaging effects of milk and dairy in 7 out of 10 of my patients for more than 35 years. It causes asthma, hayfever, eczema, sinusitis, and ear infections."

When you take kids off these products, problems clear up, says Attwood. "I have observed this hundreds, maybe thousands of times. I have been amazed over the years at the extent of benefits that occur after stopping dairy. Parents tell me that everything improves. Children don't miss school anymore. No sniffles. No colds. No congestion. No more ear infections."

How we treat ear infections

Dr. Attwood's advice on milk drinking is good. I have often found a connection to dairy consumption and ear infections, and other health problems, in youngsters. I recommend eliminating dairy from the diet. However, ear infections are certainly not limited to dairy allergy alone. I treat many breast-fed infants with ear infections whose mothers eat excellent diets.

We also look for sensitivities to grain and other common food allergens. See chapter nine. Recurrent infections — and other problems, including hyperactive behavior — may often be the result of eating allergenic foods. According to environmental illness expert Doris Rapp, M.D., "more and more individuals seem to be affected...at earlier ages because of the continued widespread chemical contamination and pollution of our food, water, and air, and our homes, schools, and workplaces."

Recurrent ear infections are signs of a weakened immune system. For this reason, we recommend the following supplements:

• Vitamin C powder, mixed in juice, is a natural anti-viral factor.

• Echinacea and goldenseal are herbs I have talked about considerably in the book. They are immune-boosting and regarded as natural antibiotics. I recommend them in the liquid glycerine-base form.

• In addition, I have had good results with Thymoglan (Thymus extract). This glandular supplement can stimulate immune function and decrease bacterial, viral and fungal infections.

• Probiotic bacteria products are natural, multiple friendly strain of bacteria. They are important for any child or adult with an antibiotic history. Probiotics replace the beneficial bacteria in the intestines destroyed by antibiotics.

• Homeopathic remedies such as aconitum 5C, especially with sudden pain, and belladonna 5C, particularly with fever, may be helpful.

There is also a popular remedy for combating ear infections topically:

• Apply garlic and mullein oil in the ear canal. You can purchase a combination product in the health food store. I recommend warming the oil slightly, then filling the ear canal. Once applied, fit a cotton ball with Vaseline or Vitamin E salve snugly into the ear canal to prevent the oil from leaking out. This home treatment can be done day or night. Garlic, used topically or orally, has known anti-viral and antibiotic effects. Mullein is a plant extract that draws fluid.

The chiropractic — ear infection connection

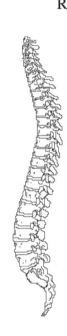

Research conducted in the U.S. and Germany has found that pediatric chiropractic manipulation can contribute to the recovery from ear infections and, more importantly, help prevent them altogether.

The so-called "atlas syndrome" refers to a misalignment of the uppermost vertebra in the neck, the so-called atlas vertebra. In Greek mythology, Atlas held up the world. In anatomy, the atlas vertebra literally "lifts up" and holds the skull in proper position.

There is considerable potential for misalignment to occur at this critical location in the body. A newborn's spine subjected to abnormal stress during birth can generate the initial misalignment that can lead to impaired sleeping, seizures, poor coordination, motor and development problems, colic, vomiting, colds, paralysis and infections.

The misalignment can also cause nerve interference that results in the tightening of a child's already narrow Eustachian tube. When this occurs, the tube loses ability to drain fluid properly from the middle ear, and the seeds of an ear infection are sown.

Manipulation to the upper neck area is often able to open the Eustachian tube and allow the body's healing mechanisms to operate normally.

G. Guttman, M.D., a German expert on the use of manipulation, has treated and reported on hundreds of cases of lowered resistance, ear infections and other problems that are helped by resolving cervical misalignments. Blocked nerve impulses at the atlas vertebra, he says, causes many problems in babies and has received far too little attention.

The preventive role of chiropractic was demonstrated in a 1989 comparative study of 200 children under chiropractic care and a similar number of youngsters treated conventionally. More than 80 percent of the medical children experienced a minimum of one ear infection episode versus only 31 percent of the chiropractic children. The latter group had a lower use of antibiotics and less incidence of other illnesses.

Brandon Juliano's case

In my clinic, the case of Brandon Juliano, 1 1/2, of Gibsonia, Pennsylvania, dramatically demonstrates the potential for

> **"The change in Brandon's personality is so dramatic he appears to be a different child."**

chiropractic care for many pediatric problems, including ear infections.

Brandon's mother, Maureen, tells his story:

"Brandon was a baby who never slept during the day unless he was held upright. He never enjoyed laying on the floor and playing with things. He hated the swing, car seat, and being held in the cradle position. He whined non-stop unless I held him upright. At four months he could hold up his head and when I put him in the exersaucer he was happy. He barely crawled before he started walking at ten months.

"I knew things were still not quite right because Brandon had five ear infections between November 1995 and March 1996. After his fifth infection, we went to see Dr. Gallagher.

"We were told that Brandon's first and second vertebrae were out causing his ears to not drain properly. This improper drainage was diagnosed as the cause of the numerous ear infections.

"After his first adjustment, I noticed a considerable change in his demeanor. He started taking naps during the day and now at 18 months he usually takes a two hour nap each day. He is happy and busy. He loves to run, jump and climb. He has even started doing somersaults.

"The change in Brandon's personality is so dramatic he appears to be a different child. Since seeing Dr. Gallagher, he has not been sick, except for a case of chicken pox. He has been exposed to numerous children with colds and has yet to come down with a cold or ear infection since treatment started."

The Newcomer girls

Debbie Newcomer, a school teacher and mother from Sewickley, Pennsylvania, had come to see me in 1993 for chronic pain and fatigue. I prescribed a regimen of

> **Chiropractic resolved not just ear infections, but fatigue and moodiness**

vitamins, herbs, whole food, and chiropractic adjustments that restored her energy and alleviated her pain.

The following year she returned with her two daughters, Annie, 14, and Sara, 9. Both had a history of ear infections since they were infants. Doctors had often prescribed antibiotics, decongestants, antihistamines, cough syrup, Tylenol and other medications for them.

Annie also suffered from chronic fatigue and sinus infections. She had been given increasingly strong antibiotics and was spending a large part of each winter in bed. After one chiropractic adjustment on her neck and mid-back, Annie's fatigue went "poof." It cleared immediately. We also put her on a program of vitamin C, zinc and spleen extract for nutritional support. She has not been bothered by infections for three years. Annie is now in college and receives maintenance treatment on her school breaks.

Younger sister Sara routinely missed school and frequently had colds, high fevers, and infections. My examination indicated a misalignment of the atlas vertebra and a need for chiropractic manipulation. The adjustments yielded some surprising results.

"We soon realized that immediately following her adjustments, there was a marked personality change from cranky and argumentative to happy and carefree," Debbie Newcomer told me. "This pattern has continued and even when Sara is ill with a cold or a virus, treatment produces an almost immediate sense of well being and improvement in her condition. The remarkable part of all this is how quickly the change is noticeable — within minutes."

Sara's changed mood was immediately noticeable to my staff and I. She would enter the treatment room moody and emerge laughing after treatment. Her elevated mood now appears to be a permanent feature. She was initially receiving weekly adjustments in the beginning and now is treated one time a month.

Sara had perfect attendance for the entire school year after she started chiropractic treatment. Like her sister, she has not taken a single antibiotic, Tylenol, or any other drug in the three years she has been under chiropractic care.

Brennon Meadows, Brandon Juliano, and the Newcomers bring home an important point. Although doctors put labels or diagnoses on symptoms and then neatly prescribe drugs or surgery to "remove" those symptoms, chiropractic and holistic healing treat the entire person. Chiropractic adjustments affect the nervous system which regulates our entire body. It is the intimate link between our body, mind and spirit.

None of the above cases were just "ear infections" alone nor did they involve neck pain or back pain. As I have said elsewhere throughout the book, back pain is not the only reason to seek chiropractic treatment.

Regardless of symptoms or lack of them, parents need to be aware of the importance of chiropractic treatment for the health and function of the body.

So many children are susceptible to illness or behavioral disorders. Antibiotics and Ritalin are not the answers. But among the real answers may be overlooked spinal misalignments.

Don't overlook your child's spinal health — or your own for that matter. Structure affects function. Function affects health. You take care of your teeth. But are you attending to your spine? Your spine is your central lifeline that contains the nerves that supply your arms and legs and vital organs and bodily functions.

For the sake of your children's best interest and optimum health, even if there are no symptoms, obtain an early chiropractic evaluation. You may spare yourself and your children much grief and expense.

Peter N. Fysh, D.C., writing in the 1990 Proceedings of the National Conference on Chiropractic and Pediatrics, called for a shift away from the conventional medical model for chronic ear infections to a new safer alternative.

"Validation of the chiropractic model as an alternative to long-term antibiotic therapy and/or tympanotomy tube insertion (surgical ear tubes) would not only help reduce the potential for hearing loss and ear drum scarring, but would also save millions of dollars in health care costs," he wrote. "The challenge is before us."

Natural Remedies for Ear Infections

- *The Gallagher Wellness Program*
- *Chiropractic cervical manipulation*
- *Identify food allergies*
- *Pulsed Diathermy to Ear (electromagnetic heat) applied directly over the ear*
- *Garlic-Mullein Ear Drops*
- *Vitamin C powder* (Directions: mix powder in juice or apple sauce. For each year of child's age, give one 500 milligram dose — one-eighth of a teaspoon. Give dosages throughout the day.)
- *Pro Echinacea/Goldenseal* .... 5-10 drops, 3 times daily
- *Thymoglan* .... 1 capsule, twice daily
- *Zinc picolinate* (Dosage: multiply age of child by 2.5 milligrams daily)
- *Probiotics (friendly multi-strain bacteria)* .... 1/2 teaspoon daily.
  Can be mixed in juice or apple sauce.

FIBROMYALGIA

About fibromyalgia

Until recently, who ever heard of fibromyalgia? Now, unfortunately, it is becoming a household word. According to the Arthritis Foundation, it is the second leading arthritis-related condition, affecting millions of Americans, and seven times more women than men.

Unlike arthritis that affects the joints and bones of the body, fibromyalgia attacks the soft tissue such as the muscles, tendons, and ligaments. Actually it is not even really a specific disease but a grouping of chronic symptoms. They can include some, but not necessarily all, of the following:

- burning, soreness, pain, and stiffness all over
- a flu-like feeling
- fatigue
- headaches
- irritable bowel
- pre-menstrual and menstrual problems
- anxiety
- depression
- intolerance to cold or damp weather.
- and insomnia, which prevents you from getting the deep rest critical to repairing your body.

Although the severity of the symptoms can wax and wane, most patients experience problems on a daily basis. Some degree of pain is always present.

Many people don't know they have fibromyalgia because it is difficult to diagnose and mimics other disorders. People may spend years seeking an accurate diagnosis.

One clue to fibromyalgia is the presence of at least 11 of 18 "tender points" on the body. These points are locations that cause pain when touched. You may not know they exist until a physician familiar with the condition applies pressure to the area.

Reports of fibromyalgia symptoms have been chronicled for a century but it was not until 1990 that the specific protocol for diagnosis was outlined. In 1992, the World Health Organization added fibromyalgia to its official list of diseases.

No one is really sure yet what precisely triggers fibromyalgia. Many patients, but not all, report having had a viral, bacterial, or parasitic infection or some kind of physical trauma such as an automobile accident, fall, or athletic injury, before the onset of symptoms.

Factors such as high sugar and high fat diets, antibiotics, steroids, birth control pills, food allergies and vitamin deficiencies may all contribute. Other possibilities include chemical sensitivities and excess toxic metals in the body.

Singularly or in combination, these stressors can trigger immune dysregulation that causes your body to attack itself. Sleeping pills and anti-depressant drugs have a negative long-term outcome on this disorder and will often lead to other drug-induced illnesses. From a conventional medicine viewpoint, there is no known cure. But alternative medicine offers both help and hope.

Carol McLean's case — 14 years on the illness treadmill

Carol McLean, 39, from Pittsburgh, lived through a horror story lasting 14 years. It started when she hurt her back, the result of lifting a half-keg of beer while doing bartending to help put herself through college. The incident landed her on disability.

> **"I wish I had found alternative medicine before I was touched surgically!"**

The medical ordeal commenced with hospitalization and traction, bone scans, cat scans, and nerve conduction testing. Her physician wasn't sure about what had occurred but said there was considerable muscle spasms and a "gray" area in the lumbar spine.

"I was sent home for bed rest with prescriptions for muscle relaxants and pain killers," Carol told me.

"A physical therapist treated me for a year but my pain and mobility were getting worse.

"I was referred to an orthopedic surgeon for a myelogram. The specialist spent 30 seconds with me after he had the results and told me there was 'nothing conclusive.' I was fine, in his opinion.

"I was referred to a rehabilitation facility at a hospital, where they applied heat packs and did little else. The doctor at rehab told me that the insurance company wanted him to sign me out of the program so I could go back to work. I could hardly walk and my pain was excruciating! He told me to 'learn to live with it.'

"Another orthopedic surgeon determined I had ruptured lumbar discs and recommended I undergo treatment at a major hospital that dealt with these kinds of problems. But after six months, there was no relief. I had bad pain, trouble standing and walking, and my legs would go numb.

"The physician suggested I have a procedure called chymopapaine injections (papaya enzyme injections) that were supposed to dissolve the protruding discs. Instead, they damaged the discs even more, and created an enormous amount of scar tissue. I was unable now to walk and the pain was so great I could not imagine living with it.

"Next, a laminectomy was performed to 'shave off' the damaged discs. Considerable scar tissue and bone tissue was removed.

"After surgery I went home to recuperate and start a rehabilitation program. But after a half-year, my pain was still out of control. It became so bad that my physician ordered an ambulance to take me to the hospital for new tests. According to the doctor, my condition was now diagnosed as arachnoiditis — scarring and inflammation of the covering of the spinal cord — which was giving me all kinds of crazy sensations and extreme pain. When I was told this, I started to cry.

"The doctor told me that I needed to come to terms with my pain and would benefit from psychiatric help. This resulted in me taking more medication. I was already taking prescriptions for the heart, high blood pressure, cholesterol, the colon, spasms and pain.

"For years I went in and out of hospitals. They did every test on me known to man. But I was not getting any better. I had become the biggest guinea pig ever. I had become depressed. And I had developed an intestinal problem that required the removal of my colon and the use of a colostomy.

"Believe it or not, this operation made me feel better in the long run. It removed the toxins that had accumulated in my colon. My skin had become grayish as a result. I felt I was going to die. So compared to that, I felt better, even though I still had my pain."

In the early 1990s, Carol began to realize that the conventional medical system would never make her well. She turned to God and prayer for help and eventually to alternative medicine for general relief. In July 1996, she decided to crawl off the medical treadmill and found her way to my office, several months after having been diagnosed with fibromyalgia.

As a result of her initial injury and subsequent treatments, Carol had many problems. She was suffering with chronic dehydration, a complication from her colon surgery; arachnoiditis, a complication from back surgery and injections into her disc; chronic neck pain and headaches; and chronic pain in the low back and legs, with numbness aggravated by any movement.

Her fibromyalgia was induced by physical trauma to her spine, muscles and discs. That in turn was followed by additional trauma from drugs and surgery.

Over the years she had taken multiple prescriptions. When I first saw her she was taking Neurontin, an anti-seizure drug, for pain control. She was also on methadone, an addictive compound with morphine-like painkilling properties that is commonly used as a substitute narcotic in the treatment of heroin addiction.

My examination revealed the presence of painful tender points throughout her muscles. She had spinal alignments at every level of her spine. She had a large scar extending from her twelfth thoracic vertebra down to the base of her spine. Drug therapy had caused a "leaky gut" and subsequent malabsorption.

Carol began a series of chiropractic manipulations three times per week, along with myotherapy, high dosages of melatonin, digestive aids, nutritional supplements designed to help repair intestinal tract damage, and intravenous administration of vitamin C and magnesium.

"My pain level has almost dropped in half, and I have started to feel like my old self again," Carol told me after several months of treatment.

Although she is permanently disabled, Carol has become increasingly functional and with much less pain. She no longer takes methadone. The Neurontin has been reduced. She is now able to sleep through the night, which she couldn't do for many years because of her pain.

Carol McLean now has a life as a result of chiropractic and nutritional treatment. She is angry at a medical system that gave her limited and painful options. She is angry because if alternative medicine was able to give her part of her life back after 14 years, she feels she might never have had to undergo the medical nightmare to begin with.

But her suffering also gave her spiritual insight. Carol is thankful that God directed her life to an awareness and participation in natural healing. She has since become a strong advocate and inspiration to others like her.

Carol says this about her experience: "Alternative medicine works. It is so much easier on the mind, body and soul. I wish I had found it before I was ever touched surgically. Just remember that it may take time to heal, because we did not get this way overnight. Our bodies need time to repair. But our bodies know what to do if given the chance and a little help and loving care. God put healing herbs and food on this earth for a reason. God knows exactly what we need and gives it to us if we ask."

Gary Kallmeyer — another 14-year treadmill case

Gary's problems started in 1977, when he was 22-years-old, with a slight pain in the heels of both feet.

> A not-so-merry-go-round of tests, antibiotics, painkillers, and anti-depressants

"Within a few months," he related, "I could not even walk without enduring severe pain in my heels. I could only take 'baby' steps that were four or six inches long." Miserable and in constant pain, Gary sought medical help in the Pittsburgh area where he lives and entered what was to become for him a 14-year medical treadmill. During this time, the severe pain spread into his fingers, arms, knees, hips, back, and then almost every joint in his body.

Gary told me he visited at least seven internists and three rheumatologists in four different cities.

"They ordered X-rays, cat scans, upper GIs, barium enemas, colonoscopies, nuclear analysis, and many other tests with names I can't remember," he said.

"I twice spent a week in a hospital for diagnoses.

"Two different doctors assumed I had a venereal disease, until they actually tested me and found out it wasn't so.

"They decided I had an 'incurable disease: arthritis.'

"They never identified the root cause of my condition.

"They prescribed various non-steroidal anti-inflammatory drugs (NSAIDs), which did provide some relief from the pain to the point I could function even though I was never pain-free.

"One internist decided I had ulcerative colitis, which was refuted by a different internist several years later."

Gary said that three different chiropractors kept him functioning with adjustments for his back pain.

By 1991, however, Gary was still having major problems and appeared to have made little headway in his quest for consistent relief.

"I had gained over 70 pounds, had developed chronic back pain, fatigue, sinus infections, constriction in almost all of my muscles, an inability to sleep most nights, and a feeling when I awoke most mornings that I had been run over by a truck," he said.

"I continued to treat my arthritis with NSAIDs and began taking significant amounts of antibiotics to fight my sinus infections. I remained active at work and in my kids' activities, but spent most of my free time sleeping in a recliner in our family room. I had no extra energy at all.

"In 1993, my condition was so bad that I spent many days at work just sitting at my desk staring at paperwork. I had no real energy to do anything at work or at home. And I hurt so bad.

"After taking more tests that I had already undergone, my physician suggested that I would be stuck taking NSAIDs the rest of my life. He recommended that I change the specific medication when it became ineffective.

"He also allowed me to take more and more antibiotics as they were less and less effective for relief of my sinus infection.

"Since I was almost in a state of physical non-function, he also prescribed an anti-depressant, amitriptyline, to help me deal with my condition. I believe this was his way of saying 'since I don't know what is physically wrong with you, it must be in your head.'

"Early in 1994, I realized that the physical aspect of my life was worse in spite of all the treatments. I made a decision to just stop them. I quit taking the NSAIDs, the antibiotics, and the anti-depressants.

"Within a week after stopping the medication, I felt better. I knew right then I was on the right track. I had, you see, been growing in the spiritual aspect of my life and had turned to God. I told Him that if He wanted me to continue to waste away to nothing and be physically worthless as I tried to raise my kids, that was in His hands. I was willing to do the best I could with however He left me."

It was around this time that Gary called to make an appointment. He was skeptical after years of the medical run-around but a friend of a friend had been through a similar ordeal and had had positive results in our clinic. The friend had recommended us.

How Gary recovered

I will let Gary describe his recovery process:

"My return to health began with interviews, observation, and diagnostics tests. The tests were definitely different. I had my range of motion, blood, saliva, and hair all tested. I had never been given the results of my tests before, much less any detailed explanations. Now I received this information and what the results meant in terms of identifying the cause of my problems.

"After evaluating the data, Dr. Gallagher recommended a plan. He told me he felt it would take at least a year-and-a-half to get my body back to where it should be. It would take that time in part just to recover from the many years of prescription drug abuse and poor diet. This seemed extraordinarily long, but after hurting for 17 years, and being told I would never be whole again, it didn't really seem that long.

"I received a lot of education to help me understand why my body was in the condition it was and how I needed to change my lifestyle to regain health.

"The treatment program began with a detox regimen and herbal/ nutritional supplements to begin attacking the candidiasis and toxins that had built up in my body. After the detox , my diet was still restricted to basically fruits, vegetables, brown rice, fish and chicken, with no dairy, sugar, or grain. When people would ask me how I could stick to that diet, I told them, 'when you hurt bad enough, it is easy to stick to this diet.'

"Some time after the detox, Dr. Gallagher began chiropractic adjustments. My body went through many changes during this process and sometimes I felt worse than ever. But Dr. Gallagher kept assuring me that this was a necessary part of the process, and encouraged me by shar- ing information about what was going on and why this process was going to be successful.

"Over the next several months, he recommended ultrasound and other electrical stimulation therapies, which did not seem to help. But I went through a Gua Sha treatment that was a marvelous cleansing process and eventually found myotherapy to be extremely helpful.

"In time, I started functioning like a human being again. I lost the 70 pounds I had gained. Almost exactly 15 months after I began treatment, my family and I went to Florida for a vacation. We spent eight days at Disney World and six at the beach, including an all day bike ride around Sanibel Island. I happened to mention to my wife that I did not think I would ever be able to enjoy the physical activity we had during that vacation.

"In 1996, my family and I skied three different times, enjoying the entire time allotted on our lift tickets with hardly any breaks at all. Prior to coming to Dr. Gallagher, I had tried skiing, but could never spend too much time on the slopes because of the pain.

"I try to stick to my diet, and for the most part I do, but I find I can enjoy small amounts of candy, cookies, cake, and ice cream without adverse affects. While I can't say I feel as good as I did in 1977, I feel as good as any 42 year old. I don't miss out on life anymore because I am too tired or hurt too bad. My muscles are still weak from almost 20 years of not being used, so I am beginning to think now about building them up.

"The treatments have given me my health back. And best of all, I have received the knowledge and tools to stay healthy. To me, the bottom line of natural health care is to enable the body to heal itself. I believe that God sent me to Dr. Gallagher to remove the obstructions in my body that kept me ill, so my body could heal itself. He did, and then I did. And I am glad."

Gary's recovery: from a clinical perspective

When Gary first consulted me, he said, "I feel like I carry another person inside of me." Most people would have given up after seeing so many specialists and would have lived on antidepressants and pain pills. But Gary prayed for help and was directed to the knowledge embodied in ancient healing systems.

I found him allergic to all gluten products (wheat, rye, oats, barley), dairy, citrus and sugar. He had misalignments in his cranium, neck, mid and low back, and hips. He had adhesions or scar tissue in his muscles. His muscles and joints hurt on movement or when touched. He was extremely toxic from his diet and drug therapy. And he was deficient in essential fatty acids and minerals.

Gary, like many of my fibromyalgia patients, had multiple causative factors that led to his diagnosis. In fibromyalgia, there is rarely one cause and one cure. It took a comprehensive healing approach to turn Gary around — chiropractic adjustments, deep muscle therapy (myotherapy), detoxification, and nutritional prescriptions. And turn around he did.

He recently traveled to remote areas of South America to carry out his missionary work. In February 1997 he told me, "I can do anything I want to do now." Not bad for a man who a few years before spent hours a day in a lounge chair, disabled, in pain, no energy, unable to move because any physical exertion made him hurt more.

Courtney Little's case

Courtney Little, a 20-year-old college student from Latrobe, Pennsylvania, is an example of a person basically cruising through life until she takes an antibiotic and then literally becomes a disease overnight.

> **"Many times I felt as if I were going to die."**

In her sophomore year of college she took Trimoxicillin, a broad-spectrum antibiotic, for an infection that developed after a tooth was pulled. Over the years she had had some back and neck pain as a result of her involvement in gymnastics, and we had helped her through chiropractic adjustments, but now, suddenly, she experienced intense pain.

"Pain started to increase very quickly," she told me two months after her symptoms began. "I had sharp pain in my stomach especially after I ate. I also experienced much anxiety and nervousness which was never severe in the past. My heart would race and my whole body would shake. I went numb on occasion from my waist down and broke into a sweat. I also lost my sense of balance and awareness of the activity around me."

Courtney said she also experienced weakness, fatigue, irritability, depression and "many times I felt as if I were going to die."

The young woman had already seen several doctors who told her the problem was totally stress-related. They had prescribed medication.

Here is a prime example of antibiotic-induced illness. The antibiotics led to a significant overgrowth of resistant bacterial and yeast strains in her body. The toxins produced by these proliferating micro-organisms adversely affected her muscles and organs. Meanwhile, her immune system became "hypervigilant" following the treatment and began reacting in an abnormal manner. As a result of antibiotics, Courtney now had fibromyalgia. She developed panic attacks, painful muscles and joints, and pain in her ribs and chest that moved to her neck, legs and arms. She couldn't sleep, exercise or pursue gymnastic and cheerleading activities. Courtney came to see me in February of 1996. We started her on a recovery program including chiropractic treatments, avoidance of allergenic foods, nutritional supplements and colonic therapy.

"I feel at least 50 percent better than when I first started," she told me six months into the program.

Courtney is not 100 percent yet, but she is recovering with natural remedies. It is a process that takes time.

The idea that natural medicine "takes longer to work" is frequently used by people who erroneously believe that drugs "cure" disease. The alternative approach "saved" Courtney from the medical treadmill. Under conventional treatment she would have been on continuous antibiotics for chronic bladder, throat and vaginal infections, Prozac for depression, and anti-anxiety drugs for panic. She would probably be taking sleeping pills for insomnia, pain pills for muscle and back pain, and cardiac medication for heart irregularities. Along with this she would have undergone endless testing and seen many specialists.

Which do you think is faster? The drugs or natural remedies? Which do you think produces side effects and more symptoms? Drugs or natural remedies?

There is no doubt in Courtney's mind. "I would probably be feeling worse than ever if I had not chosen natural health care," she told me. "Some people think this not the way to go because it involves more than just taking a pill. But people have to realize that the improvements last longer than any drug and it is worth it in the end."

How we treat fibromyalgia

Q "*I have worked in the financial field and banking for 15 years. Although my job is not physically demanding, I can barely make it through the day. I am 37-years-old and my entire body is sore, even to touch. I feel like I have arthritis all through my body. Sometimes even clothing touching my skin, or bumping into things, is extremely painful. I never seem to get a full nights sleep. I went to an internist. He diagnosed me with fibromyalgia and said to take Xanax (sleeping pills) at night and Zoloft (mood elevators) during the day. I am not a pill person, so I thought maybe natural medicine might help.*"

A I treat many cases of fibromyalgia in my clinic. Due to the severity of this problem, we recommend our comprehensive wellness program to facilitate recovery. It requires patients getting wholeheartedly behind the healing process.

Research and clinical experience have found that methods used by chiropractic physicians — spinal manipulation, exercise, dietary changes, nutritional prescriptions, physical therapies, and stress management — are often effective in helping to relieve many symptoms associated with fibromyalgia.

My recommendations include the following approaches:

• Chiropractic manipulation, especially the Activator and Thompson methods. Chiropractic care helps improve structural alignment distortions and promote drainage of stored toxins. Individuals whose symptoms appeared after a trauma may be especially benefited by manipulation, although spinal misalignments not related to trauma may also aggravate or even be a cause of symptoms.

• Physical treatments such as heat, ice, light massage, lymphatic massage and drainage techniques, Gua Sha (an ancient Chinese massage method), and warm water aerobics.

• Light stretching exercises.

• Identification of food allergies through applied kinesiology (AK) or Elisa testing is critical to defuse inflammatory reactions. Common food sensitivities include dairy, wheat and citrus products.

• Toxicity has a huge hand in this condition. For this reason, detoxification of the liver and colon is a routinely recommended starting point for most patients along with raw juice fasting and colonic hydro-therapy. See chapter six on detoxification.

• Oral intake of magnesium, calcium, manganese, bromelain, valerian root, passiflora, primrose oil, and arnica are singularly, and in combination, excellent agents against pain and inflammation.

• Useful herbal supplements include burdock root, an excellent blood purifier; milk thistle, an herbal (not a dairy product!!) known for its ability to repair liver cells; and licorice, which has natural anti-inflammatory and anti-arthritic properties.   Dandelion, alfalfa, and celery seeds are also beneficial in many cases. They have anti-arthritic properties. Turmeric, the spice that provides the typical yellow color familiar in curry dishes, has natural antibiotic effects, anti-cholesterol action, and decreases inflammation associated with fibromyalgia.

• We have made good use of German homeopathic injections at the site of fibromyalgia trigger points and intravenous vitamin therapy, especially magnesium and vitamin C.

• Lack of quality sleep is one of the most common symptoms of fibromyalgia. Using sleeping pills can cause additional side effects and for sure individuals with this condition don't need any additional symptoms to deal with. To promote sleep, we recommend melatonin, the well-known amino acid. Relaxation techniques are also beneficial for sleep and reducing symptoms.

Natural Remedies for Fibromyalgia

- *The Gallagher Wellness Program*
- *Chiropractic manipulation (Activator and Thompson methods)*
- *Lymphatic drainage*
- *Warm water aerobics*
- *Colonic irrigation*
- *Detoxification*
- *Magnesium malate (200 milligrams magnesium / malic acid 500 milligrams)* .... *1 tablet, twice daily*
- *Primrose Oil* .... *3 capsules, twice daily*
- *Milk Thistle (standardized extract)* .... *2 capsules twice daily*
- *Licorice root (standardized extract)* .... *1,000 milligrams daily*
- *Turmeric (standardized extract)* .... *100 milligrams, 3 times daily*
- *German homeopathic injections into trigger points*
- *IV vitamin infusions*

HEADACHES, MIGRAINES AND NECK ACHES

Q "*I am a migraine sufferer. I used to get them during my men strual cycle when I was in my teens and twenties, but ever since I turned 40, I have them 2-3 times a week. All the specialists have told me that it is hereditary and stress. I live on pills but nothing seems to work. I am desperate.*"

About headaches

Headache, the statistics make clear, is a major health problem that affects and disables millions of people annually. Most headaches have two primary causes — structural and/or nutritional. Whether they are of the tension or migraine variety, they are messages from your body telling you something is wrong that needs to be corrected.

The standard medical approach is to snuff out the pain — that is, stop the message — with medication ranging from common aspirin to powerful narcotics in severe cases. And while medication may indeed abort a headache or migraine and lessen its severity, it never corrects the underlying cause of the problem. Pain pills may, in fact, create new problems and undesirable side effects, including more headaches!

It is now estimated that up to 70 percent of all headaches and migraines may be induced by the same drugs that are supposed to stop it. Let us recall the admonishment of the ancient chiropractic physician Hippocrates who said, "First do no harm."

According to Seymour Diamond, M.D., executive director of the National Headache Foundation, common analgesics such as aspirin, acetaminophen and ibuprofen can cause what is called "analgesic rebound effects" when taken in excess.

Quoted in The Oregonian (November 22, 1993), Diamond said that this effect is similar to a chemical dependency. The body becomes accustomed to an analgesic for the relief of pain, so it starts to produce headaches in order to receive an ever larger dosage of the painkiller.

In the same article, Robert Ford, M.D., of the Ford Headache Clinic in Birmingham, Alabama, said that as many as 60 to 70 percent of headache patients are victims of analgesic rebound.

The experts say your headaches may be associated with

these effects if:

- they develop almost every day.
- they are present when you awake and last most of the day, varying in intensity.
- pain is mild to moderate.
- you take over-the-counter painkillers at least twice a week or every second day and for at least a month.

Such headaches are said to be between 5 and 12 times more common in women because more women suffer from chronic headaches.

Facts on headaches

- *15 to 20 percent of men and 25 to 30 percent of women will suffer at least one migraine episode during their lifetime (Scientific American, 1987).*
- *More than 10 million Americans (4 percent) experience moderate to severe disability from different forms of headaches (Journal of the American Medical Association, 1992).*
- *The prevalence of migraines increased by nearly 60 percent during the decade from 1980 to 1989! In 1980, an estimated 26 out of a thousand persons were affected. By 1989, the number was up to 41 per thousand.*
- *The greatest increase has involved women under 45 years of age (Headache, 1993).*
- *In 1974, 15 percent of 7-year-old children suffered from headaches, and 2 percent from migraines. In 1992, the numbers were 52 percent and 6 percent respectively (Headache, 1996).*

How to tell one headache from another

More than 90 percent of headaches are so-called primary headaches, that is, they are not related to an underlying disease process. They are categorized into tension, migraine, and cluster headaches.

Not that it will give you any relief, but the following will help you put a label on your suffering:

Tension type

Dull pain, bilateral (both sides) pain, no nausea, mild/moderate pain, steady pain, mild light and sound sensitivity, frequent headaches that are long-lasting, able to exercise with headaches. You can "live with it."

Migraines

Sharp, severe, throbbing and unilateral pain, nausea, extreme light and sound sensitivity, usually infrequent, short-lived headaches, exertion makes worse. Migraines are often disabling.

Cluster headaches

Extremely painful to the point of incapacitation, occurring in a series or cluster over a period of weeks or months and then disappearing for variable lengths of time. Primarily affect men over 40. Are of short duration, usually less than one hour, and located in the region of the temple on one side. They often wake the individual in the middle of the night. Alcohol and tobacco can trigger attacks.

The chiropractic — headache / neck pain connection

According to a 1994 survey of Consumer Reports readers, headache was the health condition associated with the highest level of medical treatment dissatisfaction — nearly 25 percent.

And, according to the famous 1993 Harvard study on alternative medicine in the U.S., 27 percent of headache patients seek treatment other than conventional medicine. Most frequently, the study said, they go to chiropractors.

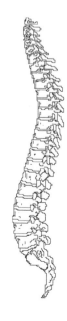

My sincere recommendation is to follow the example of these wise patients and seek a skilled chiropractor for an evaluation. There's a good chance you may find lasting relief. Many headaches originate from misalignments in the cervical (neck) spine, which conventional physicians are not trained to recognize or treat. A number of scientific studies have linked the neck to headaches. In fact, according to one authority, Craig Nelson, D.C., of the Northwestern College of Chiropractic in Minneapolis, the cervical spine of chronic headache patients is functionally different from non-headache sufferers. This dysfunction is capable of generating both head and neck pain.

We tend to overlook our neck unless it pains us. In fact, there is an anonymous poem that goes like this:

> *Alas, that pain unpleasant*
> *proclaims your neck is present.*

The neck does more than just connect your head and body. It is a vital body part. It carries great blood vessels that supply the blood to your brain. Below your skull, the spinal cord emanates downward through the neck containing the nerves that control your body. The neck also contains the pipelines that carry oxygen into the lungs and food into the digestive tract.

What concerns chiropractors the most are those seven neck bones called the cervical spine. They are no thicker than a bamboo shoot and yet they hold aloft the 10-pound weight of your head with all its heavy thoughts.

A supporting company of discs, muscles and ligaments helps the bones carry the load. Together, they facilitate the marvelous mobility that enables you to do all kinds of things that other animals can't do.

The discs are like rubbery pads between the vertebral bones of the neck and the back and serve as shock absorbers. They also cushion much of the bending action of the neck. The neck muscles and ligaments hold the bones and discs in alignment, much like a tent pole is held erect by ropes.

There are many ways this efficient arrangement becomes unhealthy. Misalignments in the neck are a great — and generally overlooked — source of grief. Misalignments, also known as subluxations in the chiropractic profession, are generated by trauma at birth and throughout life by mishaps, falls, and the way we sit, sleep, work and walk. They result in an endless array of symptoms for which the conventional medical system rolls out its standard tools of drugs, surgery, and physical therapy. Rarely, do they correct the underlying cause. Often, they cause more problems.

In the case of neck pain, I have had multiple cases of patients, who, before they came to see me, had been told they should have surgery because of poor response to medication and/or physical therapy for their neck, arm and hand pain, numbness and tingling sensations.

Over the years, such patients have been told by their medical doctors they need surgery because:

- "You have a herniated disc."
- "You have a calcium deposit (neck spur)."
- "Your discs are degenerated (or dissolving)."
- "Your neck is filled with arthritis."
- "Your bones are deteriorating."
- "You have a congenital problem in your bone structure."
- "You have a narrowing of your spinal canal."
- "You have a narrowing of the opening where your nerves come out."

Most of these diagnoses are now termed "garbage can diagnosis" because medical doctors are unfamiliar with spinal misalignments. Although caring and concerned about the well-being of their patients, M.D.s unwittingly advise them that the cause of their problem is arthritis, spurs and degeneration and the patient then begins a journey of drug treatments and invasive medical procedures that often makes things worse.

The majority of these diagnoses have been proven inaccurate as the cause of pain. These patients should be referred to a chiropractor. Fortunately, there is a trend of increasing cooperation between medical physicians and chiropractic physicians. Hopefully, this will result in more head and neck pain patients receiving a chiropractic evaluation.

Often we can relieve the pain, numbness, and tingling, along with many other symptoms caused by subluxations in the neck, through adjustments that restore normal vertebral alignment and movement.

The reason to see a chiropractic physician if you have headache or neck pain is not because of the pain alone. That may be just one symptom of misalignment. Others may include blurred vision, ringing in the ears, sinus and ear infections, post nasal drip, dizziness and lightheadedness, mood swings, problems remembering and concentrating, and mental confusion.

In 1995, a patient came to me who said he felt like a sailor on a storm-tossed ship. This patient, a man in his late 40s, said he never felt as if his feet were on the ground. He always felt imbalanced, lightheaded and dizzy. He had gone through exhausting medical and neurological exams. Following 60 days of chiropractic manipulation to the upper part of the neck, his equilibrium returned.

Scientific studies have validated the effectiveness of chiropractic manipulation for head and neck pain sufferers. Howard Vernon, D.C., dean of research at the Canadian Memorial Chiropractic College in Toronto, investigated the phenomenon of headaches and migraines and found that manipulation was successful in 80 percent of the cases.

According to a review of the medical literature by Vernon, studies have shown that patients with chronic head and neck pain achieve a "highly significant reduction in self reports of pain" and as much as a 90 cent reduction in the use of medication when they were switched from medication and physical therapy to chiropractic care, trigger point treatments, relaxation methods, and specific home strengthening exercises (Journal of Manual Medicine, 1991)

A 1996 study at the University of Colorado compared the effectiveness of chiropractic adjustments with Tylenol (acetaminophen) among patients with chronic neck pain. Specifically, the researchers analyzed the effects of manipulation to 500 milligrams of acetaminophen taken four times daily. Thirty-five patients, with neck pain for an average of 10 years, visited one of 24 community chiropractors and received 12 manipulations over a 6 week period. Thirty-four patients, the comparison group, visited a nurse and received the medication. After six weeks, chiropractic patients reported significant improvements in neck pain and function (better range of motion and strength) compared to the pill-takers, who reported no real changes. A continuing follow-up was being conducted to determine if the results were long lasting (Family Practice News, June 1, 1996)

The first-ever controlled study comparing the effectiveness of chiropractic to drug therapy for chronic tension headache was reported in 1995. In this six-week-long experiment, P. D. Boline, D.C., and several colleagues at the Northwestern College of Chiropractic randomly assigned 150 headache patients into two groups, one receiving manipulation and the other receiving amitryptyline, an antidepressant medication frequently prescribed for headaches.

The drug reduced pain somewhat more effectively. However, it generated side effects, including dry mouth, drowsiness, and weight gain, in 82 percent of the participating patients. No side effects were reported by the patients who were manipulated, other than slight neck stiffness during the first two weeks by a small percentage of the group.

The superior value of manipulation became apparent when the patients were evaluated four weeks after treatment was terminated. At that time, the manipulation group documented a reduction of 42 percent in headache frequency, 32 percent in intensity, and 30 percent in usage of over-the-counter medication. The amitryptyline group scored an improvement of only 6 percent or less in these measured categories (Journal of Manipulative and Physiological Therapeutics, 1995).

Other studies also indicate favorable results from chiropractic treatment:

• Twenty-six patients with chronic headaches were found to have neck misalignments. After manipulation, 24 out of 26 experienced significant reduction in severity and frequency of pain (Journal of Manipulative and Physiological Therapeutics, 1994).

• Studies by Parker in 1978 and 1980 found that chiropractic manipulation was effective in the management and cure of common and classical migraine (Australian Journal of Medicine, 1980).

• In a 1995 study in Italy, spinal manipulation achieved major reduction in the amount of pain and the use of medication in headaches generated by cervical misalignments. The eight week study showed manipulation was effective during the treatment period (weeks 1-4) and the follow-up period (weeks 5-8) (Journal of the Neuromusculoskeletal System, 1995).

• Karel Lewit, a Czech neurologist who uses manipulation in his practice, reported that of a total of 57 children with migraine, 48 had excellent results after manipulative therapy ("Manuelle Therapie," J.A. Barth, Leipzig, 1973).

The safety factor

If you are concerned about the safety of chiropractic neck adjustments compared to medication and surgery, just consider the following analysis conducted by the RAND Corporation:

• **Chiropractic manipulation**

Vertebrobasilar accident (stroke): 1.46 per million

Major impairment: .639 per million

• **Cervical spine surgery**

Neurological complication: 15,600 per million

Death: 6,900 per million

• **Non-steroidal anti-inflammatory drugs (NSAIDs, such as Advil, Nuprin, Motrin, etc)**

Serious gastrointestinal side effect for people of all ages: 1,000 per million

Serious gastrointestinal side effect for people 65 and over: 3,200 per million

In another published safety analysis, researchers found that cervical manipulation for neck pain is 100 to 400 times safer than the use of NSAIDs (Journal of Manipulative and Physiological Therapeutics, 1995).

A word on degeneration

People with neck pain are often told by their doctors that their problems are caused by degeneration. Degeneration may indeed be involved. In fact, almost everyone has some degeneration in the fifth or sixth cervical (neck) vertebra who is over the age of 40. By 60, degenerative changes are present in approximately 80 percent of the population.

However, the degeneration is not the cause of the pain. Rather the degeneration is a result of the misalignment. Let me explain.

The misalignment causes loss of motion of the joint. This "locks" out normal nerve and blood supply to the site, and that causes degeneration <u>and</u> pain.

You have to get the joint working normally again. Drugs won't do it. Surgery won't do it. Exercise won't do it. Usually, only a series of manipulations will restore normal motion.

Once normal motion is re-established, then rehabilitative exercise is next. But not before. If you do the physical therapy and strengthening exercises before you re-create normal motion, than you are just setting up a vicious cycle of pain and damage.

Sometimes the reason for the neck pain has nothing to do with the neck. Rather, it may be related to misalignments of the first and second thoracic vertebrae, the first joints below the neck.

Here's how to tell if that is the case:

Sit down and try to fully extend your neck back so you can look directly up to the ceiling. Simply try to lift your chin upward and as you do look at the ceiling. Can you do it without pain?

If you can't do that without pain, and without moving any other part of your back, or arching your low back, than your problem is likely in those spinal joints of the upper back.

I often encounter people with numbness and tingling in their arms and hands. It would appear to be a neck misalignment. But it may be related to mechanically-locked rib joints or the vertebrae between the shoulder blades.

Chiropractic physicians can sort out problems like this with what is called motion palpation, that is, a hands-on process that evaluates the movement of each vertebral segment.

Trouble in vagus

Two of the most common trouble spots along the spinal cord are at opposite ends — the upper neck and the lower back.

At the upper end, misalignments in the first two neck vertebrae can aggravate the vagus nerve, an extremely important piece of electrical wiring that has nothing to do with Las Vegas but a lot to do with your health.

The vagus nerve (latin, for "the wandering nerve") supplies critical organs throughout your body — the vocal cords, heart, lungs, digestive organs, urinary bladder and the reproductive system. The nerve originates in the lower brain and leaves the skull through a small opening near the joints of the first neck vertebrae.

Misalignments in this area, technically called "upper cervical vertebral subluxation complex," can trigger a vast and bewildering array of symptoms throughout the body.

Chiropractic treatment can correct these misalignments, and clear up symptoms, in a vast majority of cases.

Linda Benninger's migraine case

Ever since she was an adolescent, Linda Benninger suffered from migraines. Now, at age 50, this medical office assistant was desperate for relief from the relentless pounding which had become more intense and more frequent with the years.

> **The doctors said she had inherited migraines and told her to learn to live with them**

"In the beginning, I just took aspirin," she told me. "In high school and college I used Darvon. Later I took Fiorinal, Ergostat and Cafergot. These all helped for a little while, but caused other symptoms, and did nothing for the cause of the migraines."

By the time she was 43, she said, she was having headaches three or four times a week.

"I was taking Sudafed and Ibuprofen every night before bedtime to avoid getting up with a headache, and then again several times during the day, often needing Cafergot as well," Linda said. Cafergot is a stronger, caffeine-like medication.

But nothing stopped the migraines. The doctors told her she had inherited them. Her mother, her mother's father, along with her three sisters also suffered migraines.

"I was told to learn to live with it," she said. Each week she spent a day or two in bed in a dark room with such intense pain that it was impossible for her to move or even open her eyes without vomiting.

In September of 1993, Linda brought her son to my clinic for an allergy problem and happened to mention her migraine condition. I suggested to her that chiropractic could help in the treatment of migraines.

Linda made an appointment and we embarked on a chiropractic and nutritional program.

"Dr. Gallagher knew that migraines ran in my family but he never once told me that I had to live with them," Linda told my nurse after one of her appointments.

For sure she did not. Holistic health care holds much promise for Linda and most migraine sufferers.

"After the first two weeks of adjustments I wasn't needing drugs during the day," Linda recalls. "I decided to try eliminating them at bedtime. It was a success! I went for several weeks migraine-free! Before long, I discovered that when a migraine was coming on, a chiropractic adjustment would abort it before it got serious."

Nutritionally, we designed a supplement program specific for Linda's needs. We also eliminated foods from her diet which appeared to be insulting her system. They included white flour, refined sugar, dairy products and caffeine.

"Whenever I got a migraine, Dr. Gallagher would quiz me on what I had eaten and this resulted in the elimination of other foods, especially those containing yellow dyes, such as dairy products and cheese," Linda says.

Linda became a label reader. She bought natural cookbooks and learned to prepare food differently for her family. This action turned out to be a major success for her.

There was another benefit for Linda "going natural." In August of 1993 she had weighed 267 pounds. After two months of chiropractic treatment and nutritional modifications, she had lost 30 pounds. She kept losing about two pounds a week. Nine months later, she had lost 90 pounds.

Then the loss slowed down and stopped. Linda was concerned. But there was no need. It was merely a temporary plateau. We made a minor change in the diet and she started shedding weight again.

By the middle of 1995, Linda was down to 150 pounds. Working out on Cybex exercise equipment has enabled her to trim down and tone up and generate major improvement to her cardiovascular health.

Today, jokes Linda, "I am half the person I used to be. I gave away all those oversized T-shirts and tent dresses. I wear shorts and jeans with T-shirts that fit, and dresses that don't hide my shape."

Health-wise, she is a much different person.

"Migraines are a thing of the past," she says. "I no longer lose days of my life and I don't take medication. I've only had two migraines this year and we were able to trace both to the cause. One time it was a food allergy. The other time a neck misalignment. I now have energy that even I don't believe. I have a full-time job along with my full-time family."

The process has been a great learning experience for Linda who now controls her health — as well as helping members of her family. "I've learned how chiropractic adjustments and nutritional prescriptions (vitamins, minerals, herbs and homeopathics) can be used to handle normal family medical problems, and how a healthy body can fight off illness without using drugs like antibiotics and antihistamines."

Linda also discovered that regardless of whatever food, chemical or neck stressor brought on a migraine, chiropractic manipulation would stop it within one hour of the treatment. This is a much better alternative to drugs, emergency rooms and suffering.

Judith Walker's case of severe headaches

Judith Walker, R.N., 54, of Ford City, Pennsylvania, came to see me with great reluctance. I had helped her husband but she didn't think that I had the goods to help her.

> **She didn't believe chiropractic could help her, but happily, she was wrong**

Judith was a school nurse with many years of experience and knowledge of conventional medicine. She had obtained advanced degrees in her profession and had, as she told me, "a certain antagonism toward chiropractic care."

In 1994, she developed severe headaches, along with sharp pain in a thumb joint and in one knee. The joint conditions were restricting her range of motion."

Judith lived with her pain, along with medication prescribed by several medical doctors.

"I was extremely fearful about having my head and neck adjusted and I was angry at my husband for pushing me into this appointment, and most of all I was so miserable and in pain that I just didn't care anymore," she said after our first appointment. "But I definitely needed relief from the pain to function at work and at home."

Judith's problem was an upper neck misalignment. In addition, her thumb was misaligned! That's right. Fingers can and do misalign.

Chiropractic adjustments solved both problems.

Judith, like many nurses and medical doctors, received disinformation during medical training about chiropractic. She believed that chiropractic manipulation would harm her and she justified her attitude by recalling the unfounded warnings of her teachers and medical co-workers.

This is a travesty that affects not only the American public at large, but doctors and nurses who desperately need chiropractic treatment just like the patients they have misdirected for decades.

After a recent treatment, Judith said to me, "You know, it's been 15 months since I started here. I rarely have a headache. My thumb is functioning at 100 percent efficiency and my right knee is at 90 percent efficiency."

"How do you feel about chiropractic now?" I asked her.

"I have to admit," she said, "that after studying the concepts, seeing my husband's transformation, experiencing my personal treatment plan, and discovering freedom from my symptoms, I am a believer!"

Perhaps the most acute case of migraine I have ever treated also involved a nurse who had to be brought to the clinic laying down in the back seat of her friend's car. If she sat up, her migraine was so intense that she spontaneously vomited.

I reviewed her history while she laid flat on her back on an examination table. She told me that she had been suffering with migraines daily for a month.

I proceeded to examine her and found the problem to be a misaligned "atlas" vertebra. The 'atlas" is the first vertebra in the neck and is often the site of problems, so much so that chiropractors refer to them as "the atlas syndrome."

Following an x-ray analysis the suffering nurse received a chiropractic manipulation. We had her return daily for the next two days. On the third day I walked into the treatment room and there she sat — smiling. Following her second chiropractic adjustment, the migraine was completely relieved.

Migraines are frequently related to neck misalignment. But unfortunately many people drug their migraines and go to medical specialists who do cat scans and MRIs. They fail to look at the neck where the real cause of the problem often lies. Neck manipulation will usually resolve the problem. Moreover, studies are finding that both cat scans and MRIs are expensive procedures that cost a great deal and yield little diagnostic value for headaches.

Tammy Worley, a female patient from Butler, Pennsylvania, came to my office in 1996 because of daily migraines. They had become so intolerable that they changed her personality. She became extremely moody and depressed. She had been to multiple medical specialists who gave her diagnoses of migraines and tension headaches and placed her on various drugs.

Following three chiropractic manipulations on the upper part of her neck, in conjunction with our detoxification diet, her migraines were totally stabilized.

Charlotte Brougher's neck pain

Charlotte, a 51-year-old homemaker from Somerset, Pennsylvania, came to see me for relief from escalating neck and arm pain which she said had developed after a major cleanup in the basement of her home.

She complained of severe pain in the right shoulder, swelling of the upper arm and forearm, and

> **Rescued from a snare of conflicting diagnoses, pain and discomfort**

burning and numbness down into the fingers. The pain was constant, day and night.

"I went to a local chiropractor and had three adjustments with no relief at all," she said. "I went to my family doctor and he treated me with anti-inflammatory medications and ordered cat scans of the shoulder, X-rays, bone scans, MRIs of both shoulders and upper arm, and mammography. All showed nothing amiss. I was also having pain starting in the left shoulder and arm, and sharp pain in the back of the knees and legs. I saw an orthopedic doctor who told me it was not an orthopedic problem. Next, I went to a neurologist at a Pittsburgh hospital.

"New symptoms were starting to occur. I was having a burning and pulling sensation of my tongue. I was extremely upset. I have a sister with multiple sclerosis. The neurologist stated that I did not have the MS nor a neurological problem. He did order an MRI of the head to reassure me that I did not have the MS.

"My family doctor called me with the results and informed me that I had a herniated disc of the neck. I was then referred to a neurosurgeon who stated that I did not have a disc problem. My family doctor said there was only one option left and that is to see a rheumatoid arthritis doctor, which I declined. I was feeling very hopeless and did not know where to turn at that time. I was started on Xanax by my family doctor for anxiety."

Around this time Charlotte happened to have conversations with two acquaintances who were patients of mine. She decided to make an appointment.

Her main problems were related to neck and mid-back misalignments that had become chronic. Precise chiropractic manipulation resolved her problems and removed the pain and discomfort from her life. We also recommended a nutritional and exercise program for her.

"I am doing so much better and I am finally pain-free," Charlotte told me a year after starting a wholistic program. "I have a normal life again. The pain in my knees and legs stopped shortly after treatment began and the problem with my tongue stopped two weeks after starting the recommended vitamins. I have regained much of the use of my arms again."

Charlotte is now functioning normally as a result of chiropractic and nutritional therapy. Her case points out the need for second or even third chiropractic opinions. She had a misalignment problem but required a different approach to solve it.

Marjorie Torrance's "atlas syndrome" case

Marjorie, 52, came to see me with many problems that turned out to be neck-related. She has the "atlas syndrome," a misalignment of the top vertebra in the neck, just under the skull bone. This led to decreased blood flow to the brain. Because her brain and nervous system were not receiving adequate oxygen and nutrients due to the misalignment, she

> **"When my neck is out of place I have a hard time functioning."**

experienced disturbances to the normal functioning of her eyes, ears, nose, throat, and brain.

"When my neck is out of place I have a hard time functioning," she says. "I feel like I have a serious illness. All the energy is drained from my body. I fall asleep very easily and could sleep forever. There is a lot of pressure in my head. It feels as if there are weights on my head. My eyes feel strange and I have a hard time focusing them. After an adjustment my energy returns and I feel much better. I can see better, too. It is unbelievable what your neck does to you. I never thought it was possible."

Today, Marjorie enjoys good health through regular chiropractic care.

Elizabeth Milcheck's TMJ case

Elizabeth, a 66-year-old homemaker from North Huntington, Pennsylvania, had been a patient for more than five years when she made an appointment to see me for a medical problem that arose after dental surgery.

> **A case of trigeminal neuralgia and TMJ....."yawning, chewing and swallowing were unbearable."**

She told me that about two weeks after surgery, she started to develop swelling, along with extreme pain, on the entire left side of her face. The pain was intolerable, causing her to take up to six pain pills a day.

"Several trips to the oral surgeon were fruitless," she said. "He prescribed penicillin and stronger pain pills, and treated me for a dry socket and possible infection. He suggested that I see my family physician who prescribed stronger antibiotics and pain pills with a suggestion of an MRI and possibly a neurologist."

"I came here instead," Elizabeth told me.

My impression was that Elizabeth's neck and jaw were misaligned as a result of the mechanical pulling of the tooth during dental surgery. This led to trigeminal neuralgia, an exquisitely painful condition of the face, jaw, teeth and cheeks. Her problems was corrected with chiropractic manipulation of the neck and jaw.

Unfortunately, dentists and family doctors, unaware of the relation-ship of structural misalignments to facial, jaw and neck pain, could only offer her medication and tests.

"After 10 visits, I am taking no pain medication," Elizabeth said. "I still have residual soreness, which is tolerable. I am confidant that after a few more treatments, I will be completely healed."

Elizabeth's confidence was rewarded. She was soon pain-free with no residual problem.

Temporomandibular Joint Syndrome (TMJ)

TMJ problems such as Elizabeth's are seen routinely by chiropractors.

TMJ stands for temporomandibular joint. In case you are not familiar with the name, it is the very important joint where the temporal bone of your skull attaches to your jaw, or mandible. Just place a fingertip in front of either ear and wiggle your jaw. You'll feel an opening that changes shape. According to the American Dental Association, nearly 30 percent of Americans have TMJ problems, called TMJ Dysfunction or TMJ Syndrome. Among the symptoms are severe headache; loss of hearing; tinnitus (ringing in the ears); shoulder, cheek, jaw, or tooth pain; and nausea and dizziness. TMJ affects more women than men.

Refer to the TMJ section in the tinnitus chapter on how to do a simple test on your own to determine if your TMJ is misaligned.

Among the most common causes of TMJ Syndrome are poorly fitting braces, poor dental work and trauma. A 1987 study reported that "a child may fall on its sacrum and in time, through the adaptive body mecha-nisms, the pelvic imbalance will affect the mandible, head and neck."

Thus, spinal problems and TMJ Syndrome can often be related.

Chiropractic care may help you avoid TMJ surgery. Surgery should not be done until chiropractic and proper dental support is provided with the exception of a tumor, fracture or serious joint pathology.

In the interest of better patient care, chiropractors and dentists are beginning to work together to ensure jaw-skull-spinal health. Chiropractic should be explored by all TMJ sufferers.

How we treat headaches and neck pain

At our clinic, we look first for neck and TMJ misalignments and perform chiropractic adjustments accordingly. Resistant headache cases referred to our offices by other chiropractic physicians often have food sensitivities or nutritional deficiencies as a contributing factor.

Obviously, there are many causes for headaches other than joint misalignments and optimum treatment can really only occur when physicians consider all possibilities through a multi-disciplinary approach.

Diet and lifestyle factors are commonly linked to migraines and headaches. They include:

- Food sensitivities
- Too much or too little sleep.
- Excessive rigorous exercise.
- Missed meals.
- Bright lights.
- Loud noises.
- Strong odors.
- Emotional stress.

Food sensitivities, at the top of the list, often includes dairy products, wheat, chocolate, eggs, citrus products, red wine, chemical preservatives and food dyes. Researchers dispute the exact percentage, but suggest that anywhere from 20 to 90 percent of migraines may be linked to allergy/sensitivity factors.

In one landmark study conducted by Joseph Egger, M.D., of the Hospital for Sick Children in London, severe migraines in youngsters were strongly related to food allergies. By eliminating offending foods, nearly all of the study's 88 migraine sufferers experienced dramatic relief (and not only from migraines, but other ailments as well).

Typical of food allergy cases, most of the youngsters were sensitive to more than one type of food. Also typical was the finding that they were allergic to their favorite foods.

Severe cases of daily headaches and migraines will often need our comprehensive program that includes detoxification and food allergy elimination (see chapter six on detoxification and chapter nine on food, chemical and environmental sensitivities).

If hypoglycemia (low blood sugar) is involved, as it often is, we structure a diet built around small, frequent and nutritious meals devoid of refined carbohydrates (sugar). Please refer to the chapter on hypoglycemia.

We design a nutritional supplement program to address the particular nutrient needs of the individual. The program will often include extra magnesium, which is a natural blood vessel relaxant, vitamin B6, particularly for those with "menstrual migraines," Lyzyme, a natural lithium supplement which helps cluster headaches, and primrose or borage oils, which reduce inflammation.

Herbal remedies include capsaicin capsules or nasal ointments; Feverfew, a common botanical used in Europe to prevent migraines; and Ginger, which has a traditional history in China for aiding in the relief of nausea, vomiting, and motion sickness.

Natural Remedies for Migraines

- *The Gallagher Wellness Program*
- *Chiropractic cervical manipulation*
- *Cranial chiropractic/TMJ manipulation*
- *Remove allergenic foods*
- *Magnesium aspartate* .... 500-1000 milligrams
- *Vitamin B-6* .... 25-50 milligrams daily
- *Lithium chelate* .... 50-250 micrograms daily
- *DEPA* .... 1,000-2,000 milligrams daily
- *Feverfew (standardized extract)* .... 1,000-2,000 milligrams daily
- *Progest Cream (Progesterone)* .... 1/4 tspoon transdermally
between ovulation and menses

Natural Remedies for Neck Pain/Tension Headaches

- *The Gallagher Wellness Program*
- *Chiropractic cervical manipulation*
- *Cranial chiropractic/TMJ*
- *Trigger point therapy*
- *Stretching/relaxation exercises*

HEARTBURN
ESOPHAGEAL REFLUX AND HIATAL HERNIA

Tell a physician you have a metallic taste or an acidic, burning-like sensation in the mouth, sometimes shortness of breath, perhaps even asthmatic symptoms, pain in the stomach and esophagus, and you are likely to receive a prescription for Zantac, an antacid and anti-ulcer medication.

That's what happened to Ted Zalac, 61, from Youngstown, Ohio. His doctor diagnosed him with esophageal reflux and wanted to suppress the production of stomach acid. Just so Ted wouldn't worry about it, the doctor also prescribed Xanax, a tranquilizer, to be taken as needed.

Ted wasn't satisfied with this approach, so he came to see me.

You may not have heard the term esophageal reflux. Heartburn may be more familiar. In any case, one of the symptoms of esophageal reflux, a quite common condition, is heartburn. The tube that carries food from your mouth down to your stomach is called the esophagus. A reflux condition means that acid from the stomach migrates upward into the esophagus and sometimes as far "north" as your mouth. This can occur with or without a weakness in the valve that separates the bottom of the esophagus from the stomach. Inflammation and bleeding in the esophagus can result.

Symptoms usually develop within an hour of eating. They include heartburn, a burning sensation in the area of the heart that is sometimes misinterpreted as a heart attack, belching, and discomfort after eating.

Esophageal reflux is often associated with the presence of a hiatal hernia, a bulge of the stomach up through an opening in the muscular diaphragm that separates the abdomen from the chest.

In Ted Zalac's case, an extensive evaluation pointed to a number of problems. He had sensitivities to certain foods, was not digesting his food properly, had spinal subluxations of his neck and mid-back contributing to digestive upsets, and also had a hiatal hernia.

There was no one single "cure" for Ted's problems. He went on a comprehensive program that included a special diet to eliminate food allergens, supplementation with digestive enzymes, magnesium to relax the esophagus, aloe vera juice to help to repair the stomach lining, and chiropractic manipulation of the neck and back. In some cases, each one of these remedies is often effective.

Following this multiple approach, Ted completely stabilized and become asymptomatic. He was able to discontinue his drugs.

Linda Kohut, a 44-year-old Pittsburgh medical secretary, suffered from esophageal reflux for more than five years. Also like Ted, she had a history of hiatal hernia. Her problem started in 1990 when she first experienced severe back and chest pain, and heartburn, upon walking. Under the care of a gastroenterologist, Linda underwent a series of tests and was given a variety of medications.

"Two years of still not feeling better, I went to another gastroenterologist who put me on some different medications, Propulsid, Axid and Zoloft, which helped a little more," she told me. During this time, Linda also developed depression.

Two friends of Linda's recommended our clinic and reluctantly she made an appointment. "How could a chiropractor help me?" she admitted to me. Remember, she was a medical secretary.

Linda went through a comprehensive diagnostic workup and started a regimen of detox, weight loss, nutrition, Cybex and chiropractic adjustments.

In her own words: "The results were amazing. I went on a detoxification diet for the first two weeks and then a nutritional program. Within six weeks, I lost the 15 pounds I needed to lose. Gradually, my body started feeling better, with more energy, improved complexion, and less depression."

After six months, Linda said she went back to her gastroenterologist for a follow-up. "He was amazed at how I looked," she told me.

Many individuals like Linda, with chronic digestive upsets, are treated conventionally with anti-ulcer drugs, medication known to contribute to depression as a side effect.

Following the dietary changes, chiropractic manipulations, and nutritional therapies, Linda was able to eliminate her medication, which in turn also helped overcome the depression. The fact that she also felt better physically helped dispel her depression. Many people stuck on the medical treadmill find themselves staying sick, and if you stay sick long enough, it is inevitable that even a very cheerful person becomes depressed.

Chiropractic — An amazing remedy for hiatal hernia

During my many years in practice, I have helped thousands of patients with hiatal hernia, esophageal reflux, and related problems. Many of them were deeply concerned about their health because such disorders often generate chest pain, pressure and cardiac irregularity, as well as throat tightness, difficulty digesting and the appearance of an ulcer. Conventional medicine has no real solutions, but chiropractic and nutritional therapies may provide the otherwise elusive solutions. I strongly urge anyone with these type of problems to obtain a chiropractic evaluation.

I have had several dramatic cases involving hiatal hernia. The most memorable occurred in my first years of practice and involved a petite woman who belched continually, loudly and uncontrollably. She had had the problem for months. She had been extensively tested by gastrointestinal specialists and advised to have an "exploratory" operation to get at the source of the problem. As a last resort, she came to my clinic. I remember hearing this suffering, embarrassed lady belching about every one or two minutes in the waiting room as she waited to see me. My examination showed two misaligned vertebrae in the mid-back (thoracic spine). I administered a spinal manipulation and, additionally, a hiatal hernia adjustment.

The belching stopped immediately.

"Thank God," she said.

That was nearly 20 years ago. She hasn't had a problem since. Today, at age 80, I see her for routine checkups and maintenance and she is doing fine.

Her suffering ceased because hiatal hernia is a mechanical problem related to misaligned spinal vertebrae in the mid-back. As I have said throughout this book, misalignments can cause all sorts of misery in the body, not just pain. Mid-back misalignments can irritate the nerves supplying the stomach and diaphragm. This can result, among other possibilities, that the stomach pushes up into the diaphragm, creating mid-back pain and the other symptoms I have described above.

Chiropractic adjustments realign the mid-back vertebrae. A specific hiatal hernia adjustment frees the bulge of the stomach trapped inside the diaphragm. The adjustment involves a light touch on the area of soft tissue just below the breast bone. Patients usually experience instant relief with these remarkable adjustments. The release is somewhat akin to removing a cork from an inverted champaign bottle. And indeed the results give many patients a just cause for celebration!

Helpful tips

- Avoid alcoholic and caffeine-containing drinks (coffee, teas, colas).
- Avoid rich and seasoned foods, and particularly foods that appear to increase symptoms.
- Avoid large meals. Instead, eat 4-5 small meals instead.
- Eat slowly.
- Lose weight. Sometimes symptoms vanish below a certain weight.
- Avoid smoking.

Q "*I am a 56 year old man with a 15-year history of high blood pressure. Over the years, my doctor has tried me on a dozen different diuretics and beta blockers. He always has to switch me because I usually get side effects. I am on a new one now called Lopressor but I am starting to get dizzy and fatigued. Is there something natural for me?*"

A There is indeed. With the exception of severe hypertension, that is blood pressure readings of more than 160/115+, most cases can be brought under control using natural and lifestyle approaches.

Hypertension, or high blood pressure as it is commonly called, is not a disease. It is an effect, a by-product of other, often more serious, underlying problems.

Anti-hypertensive medications in the form of diuretics, beta blockers and calcium channel blockers are among the most widely prescribed and represent yearly sales of more than $10 billion. Pharmaceutical sales are brisk despite the fact that most medical authorities, including the Joint National Committee on Detection, Evaluation, and Treatment of High Blood Pressure, recommend nondrug treatments be used for borderline to mild hypertension. At the milder phase of the disease, the drugs offer no benefit. Quite the contrary, many scientific studies conclude they may generate a range of side effects that include a substantially increased risk of heart disease. High blood pressure IS itself a major risk factor for heart attacks and for strokes. So that means doctors are prescribing medication that increases the risk! Go figure that one out.

There are nearly 50 million Americans with high blood pressure — about one-fifth of the population. That says a lot for the health of our country. Eighty percent of them fall in the borderline to moderate range (120-180 over 90-114) and require no drug therapy at all. A normal blood pressure is 120 over 80.

High blood pressure refers to a situation where the force of blood pressing against the walls of the arteries is too great. This rise in pressure is believed to be caused by a narrowing of the arteries, which can occur as a result of plaque buildup or constant stress. The narrowing of the vessels means that the heart has to work harder and strain to pump blood through the circulatory system.

Hypertension, if not controlled, can lead to heart attacks, heart failure, stroke, brain damage, and kidney disease.

In 90 percent of cases, the cause is not precisely known and is referred to as essential hypertension. Among the factors are heredity (high blood pressure is more common and severe among blacks than whites), age, body weight, kidney infection, stress and diet.

A University of Nebraska study found that among 1,000 apparently healthy individuals one in five had elevated blood pressure due to stress. According to Robert Eliot of the Life Stress Simulation Laboratory at the University of Nebraska, "traditional risk factors account for only about half the cases" of heart disease and "stress may turn out to be the most crucial factor."

The Lucy case

Dorothy Marie Lucy, 62, a retired secretary from Uniontown, Pennsylvania, had high blood pressure and was too heavy. She didn't

> **Prescription-free and lost 40 pounds.**

feel good at all. She told me that her family physician and a specialist said her blood pressure was so high that if she didn't control it with drugs she ran the risk of a serious stroke. Dorothy had been on multiple courses of antibiotics for recurring sinus, nose, throat, ear and bladder infections. She had some digestive problems, psoriasis, and premature gray hair. Tests in our office indicated some arthritis and borderline lupus.

In May of 1994 she came to see me with her husband John, who also had high blood pressure along with back and neck pain and was experiencing side effects from prescription drugs. We started them both on the full wellness program.

"That was the beginning of a success story," Dorothy told me after several months into the program.

Since August of 1994 she has "been prescription-free with blood pressure readings normal," she says.

"I no longer take any medication or over-the-counter drugs. I lost 42 pounds and have kept it off by following a nutritional food plan, taking vitamins and mineral supplements as directed, doing toning and strengthening exercises in the rehab area of the clinic, plus chiropractic treatments twice per week.

"In December of 1996 I caught a bad cold, which turned into flu, then acute bronchitis, but was spared bronchial pneumonia. I was healed by using natural health care remedies — homeopathic medicine, supplements, diathermy, chiropractic adjustments and bed rest.

"Also, my hair which was mostly gray when I began treatments, is nearly all black and my hairdresser tells me it grows faster and is thicker."

Husband John was able to gradually stop his hypertensive medication and lose 40 pounds. Chiropractic resolved his back and leg pain.

Like a vast number of other Americans, Dorothy and John Lucy had been caught up on the illness treadmill. They had chronic illness, duly took their prescriptions, but never really felt well.

Then they discovered that chiropractic adjustments not only alleviated back pain but also lowered blood pressure and improved immune function. They learned the importance of lifestyle modification and how exercise, vitamins, herbs and proper diet can overcome serious health problems.

Perhaps their greatest benefit is that they realized that healing comes from within. They have in a sense become "spine conscious" and "nutritionally aware." They have become health activists. Instead of waiting for the heart attack or stroke, they've learned how to diffuse the bomb.

How we treat high blood pressure

Research shows that most cases of hypertension can be controlled through changes in diet and lifestyle. The focus in our clinic is on the natural remedies that address the underlying lifestyle, nutritional and structural factors.

Obesity, caffeine consumption, alcohol intake, smoking, and lack of exercise are major contributors. We recommend programs to deal with these issues.

Exercise, particularly of the aerobic type that increases heart rate, provides considerable benefits, such as lowering blood pressure and body fat, and helping to maintain proper weight (see chapter 10).

Overloads of toxic metals in the body, acquired through food, water and air, are linked with heart disease, hypertension and many other illnesses. High on this list are cadmium, lead and mercury, which we frequently see at elevated levels on patient hair analyses. Detoxification, using Nutri Tox, a toxic metal binder, and homeopathic detoxisodes, are helpful in reducing these harmful buildups.

Food sensitivities may be a possible cause of elevated blood pressure — an often overlooked connection.

Past research has indicated that a modified vegetarian diet, high in complex carbohydrates and fiber, and low in fat, helps to lower blood pressure and reduce the risk of cancer and diabetes.

In 1997, the first conclusive study was published in the New England Journal of Medicine showing that changing the overall diet will reduce blood pressure independent of salt intake, lowering body weight and minimizing alcohol. Lawrence Appel of Johns Hopkins University, and other researchers found that eating diets high in fruits and vegetables, and low in fat, can quickly drop mild high blood pressure and achieve reductions similar to medication.

"It's already known that three dietary factors — salt, body weight and alcohol — affect blood pressure, but our findings are important because they identify a fourth factor: the pattern of food we eat," according to Appel. His study involved 459 adults with systolic pressures of less than 160 and diastolic pressures of 80 to 95. The participants ate 9 to 10 servings of produce daily and 3 servings of low-fat dairy products.

The researchers concluded that if this type of diet was widely adopted, it had the potential to reduce the risk of heart disease by 15 percent and stroke by 27 percent.

Results like this make it obvious why we need to change our eating habits. Did you know that the type of fat you eat can increase or decrease your level of pain, raise or lower your blood pressure, turn migraines on or off, or promote or slow down allergies? Unfortunately, the SAD (Standard American Diet) is overloaded with the wrong kind of fat. It is known as arachidonic acid and actually accelerates pain, heart disease and allergies. This particular fatty acid is derived from meat and dairy products, and, if you want to get technical, it is converted in your body to prostaglandins and leukotrienes, substances that contribute to inflammatory processes.

To counteract this, I recommend naturally occurring fats found in raw nuts, seeds and grains and the oils found in certain cold water fish species. They have been found to lower cholesterol, help reduce migraines, PMS, menopause, prostate disorders, arthritic pain, immune dysfunction, eczema and psoriasis. The supplement I have long used is called Nutri EPA. It is derived from cold water fish, and serves as a rich source of the beneficial fatty acid eicosapenentaenoic acid (EPA).

Our nutritional supplement program also includes the following:

• Magnesium, calcium and potassium — the three most important minerals for lowering blood pressure. Deficiency of any or all of these are major contributing factors to resistant high blood pressure. Magnesium, a mineral commonly found to be deficient in Americans, is a potent vasodilator. That means it has the ability to open arteries.

• Ora Key is a nutritional formula we recommend for our cardiovascular and hypertensive patients. This product combines Co-enzyme Q10 (see below), carnitine, magnesium, hawthorn and other key nutritional factors critical for circulatory problems, angina (chest pain), hypertension, congestive heart failure and other cardiac disorders.

• The amino acid tyrosine has an anti-hypertensive effect on the body and a secondary beneficial effect on mood.

• Our herbal recommendations include SGP, a special preparation of garlic and onions, whose benefits are not limited to cooking. Taken supplementally, garlic and onions can help lower blood pressure as well as cholesterol and triglycerides. And don't worry, the formula has only a minimal odor and is well tolerated by patients.

• European herbalists have for centuries prescribed hawthorn berries for their ability to reduce angina (chest pain) and lower blood pressure. Taken as a syrup (1 tablespoon per day), this works as an excellent cardiac tonic.

• The root of coleus forskoli (5-10 milligrams), an ayurvedic remedy, produces arterial relaxation with resultant lowering of blood pressure.

The CoQ10 connection

CoQ10, short for Co-enzyme Q10, is an important fat-soluble vitamin critical to cellular energy production. Lower levels of this naturally-occurring substance are found among hypertensive individuals. The CoQ10 connection to high blood pressure is extremely interesting and worth mentioning in detail here.

Peter Langsjoen, M.D., a Texas cardiologist and CoQ10 expert, explains that the first abnormal change that occurs in any disease affecting heart muscle function is a stiffening of the heart muscle. This can develop in diabetes, coronary artery disease, mitral valve disease, or even as a result of the use of toxic chemotherapeutic agents.

The body reacts by increasing adrenaline, the stress hormone, which in turn raises blood pressure. This situation is referred to by cardiologists as diastolic dysfunction.

The rush of adrenaline makes the heart work better, but on a chronic basis, adverse secondary changes occur, including a general constriction (narrowing) of your blood vessels. That accounts for the higher blood pressure.

According to Langsjoen, the medical profession generally doesn't pay much attention to these early events until there is a pronounced problem.

"Without exception," he says, "we now see that patients with essential hypertension have this diastolic dysfunction — this stiffening of the heart muscle. When you put individuals on CoQ, you get a reverse of this abnormality back toward normal. As it improves, you see a gradual fall in blood pressure."

In a 1994 study published in a medical journal, Langsjoen described how 109 patients with symptomatic essential hypertension benefited from the addition of an average of 225 milligrams of CoQ10 daily to their existing anti-hypertensive drug regimen.
About 25 percent of them were eventually controlled on CoQ10 alone. The patients had had high blood pressure for a mean of nine years.

Within the first six months, a definite and gradual improvement in functional status was observed along with a need to reduce drug therapy. Thereafter, clinical status and drug requirements stabilized with a significantly improved systolic and diastolic blood pressure.

Langsjoen feels that such research has "tremendous implications for all the many millions of people affected by high blood pressure who are taking medication. Not only do individuals have improvement in their functional capacity and sense of well-being, and quality of life, but they would also be on considerable less drug therapy. The potential here for CoQ10 is vast. It should certainly be considered prior to embarking upon an escalating course of pharmacological interventions. Keep in mind, however, that CoQ10 doesn't address all the multiple things that may have got you into the mess to begin with. The stresses and the toxins and other causal elements are still ongoing."

The importance of stress-reduction

Tension and stress that build up in our busy lives can contribute to high blood pressure. For this reason many physicians recommend prayer, meditation, and biofeedback. These are excellent relaxation methods — validated by scientific studies. They are a fundamental part of our wellness program. Remember, "God's power that made your body, heals your body" (Refer to chapter 12).

The chiropractic connection

Keep in mind that your heart and blood vessels are controlled by the nervous system. For this reason, chiropractic evaluation and manipulation should be an integral part of a comprehensive hypertension recovery program that also includes attending to lifestyle issues such as diet, stress and exercise.

Chiropractic studies show that manipulation of the spine may indeed offer important benefits:

• Significant short-term reduction in systolic and diastolic blood pressure was achieved for 21 patients with elevated blood pressure. In this study, patients undergoing chiropractic treatment were compared to subjects receiving a placebo or no treatment at all. The findings indicated that elevated blood pressure can be decreased significantly on a short-term basis by chiropractic manipulation of the thoracic spine (mid back) (Journal of Manipulation and Physiological Therapeutics, 1988).

• Two chiropractors, G. Plaugher and T. R. Bachman, reported the case of a 38-year-old male who had a 14-year history of hypertension. In addition, he experienced bloating sensations, depression, fatigue, impotency, and side effects from the medications Minipress and Corgard.

Following three manipulations, the patient's medical doctor stopped one of the medications and reduced the second. After six manipulations, the remaining medication was once again reduced. After one more manipulation, the medication was stopped entirely. Side effects disappeared. After 18 months, the patient's blood pressure was stable at normal levels (Journal of Manipulation and Physiological Therapeutics, 1993).

• Six out of eight patients with high blood pressure experienced relief of symptoms and reduced blood pressure after chiropractic treatment.

In this study, eight patients were followed over a two-month period. Based on chiropractic analysis, all of them had the "atlas subluxation complex." This is the name that chiropractors give to a misalignment of the first vertebra in the neck, the atlas vertebra, located just below the skull. Because of its anatomically strategic position, a misalignment here can produce structural distortions and stresses throughout the body and disturb a person's sense of balance.

The patients were seen 10 times during the study period. Blood pressure was recorded at each visit. During these visits they were adjusted only if a subluxation was found on re-analysis. Thus, some subjects were only adjusted three or four times during the treatment period.

At the end of the study, blood pressure readings for six patients were lower. Systolic pressure was lowered by an average of 27 mm; the diastolic by an average of 13 mm.

In several of the subjects, other symptoms, such as low back pain, chest tightness, headaches, and general malaise, diminished following the

he greatest changes occurred with patients taking no
ropractic Research and Clinical Investigation, 1992).
.. interesting report described the effect of chiropractic treat-
..nent on the blood pressure of 75 individuals undergoing care for other
conditions. Each had blood pressure readings in the normal range. A
normalizing influence on the blood pressure was noted, most significantly
among those with higher blood pressure levels (Journal of Manipulation
and Physiological Therapeutics, 1988).

After treating thousands of patients in my own practice over the years,
I have seen this beneficial effect many times. I consistently observe a significant lowering of blood pressure with patients being treated for different
problems and whose blood pressure is considered "normal" when they started
chiropractic care. My conclusion is that many people are "relatively" hypertensive and become "truly normal" when spinal stresses are corrected.

Often I will have situations where a patient starts chiropractic care
with a blood pressure reading of , say, 130/84. Then, two months later he
or she will have a reading of 90/60.

"My headaches are gone, my energy is great, I sleep better, I can
think better, but I don't understand why my blood pressure is so low," the
patient will say. "Isn't that dangerous?"

The answer of course is that manipulations have an adaptogenic effect
on the body, that is, they help your body achieve its natural level of balance.

In cases of moderate to severe high blood pressure, patients need to
be managed through a combined wholistic and medical approach.

Natural Remedies for High Blood Pressure

• The Gallagher Wellness Program
• Chiropractic cervical manipulation
• Calcium aspartate ....1,000 milligrams daily
• Magnesium aspartate .... 500 milligrams daily
• Potassium aspartate .... 200 milligrams daily
• SGP (deodorized garlic) .... 3 capsules, twice daily
• Ora Key (CoQ10, hawthorn, carnitine) .... 2 capsules, 3 times daily
• IV chelation therapy needed in advanced cases involving arteriosclerosis
• Prayer and meditation
• Weight loss and Exercise

HYPOGLYCEMIA

About hypoglycemia

- Tired
- Nervous?
- Shaky?
- Irritable? Even hostile?
- Fatigued?
- Depressed?
- Light-headed?
- Dizzy?
- Confused?
- Mood swings?
- Poor memory and concentration?
- Low sex drive?
- Blurred vision?
- Insomnia?
- Frequently hungry?
- Crave sweets?

Welcome to the world of hypoglycemia, a collection of symptoms that contributes to widespread misery and is usually unrecognized by most conventional doctors. It underlies almost every known disease and serious ailment, and almost everyone has it to some degree.

Hypoglycemia refers to low blood sugar. By comparison, diabetes is a disease in which the blood sugar level is too high. Hypoglycemia can lead to diabetes.

Blood sugar is the primary fuel that is used by your body for mental and physical activity. It is converted by cells into energy. It operates the body just as gasoline runs your car. If there isn't enough fuel, your muscles become weak and your nervous system suffers; particularly your nervous system, I should emphasize. The brain and the nerves are the major consumers of sugar in your body. That is why, as the above list demonstrates, multiple symptoms affecting your whole body are the consequences when the fuel tank is low.

Because the nervous system is so dependent on an adequate sugar, many "nerve" symptoms can develop. The array of complaints often prompts physicians to label a patient as a "hypochondriac" or "nervous."

Under normal circumstances, you eat nutritious food and your body processes the food to provide fuel and nourishment to all the cells. All food consumed gradually breaks down into glucose (simple sugar) to supply the body. Throughout man's evolution, this process was done slowly and efficiently without stress to the human body because the food was typically raw, high in fiber, and rich in vitamins, minerals and enzymes. None of our contemporary sugar-added "junk food."

In recent times, and particularly in Western societies, we have made enormous changes in the type of food we eat; changes, unfortunately, that may be good for the financial health of fast food restaurants but not good for our own personal health.

According to S. Boyd Eaton, M.D., a medical anthropologist at Emory University and an authority on pre-historic diets, much of the food we eat today is out of sync with our genetic requirements. The less you eat like your ancestors, he says, the more vulnerable you are for coronary heart disease, cancer, diabetes and many other "diseases of civilization."

For many Westerners today, a large and unhealthy proportion of the diet consists of highly processed, refined food — cakes, ice cream, donuts, white flour, alcohol, and sodas. Such food is typically lacking in fiber, vitamins, minerals, and enzymes, but is high in sugar content that is rapidly absorbed into the bloodstream. Today, the average person eats more than six times the amount of sugar than at the turn of the century. Parallel to this habit is an increase in the illnesses of sugar — diabetes and hypoglycemia.

Blood sugar on a roller-coaster ride

The rush of sugar sets off a chain of biochemical reactions in the body. Among them is a wild blood sugar roller-coaster ride.

When sugar starts to flood the blood stream, the pancreas, a large gland in the abdomen, goes into a rapid response mode and secretes a large quantity of insulin in order to restore a normal blood sugar level. However, the excess insulin often pushes the blood sugar level downward beyond normal. Fifteen minutes to one hour later, your level is lower than when you first ate the junk food and you experience symptoms associated with hypoglycemia.

"Many people who follow such diets have fatigue and a persistent depression which is not explainable by events," according to Harvey Ross, M.D., a California psychiatrist and nutritional expert who treated hypoglycemia for many years. "Often patients tell me: 'I have everything in life to feel good about and I just feel terrible.'

Ross, in a 1988 magazine interview, pointed out what many nutritionally-oriented physicians have observed, namely that the drop in blood sugar levels that creates symptoms is highly individual. A tiny dip, deemed normal by standard glucose tolerance testing, can be troublesome for many people. This is one major reason why standard tests are not reliable measures of hypoglycemic problems.

In the same magazine article, the highly individual nature of hypoglycemic reactions was emphasized by Mollie Shriftman, Ph.D., executive director of the North Nassau Health Center of Manhasset, N.Y. "We all react differently, even people in the same family, to different foods and different amounts of food," she pointed out. "Subtle biochemical differences create wholly different reactions from one person to the next. Our experience shows that hypoglycemic reactions are the cause of problems among many people who suffer from mood swings, depression, undue fatigue, and vague apathy."

Another frequent mood accompaniment of hypoglycemia is irritability. When blood sugar drops, adrenaline is released in the body. This is the same stress hormone produced when a person is confronted with a "fight or flight" situation. Patients would often tell Ross that they had no control over the irritability. They would say they feel psychologically bad after an emotional outburst because they have overreacted, lashed out or hurt someone, but yet they feel physically better.

"In hypoglycemia, it seems, things are backward," Ross said. "You have the adrenaline first and then the fight. The hormone may be spent in the outburst and no longer creates discomfort."

Over time, uncorrected hypoglycemia can cause many chronic problems, including diabetes and obesity. Our eating pattern not only creates this, but a parallel condition we call "overconsumptive malnutrition." In other words, we are overfed but undernourished. We eat too much of poor quality food and not enough good nutrition is reaching our billions of cells. This state of cellular deficiency is a common denominator in such diverse disorders as PMS, ADHD, depression (including post partum depression), migraine headaches, angina, asthma, panic/anxiety attacks, diabetes, heart palpitations, seizure disorders, alcoholism, drug addiction and even criminal behavior.

Hypoglycemia is a good example of "you are what you eat."

Kathleen Ebersberger's case

For more than 20 years, Kathleen Ebersberger had been suffering from what she called her "weak attacks." In her first visit to me in May 1996 she described these as periods of weak-

> "Sleeping is impossible without an alcoholic drink."

ness, light-headedness and the shakes.

"They have increased in length and I am having trouble functioning," she told me. "Sleeping is impossible without an alcoholic drink."

Kathleen, a 48-year-old housewife from Latrobe, Pennsylvania, had previously seen three doctors. They all said nothing was wrong, that her blood work was fine. The last doctor gave her an anti-depressant.

"This was truly a low point in my life," she said. "I knew I did not want or need this but he insisted. The prescription worked! It was for depression and that is what it gave me."

We diagnosed Kathleen with hypoglycemia and hypoadrenia, the latter a condition of exhausted, stressed-out adrenal glands. (Please refer to chapter on stress and your adrenal glands). The adrenal glands are partly responsible for raising the blood sugar level when it is too low. If they are not functioning properly, they can contribute to a blood sugar management problem in the body. Many people have both hypoglycemia and hypoadrenia involved.

Using applied kinesiology, I also found that she had a weak pineal gland, an organ located behind the forehead that regulates serotonin and melatonin. Serotonin is a chemical messenger in the brain. A low supply is associated with anxiety, depression, pain and agitation. Melatonin is a hormone that exerts a governing role on our internal biological clock overseeing body temperature, hormone secretion, the onset of puberty, the sleep cycle, and the body's repair and rejuvenation activities when we sleep. A deficiency can cause sleep disorders and depression.

The pineal gland is connected neurologically to the upper neck. In Kathleen's case, she had misalignments in her cervical (neck) spine that were "short-circuiting" the pineal gland. The spinal stress was disturbing the production of melatonin and serotonin. Kathleen became depressed and a chronic insomniac. Misalignments in the cervical (neck) spine can create many problem in the brain, head and body, including interference with pineal function.

To help Kathleen, I recommended a series of chiropractic adjustments to correct the misalignments. I also prescribed a nutritional supplement called Adrenoglan Chelate for her weakened adrenal glands.

When Kathleen returned to the office for her third chiropractic treatment her face was beaming.

"For the first time in 20 years I am able to sleep at night without alcohol," she told me.

Prior to these treatments, she said "I was so run down that I would get depressed about it and just sit around and cry. I really wasn't depressed.

But not being able to do anything is what really caused the problems, and none of the doctors knew what was wrong or believed I felt the way I actually felt."

In addition to chiropractic, we started Kathleen on a program of supplements and dietary changes.

Kathleen argued about the diet changes. "Too hard to do," she said.

We managed to convince her about how important it was and how she would feel so much better as a result. She finally accepted the challenge. Now, she is a keen follower of better eating.

"I am now back to my old high energy self," Kathleen told me in a recent visit. "I'm happy again. Once, I just cried because I felt so good."

Although addressing the hypoglycemia and nutritional problems played a role in her recovery, chiropractic manipulation was the primary treatment that reversed 20 years of suffering. It happened with two adjustments in 10 days."

Emily Davis' case

When Emily Davis, 48, a home health aide, from Apollo, Pennsylvania, first visited my office she had been very ill for many years.

"I have seen many doctors," she told me, "but I haven't had any lasting relief and no understanding, insight or compassion. Since 1989 my health has been gradually declining. Can you help me?"

> **"I have more energy and stamina now than I think I have ever felt."**

She had been diagnosed with depression and "neurasthenia," a neurosis marked by chronic abnormal fatiguability ("sometimes exhaustion"), overall lack of energy, feelings of inadequacy, inability to concentrate, loss of appetite, and insomnia.

Initially she saw an internist who prescribed anti-depressants.

"I didn't feel in my heart that I had depression," she said. "But I do feel I have been patronized. It seems to me that when one's condition doesn't fit into what the medical books describe, then doctors tend to say you have depression."

Her condition worsened, she said, so she cut out the drugs and consulted a neurologist who advised her to immediately stop working, have complete rest, and take vitamin B-12 shots. She remained off work for four months and slept 18 hours per day. She continued the treatment for one year with no results.

"I do know this, that I can't work any longer, that I have to rest for hours every day, and that I am very nauseated, have headaches, chest pain, my back hurts, and I often feel like fainting," she told me. She also suffered from irritable bowel syndrome, urinary frequency, arrhythmic heart, and symptoms resembling fibromyalgia. She said she had to consume sweets every two hours to overcome the constant fatigue and weakness.

Emily's chiropractic and nutritional evaluation indicated multiple spinal misalignments, hypoglycemia and nutritional deficiencies. Her customary diet was a disaster for her. She routinely ate red meat, cold cereals, dairy, and lots of sugar.

I suggested a restrictive high protein, low carbohydrate diet, and recommended she avoid sugar and caffeine. I also prescribed chiropractic adjustments and a specific supplement program, including chromium, an adrenal glandular extract, and magnesium.

"The tough part was the food," she told me afterward. "I really experienced withdrawal symptoms."

By the end of 30 days, Emily was like a new person — no longer requiring 18 hours of sleep. No more constant fatigue, dizziness, weakness, irritable bowel or heart irregularities.

She continued to make great progress. Within four months she told me that she felt like a new person. She became, in a sense, not a new woman but rather the person she always wanted to be.

"I can hardly believe it," she told me. "I have more energy and stamina now than I think I have ever felt. Looking back on my experience, I can only say that why anyone would choose a drug with harmful side effects over natural alternative medicine is beyond me."

So much for depression and neurasthenia!

How we treat hypoglycemia

As I said a moment ago, there is no accurate test for hypoglycemia. I tell patients they have to go on the comprehensive program to see if it makes a difference. Generally speaking, it not only helps them maintain stable blood sugar levels throughout the day and night, but also it helps them attain the best possible level of energy and health. What I say to my patients is this: "The worse that can happen is that you will feel better."

The persistent mood changes and energy deficits that develop from low blood sugar over a long period of time generally take about two or three months to be relieved after the start of a corrective program, Harvey Ross, the California expert on hypoglycemia, noted. That has been my observation as well.

During the treatment of hypoglycemia, many patients will cut out sugar and refined carbohydrates and experience only partial relief. They may even feel worse — a withdrawal symptom to the sugar — or perhaps feel refreshingly "up" for days or parts of days. But the improvement doesn't last and they still experience mood swings.

Such people may need more than just eliminating sugar. In order to make progress, we recommend wholesome snacks of protein or complex carbohydrates every couple of hours to prevent blood sugar dips along with B complex vitamin supplements which help bolster the nervous system.

I often prescribe "Pro Equalizer" to my hypoglycemic patients. This is a high energy shake product that you take upon awakening. The drink is composed of brown rice powder, vitamins, minerals, enzymes and fiber that can be mixed into rice milk, soy milk or juice. It is a great way to raise your blood sugar without side effects.

I also recommend the following:
- small frequent meals
- high-protein, low carbohydrate diet
- avoid processed foods as much as possible
- avoid caffeine and alcohol
- avoid food allergens

The chiropractic — hypoglycemia connection

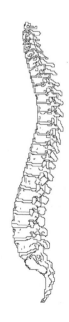

The nervous system controls and coordinates all our activities and functions. If there is a single or multiple subluxation complex in the spine, the nervous system malfunctions. D.D. Palmer, the founder of chiropractic, said that "disease is caused by too little or too much nerve energy." This concept is not unlike the oriental medicine concept that health requires a balance of yin and yang, that is, of positive and negative energy.

In the case of hypoglycemia it is sometimes difficult to separate the wheat from the chaff. Misalignments cause the nervous system to malfunction, which can trigger the body's hormonal system to malfunction. The scenario of possible effects includes how the body handles sugar.

On the other side of the coin, we may have a spine and nervous system functioning optimally. However, a diet high in "junk food" triggers many unhealthy reactions and stresses within the body. Such chemical stress has the potential to generate spinal subluxations and multiply a person's health problems.

Moral of the story: Eating poorly can do you in many ways. In the words of Arthur Kaslow, M.D., a California expert on nutrition, "you don't catch disease, you eat it."

Natural Remedies for Hypoglycemia

• The Gallagher Wellness Program
• Chiropractic spinal manipulation
• Identify food allergies
• Small frequent meals
• Pro Equalizer .... 1-3 tablespoons daily
• Ultra Preventive (high-potency multi vitamin) .... 2 capsules, 3 times daily
• Chromium GTF .... 2 capsules, 3 times daily
• Adrenogland Chelate .... 2 capsules, 3 times daily

HYPOTHYROIDISM (LOW THYROID)

About the thyroid

In front of your throat, between your Adam's apple and top of your breastbone, is a small, butterfly-shaped gland weighing less than an ounce — your thyroid.

Minute secretions from this gland, less than a spoonful a year, affect the body in many important ways.

The thyroid controls metabolism, the process by which food is transformed into energy. It regulates heat production in the body, and influences the circulatory system, sensitivity of the nerves, and muscle health.

If your thyroid doesn't manufacture enough of its critical hormone output, you will feel the consequences in many possible ways. Replacement with thyroid hormone is necessary. The condition is called hypothyroidism.

Extreme low thyroid production is rare. But, according to many experts, mild hypothyroidism is fairly common, and is enough to throw the body out of balance. Among them are Broda O. Barnes, M.D., who years ago wrote an important, well-detailed book on low thyroid still available in many health food and book stores. It is appropriately entitled "Hypothyroidism: The Unsuspected Illness" (Harper and Row, New York, 1976).

During more than 35 years of treating and studying this problem, Barnes found that many symptoms and conditions are related to an unrecognized and underactive thyroid. They include fatigue, depression, weight gain, hair loss, menstrual difficulties, impaired memory, mental illness, intestinal problems, low blood pressure, and heart disease, just to name a few.

Barnes was convinced that untreated low thyroid was responsible for or involved in as many as 64 common ailments affecting 40 percent of the population. A healthy functioning thyroid, he believed, was central to the health of the whole body.

According to Stephen E. Langer, M.D., a California wholistic physician and contemporary expert on thyroid, "when the thyroid is underactive, everything in the body gradually becomes hypoactive as well, from circulation to libido."

The "cure" for low thyroid is simple and inexpensive — a prescription for thyroid hormone. With the help of a knowledgeable physician, hormonal adjustment can be readily made without upsetting the system.

Writing in Alternative Medicine Digest, Langer tells the story of a patient who had been depressed for 60 years. "Yet when he took thyroid hormone, his depression was gone within a month," said Langer. "Whatever his previous physicians prescribed focused on his depression but missed the underlying thyroid cause, so he was miserable for most of his lifetime."

Wilson's Syndrome, often overlooked as a cause of serious health problems, is a thyroid disorder in which a person produces enough thyroid but the cells cannot use it properly.

The thyroid function test

Barnes' work, among other important contributions, brought attention to the deficiency of standard laboratory blood tests for thyroid function. Such tests are relatively inaccurate. In spite of all the complex evaluations and cross-evaluations, the true status of the thyroid is elusive.

Functional tests, such as the underarm temperature test, reveal more about individual patient status. Barnes felt this simple procedure, which anyone can do at home, was more accurate than blood tests. Many people, whose blood tests show normal thyroid function, often have low thyroid as indicated by the underarm test and benefit when they are supplemented with thyroid hormone or natural substances.

Barnes instructed his patients to do their own underarm temperature tests. Many prevention-oriented health professionals do likewise. We have recommended this easy-to-do test for years to our patients.

Here's how to do it yourself. All you need is a standard thermometer.

• Upon retiring, put the thermometer next to your bed on a handy night table or chair.

• Shake it down. This is important.

• When you wake up, before doing anything, reach over and put the thermometer under your armpit. The thermometer must be placed under your bare arm. Once done, press your arm against your body, with no clothing between. Hold it there for a full ten minutes. Lay in bed as you do this.

• Make a note of your reading. Be sure to read it accurately. It is your accuracy which determines the value of the test. Mark down the date.

• Do this for a week.

The normal reading when taken this way is between 97.8° and 98.2°. If the temperature is consistently low, then there is underfunction of the thyroid, no matter what any laboratory analysis says.

In our clinic, the record of this early morning basal temperature acts as a great aid in making a proper diagnosis.

Family history of low thyroid

Q *"I'm 35 years old with a family history of low thyroid. Over the past year, I have gained 15 pounds, my skin has become very dry, and I am always tired. My family doctor tested my blood for thyroid and anemia and said I was normal. I know I am not imagining these symptoms, so what can I do?"*

How we treat low thyroid

There are a number of ways to help promote and support thyroid health. Among them: kelp, iodine drops, and Irish moss (a herbal).

The major thyroid hormone (thyroxine, which accounts for 93 percent of the gland's hormonal activity in the body) relies on proteins, the amino acid tyrosine, iodine, vitamins A and B-6 as important raw materials. For this reason, I usually prescribe a complex of these nutrients.

It is definitely a good idea to have a nutritional evaluation to determine whether you have enough of the primary "raw materials" in your body and diet to make thyroid hormones. These nutrients give individuals who are slightly hypothyroid the necessary building blocks that allows their own thyroid hormones to make what the body needs.

Given the inadequate way that many Americans eat, I suspect there are millions of individuals, especially women, who have nutritionally-induced hypothyroidism. Their thyroid glands are simply missing the needed ingredients. For the most part, conventional doctors do not look for these factors. Many people are probably — and unnecessarily — put on a lifetime of replacement hormone therapy as a result.

Many patients, however, do require a thyroid replacement despite supplementation. Some have thyroid glands that are no longer active due to disease or surgery.

The replacement choices are Synthroid, a standard synthetic prescription, or a natural bovine glandular compound such as Armour Thyroid.

There have been some problems associated with the synthetic form, in particular a depletion of bone tissue that may contribute to osteoporosis. Studies have not been done to date comparing the two. Armour may have the edge, because it contains both T3 and T4 (the two major thyroid hormones) and Synthroid offers only a synthetic dosage of T4.

Improving liver function with detoxification and herbal remedies, especially milk thistle, along with a supplementation program, often corrects thyroid imbalance.

Marian's case

When she first came to see me, this 59-year-old female patient had no energy.

No Energy

Her condition was so pronounced and so chronic that she had actually figured she was living only a third of a day every two days. She was too tired the rest of the time to pursue normal activities.

"A lifetime of hard experience has taught me that there is no help to be found in the medical community, that is, the standard medical community, which is the only one I have known. I feel pretty hopeless," she said.

Marian had a history of thyroid problems beginning as a teenager. She suffered hyperthyroid and goiter and at the age of 17 had her thyroid totally removed. Despite faithfully taking her thyroid replacement pills, she never had the energy of a normal person and often experienced constant fatigue.

"Complaints to the doctors brought no relief, and their tests didn't show anything" she said. "Mostly, I was told I was just depressed and should get more exercise. I was ignored when I protested that if I was indeed depressed it was because of constant exhaustion and the inability to do anything. If I went for my prescribed walks, I was afraid that on crossing a street I might not be able to pull myself up onto the curb on the other side and would end up stuck in the street or sitting on the curb until my husband came to get me."

At the insistence of her daughter, Marian came to see me in mid-1996. Together with one of my medical associates, her thyroid medication was changed to a more natural form. I recommended a diet that eliminated certain foods which we felt were having an adverse effect on her body, and prescribed a series of chiropractic manipulations and trigger point therapies.

Although most people are unaware of the role of chiropractic on the hormonal system, spinal adjustments indirectly influence the secretion of pituitary and thyroid hormones via the nervous system. In Marian's case, part of her severe energy loss was in part due to spinal stress.

Marian's improvement was rapid. In an assessment of her condition during a follow-up six months after starting on her program, she told me she was making great progress.

"I no longer have to put off doing things that require a climb to the second floor," she said. "I just walk up the stairs. I no longer have to steel myself and take a deep breath before pulling myself out of a chair. I just stand up. I have taken on a small consulting job and am more active in my church. With each month of treatment, I have more energy and I feel myself continuing to improve."

Millions of unfortunate people are stuck in low gear because their thyroid glands are functioning below par but are not outright diseased. Such people pass the standard medical tests but never can seem to get up to speed. Marian, however, discovered a way off the sickness treadmill and onto better health.

The chiropractic — hypothyroid connection

A direct link between spinal or cranial misalignments and hypothyroidism has not yet been scientifically investigated. However, my clinical experience leads me to believe that this connection will likely be proven someday. A preliminary study in the Journal of Manipulative and Physiological Therapeutics in 1996 points to a potential relationship.

In the study, Arthur C. Croft, D.C., director of the Spine Research Institute in San Diego, and Keith W. Schnert, M.D., a private practitioner in St. Louis Park, Minnesota, studied 101 consecutive patients who had whiplash trauma.

Their rather startling conclusion, based on both standard laboratory testing for thyroid function and basal metabolic temperature (the underarm test), was that "whiplash seems to result in a form of hypothyroidism suggesting direct injury to central tissues."

An automobile collision with rear impact is known to generate forces in the head and neck of occupants riding in a vehicle that can be several times greater than the force absorbed by the vehicle itself. Animals subjected to similar trauma have developed inflammation or hemorrhage involving 50 percent of thyroid gland tissue.

Croft and Schnert, the researchers, theorized that "because the thyroid gland can store enough thyroglobulin to last for three months, a delay of onset of frank hypothyroidism-like symptoms would be possible." In other words, physical stress, in this case trauma from a rear-end collision, might destabilize the thyroid and cause symptoms once the gland has used up its internal biochemical reserves.

The question begging an answer here is whether chiropractic adjustments, which have a beneficial effect on neck pain and headaches, might also play a supportive role in improving the course of hypothyroidism.

After reviewing this study, I recalled the case of Claudia, a patient in her early forties, who had complaints of fatigue, mental dullness, tightness in her throat and nervousness. An Applied Kinesiology (AK) examination pointed to a thyroid imbalance. With just two chiropractic adjustments of her C5 and C6 (cervical spine vertebrae), her problem cleared up.

Over the years I have found that the thyroid often mimics other disorders. For instance, you may have weak adrenal glands or a malfunction of your pineal or thymus glands, but the problem will manifest as a thyroid disorder. Chiropractic evaluation and reflex testing are natural "high tech" methods of identifying hidden and confusing weaknesses. Once identified, they can often be corrected with manipulation and nutritional prescriptions.

Natural Remedies for Low Thyroid

- *Gallagher Wellness Program*
- *Chiropractic cervical manipulation*
- *Basal temperature test (97.8° - 98.2°)*
- *Tyrosine* .... *500 milligrams daily*
- *Beta carotene* .... *50,000 IU daily*
- *Milk thistle (standardized extract)* .... *300-600 milligrams daily*
- *Kelp* .... *2 capsules daily*
- *Prescription Armour Thyroid if hormonal replacement therapy is needed*

MALE SEXUAL DYSFUNCTION (IMPOTENCE)

Jim, a patient in his 30s, came to me with low back pain that had persisted for years. Following a series of lumbar adjustments his back pain was over — as well as an additional problem with erectile dysfunction.

Jim's case is an all-too-common story that affects many men. Most, however, are too embarrassed to speak about it. Erectile dysfunction (ED), usually and inappropriately called impotence, includes a wide array of disorders, such as difficulty getting or maintaining erections, premature ejaculation, and inability to ejaculate.

For decades, the conventional medical field has perpetuated the idea of a psychosomatic origin to this problem. In other words, it was said to be largely psychological and had little to do with physical causes. Currently, experts think the opposite, and believe that 70-80 percent of cases are related primarily to physical factors.

This is an important difference, because physical problems can be more easily identified and treated than psychological causes.

Prominent physical causes cited by experts include these:

• Blood flow problems. Normal erections require that blood flow readily into the penis, where it becomes "captured" in erectile tissue long enough to sustain the erection. Afterward, it has to be able to flow out. Difficulties are often created by abnormal flow of blood in or out of the penis and "leakage" of blood within the penis.

• Erectile tissue that has lost its elasticity and capacity to relax adequately.

• Any trauma, such as pelvic surgery (examples: hernias, prostate, colon, or rectal cancer), injuries from vehicular or industrial accidents, and gunshot wounds, can affect the ability to develop and maintain an erection. Such traumas can have a negative effect on blood flow and nerve conduction.

• Diseases affecting the nervous system can cause erectile difficulties. Among them are tumors of the brain and spinal cord, epilepsy, Parkinson's disease, and multiple sclerosis (MS). Damage to the nerve circuits serving the penis occur in about 25 percent of all MS cases.

• Diabetes can interfere with the nerves and blood vessels that control blood flow, or produce an increase or decrease in the sex hormones. The physical impact on sexual function can take many years to develop, however, not all men with diabetes are affected.

• More than 200 prescription drugs create erectile problems. Among them are sedatives, tranquilizers, anti-depressants (SSRI class drugs) and drugs used in treating cardiovascular conditions.

• Street drugs in general, uppers and downers like cocaine, speed, and Quaaludes, may at first raise the desire for sex, but with regular use they decrease a man's potency.

• The steroid drugs used by some body builders and athletes to aid in muscle building and competition may initially generate a powerful sex drive. With time, however, testosterone levels are adversely affected, resulting in decreased sexual desire and performance, and, frequently, depression.

• A small amount of alcohol stirs up desire and reduces inhibitions. Continued drinking, however, decreases desire and the ability to perform sexually. Regular drinking produces hormonal changes in the body that impair sexual responsiveness.

• The harmful effects of smoking on general health are well known. Less known is the fact that smoking can impact sexual function. Nicotine causes a constriction of the blood vessels. This means that less blood flows into the penis. Long-term smoking contributes to hardening and narrowing of the arteries, a cause of physical impotence.

The combination of chronic smoking and drinking increases the likelihood of erectile dysfunction.

The missing links —
nutritional deficiencies and spinal misalignments

Men with ED often go to urologists for help and undergo a battery of standard diagnostic tests, including prostate examination, hormonal tests, and penile vascular tests (blood flow studies). If results are normal, and no disease process has been found, conventional medicine leans towards a psychological verdict. That means an individual is left to live with sexual dysfunction and the blame, shame, and guilt associated with "not being a man." There is, of course, the option of "talk therapy" and exploring the psychological undercurrents of why functioning sexually has become a problem.

After all the tests, doctors and talking, many men still face continuing dysfunction, along with depression.

The problem with the conventional approach is that it almost always overlooks two factors that may be involved — nutritional deficiencies and spinal misalignments.

The fields of chiropractic and nutritional medicine recognize that many cases of ED are functional. That means you don't have a disease but something isn't functioning right. Something is missing or lacking. That something could be inadequate nerve or blood supply, caused by a spinal misalignment, or it could be nutrients that are deficient because of a poor diet.

In one study conducted years ago, researchers found that of 43 men who had lower back problems due to industrial injury, 63 percent also experienced sexual dysfunction. Research and chiropractic experience have demonstrated that spinal misalignments in the lower back can produce not just pain but also a wide array of organic and functional problems, including sexual difficulties.

Chiropractic adjustments release blocked nerve and blood supply to dysfunctional reproductive organs. Thus, chiropractic evaluation is a worthwhile measure to consider for erectile dysfunction problems.

Nutritional supplements such as vitamin C, zinc, and vitamin E improve sperm counts, sperm motility and decrease the size of enlarged prostates.

Some herbal medicines such as Siberian and Korean Ginseng, in addition to reducing fatigue and improving depression, are known to increase fertility and libido. Ginkgo biloba, the well-known traditional Chinese herb, increases penile blood flow even among advanced diabetics suffering from ED.

Potency wood, a Brazilian folk medicine and Yohimbe, an African fertility medicine, are often helpful either individually or in combination, for male functional health problems.

My message is this: There are good options available outside of what conventional medicine offers. Don't learn to live with your problem without trying all the options. Explore natural medicine. You may discover that it's not "in your head," but in your spine or in your diet instead.

The following cases demonstrate my point:

• Tom Diffendafer, 48, of Pittsburgh, came to see me complaining of low energy, back pain and sexual dysfunction. I prescribed healthy diet, a vitamin program, and chiropractic manipulations.

The combination worked to alleviate his problems. During a recent visit to the clinic, Tom said, "my job as a custodian puts demands on my back. I often have to lift heavy objects that put my back out. But the manipulations put things right back in place. With chiropractic care, the vitamins, and eating the right foods, my low back pain has disappeared, my health improved dramatically, and my sex drive has returned."

• A 72-year-old male patient experienced sexual dysfunction associated with diabetes. An examination of his lower back determined that he had a subluxation to the fifth lumbar vertebra.

We started him on a series of spinal manipulations. In addition, he was placed on a high complex fiber diet consisting of raw fruits and vegetables, grains, nuts, seeds and small amounts of animal protein. A supplement program included glucose tolerance factor and vanadyl sulfate, to help with lowering his blood sugar, and ginkgo biloba, a herb that improves circulation.

Following his first month of chiropractic and nutritional therapy, he reported that his erection response was improving. At the end of four months, he said his condition had completely normalized.

Natural Remedies for Erectile Dysfunction

- *Gallagher Wellness Program*
- *Chiropractic lumbar manipulation*
- *Ginkgo biloba (standardized extract)* ....*160 milligrams daily*
- *Ginseng* .... *500-1,000 milligrams daily*
- *Yohimbe (standardized extract)* .... *15-40 milligrams daily*
  (avoid if hypertensive, or if have history of cardiac problems)
- **Potency wood (standardized extract) 1,000-1,500 milligrams daily**

MEMORY PROBLEMS FROM EVERYDAY MENTAL MALFUNCTION TO ALZHEIMER'S DISEASE

Who among us, young or old, hasn't had a lapse of memory or days when we don't seem to be all there? For some people it's a now and then thing. For others, well, fogginess and confusion is a way of life. Such people often wonder, "Am I getting senile? Do I have Alzheimer's?"

There are major differences between such everyday mental malfunction and the mental deterioration — such as age-related senility and Alzheimer's disease — that afflict many in later life.

This chapter is designed to explain the differences and provide some fresh perspectives about dealing with loss of mental fitness.

About everyday mental malfunction

"I can't concentrate."

"My mind feels like it's in a fog."

"My brain just doesn't work right and I don't know what's wrong."

"I have words on the tip of my tongue but I can't get them out."

"I'm fine one day, in a state of confusion the next."

"I have friends in their 70s with better memories than me."

Patients make these comments all the time. Men. Women. All ages. All professions. Some patients genuinely fear they are getting Alzheimer's. Often they have been tested by conventional medical doctors and their results are normal.

I have spoken to other physicians around the country and they tell me these are common complaints among their patients as well. This leads me to believe that there are probably millions of individuals functioning with much less of their God-given mental power.

The typical complaints are:

• Difficulty in thinking, focusing, concentrating and learning
• Confusion
• Mixing up words
• Forgetfulness and problems remembering
• Personality changes
• Losing track of conversation when talking
• Mild anxiety and depression

The causes of everyday mental malfunction

In my practice I have often found the cause of these problems to be:

• Decrease of blood flow to the brain because of subluxation of the neck. (see the chiropractic — mental malfunction discussion later in this chapter)

- Toxic metal syndrome
- Nutritional deficiencies
- Food allergies
- Drug side effects
- Hypoglycemia
- Excess stress
- Not enough rest

About Alzheimer's and age-related memory loss

Alzheimer's Disease is the most common type of dementing illnesses, causing progressive impairment of memory, thinking and behavior, and eventually leaving its victims unable to care for themselves. This situation increasingly forces family members into draining caregiver roles. They become, in essence, "second victims."

Alzheimer's strikes older people more frequently. Currently about 10 percent of Americans over 65 and nearly 50 percent of those over age 85 are said to be affected — a total of more than four million. By 2020, that number may rise to 14 million.

The differences between Alzheimer's and age-associated memory loss are significant.

Alzheimer's

• Memory loss increases.

• Begins to interfere with normal activities of daily life.

• May also change mood and personality, impair ability to use words, work with figures, solve problems and use reasoning and judgment.

• Patients gradually unable to use reminders or notes, handle money, dress themselves, read or write, and use the simple tools of daily life such as a key or television.

Memory loss

• Normal forgetfulness comes with aging.

• Memory problems may remain unchanged for years.

• Most people can compensate with reminders and notes.

No one knows for sure how Alzheimer's is caused. Scientific investigation has looked at neurological damage, biochemical deficiencies, viruses, genetic abnormalities, toxicity from metals such as aluminum, mercury and lead, and malfunctions in the body's defenses.

There are no clinical tests for Alzheimer's. Diagnosis involves ruling out all other causes of memory loss. A positive diagnosis is only possible by autopsy. Post-mortum findings reveal damaged nerve cells and other abnormalities in the area of the brain that governs memory and thinking.

Even when the health of ex-presidents like Ronald Reagan is at stake, the big guns of mainstream medicine have little firepower to bring up against the relentless loss of faculties and function caused by Alzheimer's.

There is no definitive cure. No definitive treatment. Two approved drugs, as of the end of 1996, do not stop the progression of the disease.

Outside the mainstream, however, there are a number of viable options available that physicians and researchers say may delay progression of the illness and in some cases even generate improvements. Many of these measures are also highly effective in combating lesser conditions that mimic signs of Alzheimer's.

Vilma Ramicone's case

The alarming case of Vilma Ramicone illustrates the point that progressive memory loss and confusion symptoms may be altogether something quite different than Alzheimer's.

> A mother's ordeal, a daughter's nightmare

Pat Ramicone, of Oakmont, Pennsylvania, was frantic when she brought her 77-year-old mother Vilma to see me. Her story was a genuine medical nightmare.

"My mother had tripped on a curb, fallen, and stubbed her thumb," Pat related. "The thumb stayed swollen for months, so we went to see a doctor to determine if it was infected.

"He said the problem was an infection and wrote out a prescription for Keflex (an antibiotic) to be taken for 10 days. After two days, my mother was confused and unable to sleep or relax.

"'I know something is wrong,' she phoned to tell me. 'I am so tired and usually I have lots of energy.'

"My mother called the doctor to report her discomfort. He said to keep taking the Keflex. A day or so later she complained of burning feet and upset stomach. She didn't feel well enough to attend a family party.

"I called the doctor to tell him that the thumb wasn't improving. He ordered an X-ray, saying there might be a bone infection. The X-ray showed a healing fracture, but no sign of infection. The Keflex was discontinued and a splint applied. Still, my mother was becoming more anxious and confused, seemingly by the minute. The pharmacist who filled her prescription assured me there was no connection to her behavior and the Keflex, even though I could see a direct correlation between the start of the drug and the onset of her symptoms.

"My mother then had a blood test. She was told that her sodium level was low, indicative perhaps, of cancer. That was a shock since my father had died from cancer just nine months before. She was advised to drink 'Gatorade' for three days and be retested.

"A few days later, my mother was rushed to the hospital. When I got there she was highly agitated, extremely confused and talking about dying. They told me she was having a 'psychotic episode.' She was put through many tests, including blood work that left her arms black and blue.

"Low sodium was the only finding. She was given Flexiril for leg cramps, the tranquilizer Ativan for agitation, and Zoloft for depression. Zoloft was changed soon to Luvox, an anti-psychotic drug. They also gave her Resperdal to help her sleep and, of all things, a low sodium diet. The diagnosis she finally received was "syndrome of inappropriate anti-diuretic hormone! No cause for her situation was given.

"For six days or so she remained in the hospital. Her sodium level actually went down during this time! She was extremely obsessive, compulsive, and even paranoid, not the mother I've always known. She was finally discharged with a recommendation for three weeks' of treatment in a psychiatric facility.

"When she was released she was unable to make any decisions or think clearly or focus for any length of time. It was the most frightening thing I've ever gone through. I can't imagine how it was for her to be so utterly helpless."

When Vilma was brought in to see me, my evaluation was drug-induced immune system dysfunction. I recommended a yeast detoxification program, spinal manipulation, a multi-strain probiotic, along with high doses of vitamins, enzymes and amino acids.

"My mother was so bad that she was unable to dole out the correct vitamin tablets for herself," said Pat. "I had to make sure she took them as recommended. To watch a once extremely independent woman be unable to count pills is most disheartening."

But within a few days the positive news started arriving.

"By the fourth day there was noticeable improvement," Pat reported to me. "By the sixth day she was counting out the vitamins herself."

The improvement continued. Within two weeks, Vilma Ramicone was back to her old self again. She was preparing her own meals, washing her own clothes and reading again. She soon began digging in her garden, playing cards with friends, riding the bus, and doing her own shopping again. Her previous energy level had returned. She hasn't had one drug since leaving the hospital.

After she recovered I received a poignant note from her daughter that said: "I shudder to think where or how my mom would be today if I followed the psychiatrists' recommendations. I am truly sickened by the thought of how many other people are in similar straits who have never been introduced to alternatives."

Vilma Ramicone did not have a mental illness. She had the disease of modern medicine. She started with one problem and received an antibiotic for it. That led to a drug reaction of anxiety, fear, confusion and depression. That, in turn, led to hospitalization and a barrage of psychiatric drugs. Here's a striking example of iatrogenic illness — problems triggered by medical treatment.

Fortunately, with natural prescriptions we were able to repair her traumatized body and bring her back in balance. Fortunately, too, she had a courageous and loving daughter who was aware of alternative medicine. Without the compassion and knowledge of her daughter, Vilma could have wound up in a nursing home wearing a "chemical straitjacket."

I wonder how many millions of elderly people are diagnosed with dementia or Alzheimer's or similar disorders that are, in fact, related to the complications of modern medicine?

Prescription drug-induced dementia, or what appears to be attention deficit disorder, mental confusion or even Alzheimer's disease, has been attributed to a variety of different medications. For instance, one investigation at the Mayo Clinic found that some elderly patients may be misdiagnosed as being senile when they are actually suffering from addiction due to prescription drugs.

How we treat these problems
The chiropractic — mental malfunction connection

There is no doubt in my mind that spinal structure and alignment affect brain function, and that misalignment can cause malfunction. I know this first-hand from my patients. Many tell me they feel like there is a coating around their brain, or that they just can't seem to think clearly, or remember names. They may have concentration or learning difficulties, headaches, clumsiness, mix up their words, experience visual disorders, anxiety and depression. They may say such things as "I know what I want to say, but it doesn't come out." One such person is Cindy Berkebile, an attractive 40-year-old woman from Windber, Pennsylvania. She receives periodic adjustments for her neck to protect her clarity.

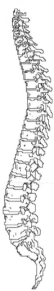

"When my neck is misaligned," she says, "I can look at an object and know what it is but I can't say what it is. Right after I get adjusted, my mind clears and there is no fumbling for words."

For decades, chiropractic patients around the world have been telling their chiropractic physicians that adjustments enable them to concentrate, learn and remember better, have more attention span, and improve their general feeling of well-being. Some patients whose jobs involve detailed calculations find they are able to maintain their required sharp focus as long as they have periodic adjustments.

Research in China and Australia has started to give us a clearer scientific picture of how chiropractic can help create better brain function for people like Cindy Berkebile and perhaps millions of others with varying degrees of spinal subluxation.

The image that is emerging is that cervical (neck) subluxations cause a decrease of blood flow to the brain, causing the brain to operate in a less-than-normal state. The brain still works. It's not like a stroke. But you never function properly. The new studies are proving what we chiropractors have long known empirically from seeing the improvements in our patients — that manipulative treatment restores blood flow. Refer to chapter 13 for more details.

The implications are truly massive: for education, enhanced learning and daily performance, and for the fields of psychology and psychiatry. Large scale research is needed to firmly establish the theories that have been advanced and the clinical results chiropractic physicians are observing every day in their practices. If we can solidly link misalignments to what are often baffling and treatment-resistant behavioral or mental problems, we will have performed a great service to the medical arts and to society at large.

Your problem may be "brain hibernation"

Chiropractors are starting to talk in terms of "brain hibernation," a phrase coined by Australian chiropractic researcher A. G. J. Terrett. It refers to an inadequate supply of nutrients and oxygen reaching the brain cells due to decreased circulation. The cause is misaligned vertebrae in the neck. The situation is chronic undersupply of nutrition to the brain as compared to an acute incident of stroke or injury, where brain cells are irreversibly damaged.

"Brain hibernation" is a described by Terrett as a "cerebral gray area" resulting in a wide variety of signs and symptoms that have been ignored or unrecognized in conventional medicine.

"Since those who are in the gray area pass most of the conventional medical tests (MRI, scans, arteriograms), they are often given a psychological label, and often medicated, told they are growing old, called hypochondriacs, or labeled hysterical," says Terrett. "Their disability is largely ignored because they don't have abnormal tests, they don't respond to usual methods of treatment and the absent functions are highly sophisticated and not important to the basic business of existing. They go about day-to-day activities but everything is an effort. They have to use increased willpower in order to accomplish tasks."

We know that orthodox medicine works best when a condition is clearly definable, as Terrett mentions, through biopsies, blood tests and other diagnostic tools of the trade. In chiropractic we often deal with abstract conditions that elude the ability of these tools to quantify them. Pain, achiness, dizziness, and numbness are examples. They are hard to measure but can be nevertheless disabling.

"Neurologists understand the effects of vascular occlusion and the resultant ischemic and stroke syndromes," adds Terrett. "The signs, symptoms and syndromes that this (brain hibernation) theory addresses are not listed in standard neurology texts because the signs and symptoms are not so devastating as strokes but they still cause severe health problems to the patient."

Nutritional therapy

Many people become categorized with confusion, memory lapses, Alzheimer's or pre-Alzheimer's. Their problem may be a misalignment, a nutritional problem, impaired circulation, toxic metal, or a side effect from a drug. We look for all these possibilities in our clinic.

Studies continually find the elderly population suffering from malnutrition, failing to get proper amounts of nutrients because of malabsorption, altered gastrointestinal function, multiple drug use or imbalances in food or diet.

Patients with dementia and Alzheimer's are more likely than others to be nutritionally deficient and because of this we strongly recommend a comprehensive nutritional supplementation program. See details in the section on the Gallagher Wellness program.

• Key nutritional elements related to dementia include the B complex vitamins, which have frequently been found deficient in Alzheimer's. Those of particular interest are choline and inositol, two lesser-known B vitamins found in lecithin, an extract of soybeans. They are known to lower blood fats and exert protective effects on brain and nerve cells.

- Vitamin C and B complex help to normalize abnormal brain wave patterns often found in patients with dementia, senility and Alzheimer's.

- Vitamin B-1 taken in megadoses of 1-2 grams daily, and phosphatidyl serine, an interesting brain nutrient also derived from soy, are often critical in difficult cases.

- B-12 deficiency is common among individuals with poor concentration, memory lapses, dementia, and dizziness.

- In 1997, the results of a major two year study conducted at multiple university treatment centers found that vitamin E can slow the progression of illness in patients with moderately severe Alzheimer's disease. In the experiment, researchers compared the effects of a high dose of vitamin E (2,000 IU), the anti-Parkinson's drug Selegiline (10 milligrams) and a placebo on a test group of 341 Alzheimer's patients. Vitamin E emerged slightly ahead of the medication in retarding progression toward institutionalization and also extending the functional ability of patients. Both the vitamin and the drug have antioxidant properties, reinforcing the theory that oxidation damage plays a role in Alzheimer's disease.

The study, published in the April 24, 1997 issue of the New England Journal of Medicine, said the findings should be of particular interest since, to date, "no treatment for Alzheimer's disease has shown similar benefits..." The researchers concluded that both vitamin E and Selegilene "should be considered for use in patients with moderate dementia." A similar statement was subsequently issued by the American Psychiatric Association as part of a treatment guideline for physicians.

- Decreased circulation in the brain is quite common among those with memory loss and confusion. I have found that such individuals are often helped by Ginkgo biloba, a Chinese herb. Nutri Smart, a supplement I use in my clinic, contains Ginkgo and many synergistic factors that act as natural brain antioxidants and help improve circulation not only to the head but also to the heart and extremities.

Studies on patients who have had head injuries with decreased attention span and lowered IQ have shown significant improvement with ginkgo alone. It has also been shown to have a beneficial effect on a patient's sociability, alertness, mood, memory and intellectual efficiency.

- The European bilberry, a herb used by World War II American fighter pilots to enhance night vision, along with Butcher's Broom, a German herb, act to promote the relaxation and strengthening of blood vessels. This is particularly useful for those whose condition is associated with decreased circulation.

• A recently developed nutritional supplement discovered in Austria called Enada may provide benefits for patients with dementia, Alzheimer's, Parkinson's and depression.

Enada stands for NADH — short for nicotinamide-adenine-dinucleotide, a major biochemical co-enzyme in the energy production of all living cells. Derived from brewer's yeast, this new supplement may help reduce some symptoms of mental illness. It was developed by Georg Birkmayer, M.D., director of the Neurochemistry Laboratory at the University of Graz in Austria. Birkmayer, a well-known European researcher in the field of Parkinson's Disease, found in a preliminary study of 17 patients with Alzheimer's that NADH not only stops the progression of dementia symptoms but also improves cognitive and behavioral dysfunction.

Chelation therapy

Many of our patients receive chelation therapy. Developed in the 1920's in Germany to help remove toxic metals in industrial workers, this treatment strategy has been found to be a safe and effective treatment for heart disease, circulatory problems and many brain related disorders.

In California, H. Richard Casdorph, M.D., has reported treating many Alzheimer's patients with a combination of chelation therapy, diet and nutritional supplementation, just as we do in our clinic. A summary of his work is contained in "Toxic Metal Syndrome: How Metal Poisoning Can Affect Your Brain" (Avery Publishing, 1995), co-authored with Morton Walker, D.P.M..

This fact-filled book covers research showing how toxic metals such as aluminum, mercury, lead, and cadmium accumulate in our bodies, damage brain cells, and over time may contribute to a variety of disturbing symptoms, including memory loss and Alzheimer's.

Chelation therapy is an extremely safe and effective method of cellular detoxification and arterial clean-up that has been performed in physician's offices for decades. In chelation, a synthetic amino acid called ethylene diamine tetraacetic acid (EDTA) is introduced into the body through a series of intravenous infusions. Metallic pollutants in the bloodstream or brain fluids are "grasped" by this substance and then eliminated by the body. This process works exceptionally well for circulatory problems by removing the calcium-based "glue" that holds together cholesterol-formed proteins and other artery-clogging substances.

"At least 50 percent of elderly people with senility and dementia problems are documented as showing greater mental keenness, memory retention, intelligence quotients, and other improvements after receiving chelation therapy," says Casdorph. "Chelation works in multiple ways by improving blood flow, exerting an anti-oxidant effect, and removing toxic metals that have lodged in the brain."

Avoid aluminum

Donald R. McLaughlan, M.D., director of the Centre for Research in Neurodegenerative Diseases at the University of Toronto, has published numerous scientific papers on the role of aluminum toxicity in Alzheimer's. Aluminum damages the nuclei of cells, preventing them from carrying out their function.

Because of the Alzheimer's-aluminum connection, we recommend avoidance of products containing aluminum. Common products include toothpaste, underarm deodorants, antacids, buffered aspirin, anti-diarrhea drugs, baking powder, and aluminum cookware. Read labels and choose from products that contain no aluminum, the physicians advise.

Natural Remedies for Alzheimer's

- *The Gallagher Wellness Program*
- *Cervical (neck) manipulation*
- *Cranial manipulation*
- *Nutri Smart (includes Ginkgo biloba,*
      magnesium, and choline) .... 2 capsules, 3 times daily
- *Bilberry/grape seed extract (95% polyphenols)* .... 200 milligrams daily
- *Enada (NADH)* .... 2.5 to 10 mg daily before meals
- *Co-enzyme B Complex* .... 100 mg, twice daily
- *Vitamin B-12 sublingual* .... 1,000 micrograms daily with folic acid
- *Chelation therapy*

Natural Remedies for Mental Confusion and Memory Loss

- *The Gallagher Wellness Program*
- *Cervical (neck) manipulation*
- *Cranial manipulation*
- *Nutri Smart* .... 2 capsules, 3 times daily
- *Cognit (phosphatidyl serine)* .... 2 capsules, 3 times daily
- *Co-enzyme B Complex* .... 100 milligrams, twice daily
- *Test for hidden food allergies*
- *Avoid sugar, alcohol and caffeine*

MENOPAUSE

About menopause

Menopause, usually occurring between the ages of 45 and 55, represents a dramatic change in a woman's body. For most women, the early indicator is irregular periods. Later, as the production of the female hormones estrogen and progesterone decline, many women begin experiencing more dramatic symptoms including hot flashes, crying spells, depression, bone and muscle pain, vaginal dryness, insomnia, thinning hair, heart palpitations, and lowered sex drive.

The medical establishment and pharmaceutical industry approach menopause as a virtual disease, promoting drugs such as Premarin or other estrogen and progesterone compounds. Although there are certainly benefits to ERT (estrogen replacement therapy) including prevention of osteoporosis and heart disease, there are also increased risks of endometrial and breast cancer. Other well known complications include gallstones, hypertension and blood clots. Many woman share justifiable concerns about these side effects.

Unfortunately, like most other conditions treated conventionally, women are only given two options — drugs or surgery (hysterectomies). However, an increasingly larger number of American women, educated about alternative medicine, are choosing natural approaches.

Q *"I am 50 years old and going through the change of life. My doctor wants to put me on Premarin but I am concerned about the side effects. Are there any herbs or natural remedies for me?"*

How we treat symptoms of menopause

There is much more available to menopausal women with symptoms than just drugs or surgery. There is, in fact, a full menu of natural prescriptions to help get you through this transition period without developing the complications associated with conventional therapy.

Chinese botanicals including Dong quai and Panax ginseng exert mild but effective estrogen-like activity as does the North American herb Black cohosh.

Those three herbs, along with Licorice root and Chasteberry, are probably the most effective herbs for controlling hot flashes.

Dong quai has long been revered in China and Japan for its ability to reduce hot flashes. It also contains compounds that help a variety of menopausal complaints.

Black cohosh, widely used by Native American Indians and later by American colonists, has a significant estrogenic effect. Several studies have confirmed that Black cohosh has at least three types of active compounds offering substantial relief in menopause.

Licorice root, historically used for both culinary and medicinal purposes, is considered a major female tonic. Well-known for its anti-ulcer and anti-arthritic properties, licorice contains glycosides, natural compounds that have a similar structure and activity as adrenal steroid hormones. The adrenal gland is often considered a backup ovary since it also produces a small amount of estrogen.

Panax or American ginseng was traditionally consumed by American Indians as a general tonic and restorative, and to help the mind. Today, American ginseng is known for its adaptogenic properties — its ability to bring balance to a distressed system. Panax is considered by the Chinese as the most sacred of all herbs. Unlike Siberian or Korean ginseng which have more stimulating effects (Yang), American Ginseng is more sedative and relaxing (Yin energy) in its action.

Chasteberry has been used since ancient times as a female remedy, controlling and regulating the female reproductive system. Modern research has confirmed chasteberry's female hormonal activity thereby helping menstrual, menopausal and PMS symptoms.

Primrose oil and bioflavonoids help reduce change of life symptoms. Primrose, a source of gamma linoleic acid (GLA), has been found useful for PMS, cystic breast disease and menopause. Bioflavonoids (vitamin P) contain chemical structures similar to estrogen.

Vitamin E, which not only helps decrease excessive menstrual clots and painful periods, offers benefits as well here in relieving menopausal symptoms. Dosage varies from 400 international units up to 2,000 units per day.

We have found that a remedy known as Dr. Wise's #47 Homeopathic Female Tablets, works well for some women with milder pre-menopausal or menopausal symptoms. Each quarter-grain tablet contains pulsatilla, ova testa, and lilium. Five tablets can be taken four times daily for the first month with a gradual reduction of dosage depending on response. More serious symptoms usually require stronger therapy.

Progesterone creams (from Mexican wild yams) can be rubbed into the skin (a quarter to a half teaspoon) on a daily basis, or particularly between ovulation and menses. For menopausal women, combinations of phytoestrogens and progesterones in tablet form or creams can be used with great benefit. I have hundreds of women who currently opt for this natural approach.

These are some of the many "natural options" we use with good results and without the risks frequently attributed to drug therapy.

The influence of diet

The incidence of menopausal symptoms and breast cancer in Asian women is much lower than their American counterparts. An explanation for this may be diet. The traditional Asian diet emphasizes soy, vegetables, and much less fat and animal protein.

In his 1995 book "Eat Right, Live Longer," Neal Barnard, M.D., the president of the Physicians' Committee for Responsible Medicine, points out that two-thirds of women in America and Western countries experience hot flashes as they pass through menopause and even beyond. In Japan, only 10 percent of women report hot flashes. Hot flashes are so rare in Japan that there is no common word for them.

Says Barnard: "Throughout their lives, Western women consume much more meat, about four times as much fat, and only one-quarter to one-half the fiber as do women on Asian rice-based diets. The result is a chronic elevation of estrogen levels."

At the time of menopause, the manufacture of estrogen in the ovaries comes to a halt and the adrenal glands continue to secrete a small amount of the hormone as they always have. The end of ovary production represents a major loss of estrogen for Westerners, but not for Asian and other women on largely vegetarian diets. For them the drop is much less dramatic, with resulting symptoms milder or even nonexistent, says Barnard.

"Those who enter menopause on a low-fat, vegetarian diet often breeze right through it," he adds.

Among the vegetable recipes popular in Asia are tofu dishes. Tofu is curded soybean and soybeans are a rich source of phytoestrogen — naturally-occurring estrogen. One cup of soybeans, in fact, provides the equivalent of about .45 milligrams of conjugated estrogens, or one tablet of Premarin. There are at least 3,000 foods that contain natural estrogens, including celery, leeks, parsley, fennel, nuts and seeds.

According to James Zhou, Ph.D., an expert in Chinese medicine associated with the department of pharmacology at Yale University, says that "for 2,000 years, foods made from soybeans, such as tofu, fuzu and roasted soybeans, have contributed to hot flash-free menopause in China and other areas of the Orient."

Gregory L. Burke, professor of public health science at Wake Forest University, reported at a major medical conference in 1996 that women suffering hot flashes report significantly less intense symptoms after eating soy protein, the main ingredient in tofu. Burke conducted a study involving 43 women, aged 45 to 55. All suffered at least one episode of hot flashes or night-sweating daily.

In his study, the women added 20 grams of powdered soy protein to juice or cereal for a period of six weeks. Then for another six weeks, they used another powder, but one containing carbohydrate.

Results revealed that the soy protein decreased the intensity of the hot flashes but not the frequency. A recent study in England indicates that soy may indeed reduce the frequency. Burke is planning a larger study with 240 women and a larger amount of soy.

Although the research with soy protein is preliminary, experts are saying that it fits in with much anecdotal evidence as to why hot flashes are so rare in Asia.

Moreover, experts say there is no evidence that the forms of estrogen found in soy products carry the same risks that are found with pharmaceutical estrogens.

Asian women, who have the lowest rates of breast cancer among industrialized countries, consume 30 to 50 times more soy products than American women. In fact, soy products are protective against colon cancer and coronary artery disease. One of the active compounds in soy, known as genestein, was found in low dosages, to be equivalent to the current drugs (Premarin) in maintaining bone mass in animals.

The good news is that soy is not selective just for women. Phytoestrogens protect men from prostate cancer.

DHEA

DHEA, which stands for dehydroepiandrosterone (pronounced dee-hi-dro-epp-ee-ann-dro-stehr-own), is a hormone that has been making nutritional headlines since the mid-1990s. It is made in the adrenal glands, and is used by the body as a raw material to make other important hormones, such as testosterone, estrogen, progesterone, and corticosterone.

Production of DHEA is known to decrease sharply with age. By 65, we have 10 to 20 percent of the amount a 20-year-old has. This drop in production is theorized by many experts to represent an important factor in numerous degenerative and age-related diseases.

Low DHEA levels are associated with menopause and subsequent reduced bone mass in women. DHEA deficiency may be part of the explanation of why osteoporosis afflicts so many women after menopause. One study showed the average plasma DHEA level in premenopausal women to be 547, in postmenopausal women 197, and only 126 in women whose ovaries were surgically removed. The lower a woman's DHEA level, the lower her bone density and the higher risk of osteoporosis.

Promising research has created an expectation that this substance may possess real medical value in the treatment of many age-related conditions. Research also suggests a hormone replacement role that might generate major prevention and anti-aging benefits for individuals as they get older. Both researchers and physicians alike who are familiar with DHEA say that in appropriate dosages it can boost energy, elevate the sense of well-being, and activate the immune system. There is much excitement about DHEA.

Experts, however, also add a word of caution. Previously available only through a physician's prescription, a 100 percent synthesized version of DHEA can now be purchased over-the-counter. There have been no long-term studies with the use of DHEA. Therefore, "appropriate dosage" is an important consideration. Too much DHEA has been associated with increased levels of male hormones among women. There have been reports of facial hair developing among women, a situation that disappears when DHEA is reduced or eliminated.

At this stage of our knowledge about DHEA, it is prudent to use it under the guidance of a health professional. Laboratory tests should be conducted to determine initial levels of DHEA, to help indicate an appropriate individual intake, and later on as well to see how supplementation is affecting levels in the body.

DHEA levels can be obtained reliably through a blood test. Wide individual variables are common at all ages and the normal range for DHEA is extremely broad. There also appear to be important genetic differences. For instance, Japanese men have significantly lower levels than American white men.

In addition to the blood test, a new and less expensive method has been developed that measures DHEA in the saliva. I currently prefer the saliva test and have found it to be more reliable than the blood test. I also check the salivary levels of estrogen, progesterone, and testosterone in women.

If you are self-dosing with DHEA, it is wise to start low (5 milligrams) and gradually increase, if needed, each month.

Pre-menopause

I have found phytoestrogens and herbal therapies extremely beneficial for menopause as well as perimenopause. For many women in their thirties and early forties, symptoms similar to menopause can occur and become problematic. Before the cessation of the menstrual cycle, the body naturally goes through a transition period. Known as perimenopause the period is short-lived for some women but prolonged for others. Hot flashes, depression, decreased libido, mood swings, anxiety attacks, hair loss and thinning, cracking nails and much more are common to patients who come to our clinic.

While gynecologists recommend low dosage birth control pills for this condition, I and many other alternative doctors have found natural progesterone creams along with herbs and vitamin therapies to be extremely safe and effective.

The chiropractic — menopause connection

Jeannette, a 50-year-old mother of two, had been experiencing extensive menopausal symptoms when she came to my clinic for a consultation several years ago. She had previously taken Premarin and Provera, the traditional estrogen/progesterone prescription drugs, but developed severe

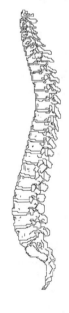

breast sensitivity and painful veins. She stopped taking the drugs. She then experienced heart palpitations, mood swings and continuous hot flashes which interfered with her sleep.

A chiropractic evaluation determined that Jeannette had misalignments in her spine. Following her first manipulation, she reported that the hot flashes stopped for three days. With further manipulations, she had a reduction in the severity and intensity of hot flashes and associated symptoms. She was able to begin sleeping again through the night.

You won't find anything written about the chiropractic-menopausal connection in the medical literature, even in the alternative medicine field. It is not well-known, well understood, or even generally considered in the chiropractic profession. But the fact is that chiropractic manipulation can often be very beneficial for menopausal women. That is my experience over the years. I have had gratifying results in quite a few cases.

Some patients have reported complete menopausal control with chiropractic manipulation alone. Since the body's hormonal system is governed by the nervous system, it just makes sense that mechanical misalignments of the spine, which can block or distort normal nerve impulses, may also contribute to a variety of menopausal symptoms.

During a major interdisciplinary conference of medical and chiropractic researchers in London, the comments of a prominent British orthopedic surgeon caught my eye. John O'Brien, M.D., was quoted as saying that "thousands of hysterectomy operations are performed annually following misdiagnosis of referred pain from the lumbar spine which would generally respond excellently to skilled chiropractic manipulation."

Natural Remedies for Menopause

- **Gallagher Wellness Program**
- **Chiropractic cervical and lumbar manipulation**
- **Vegetarian diet with tofu and other soybean products**
- **Osta B3 (phytoestrogen/progesterone)** .... .625 milligrams daily
- **Vitamin C with bioflavonoids** .... 1,000 milligrams, 4 times daily
- **Vitamin E** .... 1,000-2,000 IU
- **Primrose oil** .... 2 capsules, twice daily
- **Osteocaps** .... 2 capsules, 3 times daily
- **Dong quai, Black cohosh combination** .... 2 capsules, 3 times daily
- **DHEA** .... 5-100 milligrams daily

                                        (preferably with professional supervision)

MULTIPLE SCLEROSIS (MS)

Q "*I am a 55-year-old woman with a long history of multiple sclerosis (MS). Over the years, I have been to the best neurolo gists and clinics hoping to find the answer. I have been on Prednisone (steroids) too many times to count and on a drug called Imuran. I have even tried the new shots for MS but I am getting progressively worse. I have numbness, weakness, blurred vision, difficulty walking, dizziness, neck pain, and bladder problems. I keep hearing about alternative medicine, so I am hoping that you can help.*"

About multiple sclerosis

The woman calling in during one of my radio talk shows had many of the typical multiple sclerosis symptoms.

The symptoms of this progressive nervous system disorder are numerous and also include:
- loss of coordination and a tendency to drop things.
- nausea and vomiting.
- unpredictable mood swings.
- double vision and blindness.
- a feeling of constriction or "pins and needles."
- heaviness and stiffness.
- sexual dysfunction.

The entire complex of symptoms is vast. Patients may experience many or just a few, and with varying degrees of intensity. In two-thirds of cases, MS develops between the ages of 20 and 40. More women than men (60/40) are patients.

In modern medicine, MS has been viewed as a destructive process that targets the protective sheath — the myelin sheath — around nerves within the brain and spinal cord. Areas of damage vary in size and loca-tion. The body naturally attempts to heal the "demyelinated" tissue and in this process hardened plaque may develop at the site. This process is known as sclerosing, from which the disease gets its name. When the integrity of the sheath is affected, impairment of bodily functions are believed to occur. However, autopsies have found that some people with evidence of "demyelination" never had symptoms of MS.

The precise cause of the disease remains unclear, although many contributing factors have been put forward by researchers. They include viruses, autoimmune factors, hormonal influences, and diet.

Contemporary research focuses on the following theories:

• An auto-immune disease in which mutant immune system cells turn on a certain protein involved in the production of the myelin sheath.

• Exposure to a virus — as yet undiscovered — that is activated by stress and other environmental factors.

• A deficiency or absence of a mysterious "X" factor in the blood that is depleted when individuals eat a high fat diet. This factor is thought to help protect myelin tissue.

There is no known prevention or medical cure for MS. Treatment largely centers on relieving the symptoms during flare-ups. The conventional medical prescription focuses on the use of steroids to decrease inflammation associated with MS "attacks." In addition, considerable resources are being spent currently on the use of immuno-suppressive drugs.

The potential is high for serious side effects using these approaches.

Recently, an interesting hypothesis and treatment has emerged that focuses on the pineal body, a pea-sized gland behind the forehead. Rueven Sandyk, M.D., of Touro College in New York, has suggested a connection between MS and calcification of the gland. All MS patients have such calcification, although many other individuals may have it as well who do not exhibit MS symptoms.

Sandyk believes calcification results from a viral infection occurring around the time of puberty and a subsequent inflammation of the gland. This development is thought to affect the supply of serotonin, an important brain chemical (neurotransmitter) that contributes to proper communication between nerve cells. The pineal contains the brain's highest concentration of this critical substance. A low supply of serotonin has been associated with many of the symptoms of MS such as depression, anxiety, sleep disorders, fatigue, and carbohydrate craving.

Sandyk uses magnets (with a strength of 7.5 picotesla) placed at the temples for 30 minutes to stimulate serotonin production in the pineal gland. He claims that all MS patients improve with this method, and 60 to 70 percent experience "marked improvement." The most serious cases have the least improvement.

Dawn Beals' case

In 1993, Dawn Beals, a 37-year-old leasing administrator from Somerset, Pennsylvania, came to our clinic. She had been diagnosed with MS in 1987

Exhausted and sick no more!

and suffered from chronic fatigue, a constant sore throat, bodily aches, and recurring ear and bladder infections.

"My health is rapidly declining," she told me. "I work full-time but that is a massive feat for me. I come home exhausted and sick, eat dinner, fall into bed and wake up the same way. All my social activities have ceased to exist."

Dawn was somewhat skeptical of alternative medicine, but she was desperate. Conventional medicine wasn't helping her.

"My neurologist told me there was nothing I could do for my MS, and my physician has no solutions for my many problems other than to pump me full of antibiotics," she said.

We did a thorough workup on Dawn and discovered that many of her problems were related to a yeast infection, the result of taking many antibiotics.

For starters, we recommended a drastic change in her diet along with a supplement program. We told her to cut out wheat, dairy, sugar, simple carbohydrates and any foods containing yeast.

After hearing what she had to give up, Dawn was shocked. But she said she would give the program a try for six months. If she didn't feel better she would go back to her old way of eating.

We also prescribed a course of colon hydrotherapy to help detoxify her colon.

A chiropractic evaluation of Dawn also revealed misalignments in her neck and low back. I began a series of adjustments to correct these problems. Cervical (neck) adjustments helped to relieve her blurred vision, recurring sinus infections and dizziness. Lumbar (low back) adjustments were effective for her low back pain and recurring bladder infections. These manipulations also helped stimulate endorphin release, that is, the body's very own natural painkillers, as well as melatonin production. The result was less overall pain, better sleep, and improved immunity.

Dawn didn't have to wait six months to feel better. Within two months she started feeling substantially better. Her energy improved. Her bladder pained her less.

"I was beginning to see the light at the end of the tunnel," she told me.

Today, Dawn maintains her health with chiropractic manipulation, supplements, and adherence to a diet that avoids foods she does not tolerate well. She takes no drugs and she no longer waits for attacks to occur. She is off the medical treadmill. She understands that she needs to maintain this lifestyle and she's elated that she discovered it.

"My health has improved to the point where I not only work full-time but travel extensively and enjoy a normal range of activities outside of work," she says. "My attacks are few and far between and always manageable. I shudder to think where I would be had I stayed with conventional medical treatments."

Stacy Stratigos' case

In October 1996, this 38-year-old housewife from White Oak, Pennsylvania, came to see me.

"I was diagnosed as having multiple sclerosis in 1984," she said. "For the next 11 years, nothing significant happened. But in July of 1995, I had numbness and tingling in both my hands and numbness in the front part of my legs and down into my feet. I was put on a course of Prednisone by an internist and the symptoms eventually ceased.

> **Slurred speech and numbness decreased after a few treatments**

"In June of 1996 I was again battling another flare-up of MS. Only this time, it was worse. I had numbness and weakness on the left side of my body. I was slurring my speech and was unable to grasp things with my left hand. Dizziness had become a part of daily living. This time, the symptoms didn't disappear with Prednisone. Also, the MRI of 1996 compared to an MRI of 1995, showed the development of significant new anomalies in the brain."

A friend told Stacy about my wholistic approach and she decided to give it a try. Her clinical workup showed she had spinal stress in her upper neck. In addition she was extremely toxic from prescription drugs and an unhealthy diet.

I recommended a 10 day detoxification diet (see chapter six) and cervical manipulation.

Stacy told me that the slurred speech and numbness started decreasing after a few treatments. She is currently stable on a chiropractic and nutritional program. She takes no drugs. "Overall, there has been a tremendous improvement in my body," she reported during a recent treatment.

How we treat multiple sclerosis

In our clinic we integrate a variety of natural alternatives for MS patients. They include the following:

• B vitamins, especially niacinamide (B-3), B-6, choline and inositol. These vitamins are essential elements in the formation of serotonin, a brain chemical (neurotransmitter) that has a mood elevating effect on the body.

• Parasitic and fungal infections are often associated with this disorder. As in the case of Dawn Beals, many MS patients have a malfunctioning immune system due to having taken many antibiotics. These medications indiscriminately destroy good and bad bacteria in the body, and open the door to yeast and parasitic infections (see the chapter on yeast infections). These opportunistic micro-organisms proliferate rapidly and discharge toxins that can seriously affect your health and energy. If such infections are determined, we recommend special nutritional plans plus colon hydrotherapy to clear the intestinal tract.

• Myelin Sheath, a nutritional supplement, that contains an actual extract of the nerve covering, serves as a repair factor for damaged nerves.

• Anti-oxidant supplements are important because they counteract free radical activity. (see chapter 11 for discussion of how free radicals contribute to many disease conditions). In multiple sclerosis, this activity is involved in nerve membrane damage. Of particular significance are Ginkgo biloba, a "brain antioxidant" and vitamins C and E.

• Essential fatty acids are frequently deficient in MS patients and, when taken supplementally, act as nerve cell guardians. The best types of supplements are raw flaxseed oil, borage oil and fish oils. All are rich in beneficial omega-3 fatty acids.

• A modified version of the "Swank diet," originally developed by Roy Swank, M.D., a professor of neurology at the University of Oregon Medical School 50 years ago. The diet is low in saturated fat, particularly saturated fats associated with meat and dairy. When the "Swank Diet" is followed over a long period of time, it reduces the severity and frequency of MS attacks.

The Swank Diet

• *Saturated fat — less than 10 grams daily.*
• *Polyunsaturated oils — 40 to 50 grams daily.*
• *Reduce or eliminate all animal foods except fish. Eat fish 3 to 4 times a week, especially coldwater fish (such as salmon, cod, bass and perch)*
• *Emphasize raw and fresh whole foods, especially fruits, vegetables, legumes, and grains.*
• *No dairy, margarine, shortening or hydrogenated oils.*

The chiropractic — multiple sclerosis connection

Experts and patients alike have overlooked one important contributing factor to MS: spinal misalignments. They don't think of a chiropractic role in multiple sclerosis. But they should.

Remember that structure affects function. If the structure of the vertebral column has misalignments at any single or multiple levels, this can affect the function of the nervous system. Remember, also, that the spinal cord, containing all the nerves that supply your body, runs down your neck and back and is protected by the spinal column. It is within this cord that the deteriorating process of multiple sclerosis occurs.

As I have said in many places in this book, misalignments do not just cause pain. Because they impact the nerve and blood supply, they can cause local degeneration, loss of motion, interference in multiple physiological functions and literally countless different symptoms throughout the body.

Initial research has indicated that long-term subluxations in the spine may irritate or compress nerves and cause degeneration of their protective myelin sheath. However, there is little direct research on multiple sclerosis. Chiropractic literature contains virtually no mention of multiple sclerosis. However, two interesting case histories have been reported that are worth mentioning here:

• A 32-year-old male, with a family history suggestive of MS, suffered from fatigue, gait imbalance, double vision, and numbness in the legs.

Originally, his tiredness, imbalance and visual problem were thought to stem from an ear infection following a bout of flu. This connection was reinforced when the patient quickly recovered after antibiotic therapy. It wasn't so simple, however. Three months later, the same symptoms returned, only now they were accompanied by nocturnal incontinence, muscle weakness, and eye twitching, and soon afterward by abdominal bloating and numbness in the legs. A neurologist and radiologist both confirmed the presence of myelin sheath damage and felt that MRI findings were consistent with MS.

Subsequently, a chiropractic evaluation also suggested the presence of spinal subluxations. Chiropractic adjustments were administered. Minutes later the patient reported that all symptoms had subsided. Two more manipulations were conducted over the next few weeks after which the patient discontinued them for several months. During that time, there were no return of symptoms.

It is well-known that MS patients experience cycles of remission and intensity. The quick response in this case prompted the researchers to suggest that correction of the subluxation triggered immediate neurological improvement (Journal of Manipulative and Physiological Therapeutics, 1993).

• The second case involved a 24-year-old women who was diagnosed by a neurologist as probable MS. Her symptoms developed gradually and included burning, prickly sensations, tingling in the arms and legs, stiffness in the left arm, chronic fatigue, spells of depression and dizziness. A low-fat diet and a prescription of Prednisone provided no relief.

Three months after the onset of symptoms the patient sought a chiropractic opinion. X-rays and chiropractic evaluation revealed misalignments in her neck and upper back. Chiropractic treatment included 14 upper cervical adjustments over a period of four months. The patient was monitored for an extended period of 10 months in order to carefully assess the progression of the disease and the effect of chiropractic care. By the end of the monitoring period significant improvement had been documented. Extremity numbness, energy level, emotional well-being and general health all increased.

This particular study was undertaken to test the hypothesis that subluxations may either originate or exacerbate MS symptoms. The researcher, Scotty L. Kirby, D.C., of Marietta, Georgia, concluded that this case "demonstrates improvement of symptoms related to MS through management with specific chiropractic adjustments. While these improvements are encouraging, additional investigation is needed before specifically linking this condition to a subluxation-based problem. Hopefully, this study will pique enough interest to initiate more research in this area."

Commenting on this study, "Neurological Fitness," a chiropractic newsletter, pointed out that the late Clarence Gonstead, D.C., a prominent chiropractic educator, "emphasized the importance of correcting cervical (neck) subluxation" and restoring the normal cervical curve in the MS patient."

This possibility is certainly worthy of large-scale research. It stands to reason that chiropractic evaluation and care should not be overlooked and can play a primary role in treatment and recovery. Manipulation is extremely beneficial to improve coordination, reduce numbness, and enhance immune function.

In my experience with many MS patients over the years, I have consistently observed improvement and in some cases reversal of the disease process. I should qualify that by saying that I have not reversed wheelchair-bound patients with severe disease, although they do get relief of many symptoms.

I remember one dramatic case that involved a 40-year-old musician from Pittsburgh who was previously diagnosed with MS by a neurologist. Everytime he played the horn, he would experience numbness throughout his body. He was facing retirement from music, which was his great passion in life.

He decided to try the alternative approach and came to me for evaluation. We tailored a chiropractic and nutritional program and within 30 days all signs and symptoms of MS were gone. I see him now once a month for maintenance care. He is back to the horn and the band — with no side effects.

Like Dawn Beals, Stacy Stratigos, and the musician, MS patients need to catch the chiropractic/nutrition wave. Conventional medical care has little to offer and what it does offer is usually toxic.

Although the medical establishment has become obsessed with the idea that a virus is involved in MS, and is intensely searching for an immunizing drug, most experts would agree that this condition is truly a multi-factorial illness. Diet, chemical exposure, vitamin deficiencies, yeast and parasite infections, spinal subluxations, pineal calcification, electromagnetic fields and other factors can enter into the MS equation as triggering or exacerbating elements.

My experience points to an integrated appraisal, taking all of these factors into consideration, and especially the most overlooked — chiropractic and the correction of subluxations that may be adversely affecting the nervous system.

Natural Remedies for Multiple Sclerosis

- *The Gallagher Wellness Program, especially detoxification*
- *Chiropractic manipulation*
- *Colon hydrotherapy*
- *Modified Swank Diet*
- *Anti Parasitic/Fungal Program*
- *Niacinamide* .... 500 *milligrams, twice daily*
- *Vitamin B-12 sublingual with folate* .... 2,000 *micrograms daily*
- *Melatonin* 3 *milligrams before bedtime, although higher doses may be needed*
- *Primrose oil* .... 3 *capsules, twice daily*
- *Myelin Sheath* .... 2 *capsules, 3 times daily*

OSTEOPOROSIS

Q *"I am a 54 year old grandmother. I have been active my whole life. Over the past two years I have gotten deep bone aches, low back pain, knee pain and I do not have the stamina I once had. I have had low thyroid since my early twenties and I went through the 'change' when I was 48. I take Synthroid and Premarin and now my doctor said I should take the new osteoporosis drug (Fosamax). I try to eat right, exercise and take calcium but something is missing. Could it be vitamin deficiencies?"*

A Osteoporosis affects 25 million Americans, three-quarters of them women. The term means "porous bones." About 25 percent of post menopausal women are osteoporotic, although rapid bone density loss is common after age 40. The areas of the body most commonly affected are the hips, spine, ribs and the weight bearing bones. Loss of height, back pain, leg pains, spinal and hip fractures, are frequent catastrophic consequences.

Osteoporosis drugs such as Fosamax have caused a worldwide alert over the severe side effects associated with their intake — including ulceration of the esophagus.

Dairy products, calcium supplements and fluoride, long touted as "osteoporotic cures," are being scrutinized in light of current information that their overuse can harden the outside of the bone but weaken the internal bone structures.

Let's look for a moment at the dairy connection.

Isn't dairy a good source of calcium? Most of us think so, including most nutritionists. It seems, however, we have all grown up with a massive myth, pushed upon us by dairy industry propaganda for decades, linking milk, calcium and bone density.

"Trying to cope with bone loss with dairy products or calcium supplements is like trying to make up for money that falls through a hole in your pocket by taking a second job. It is better to sew up the hole," says Neal Barnard, M.D. author of "Eat Right, Live Longer" (Harmony Books, New York, 1995).

It turns out that nations with the highest consumption of milk invariably have the highest incidence of osteoporosis, such as England, Sweden and the United States. And on the other side of the coin, according to such experts like Mark Hegsted, formerly of Harvard University's School of Public Health, places like Japan and China, where less dairy and protein are eaten, have little osteoporosis.

Something less than 30 percent of the calcium contained in dairy is absorbed. Moreover, milk and other dairy products, even though they are high in calcium, are also loaded with animal protein, which has been determined to promote calcium loss through the urinary tract.

This may help you understand why countries with the highest dairy and meat consumption have for the most part the highest rate of osteoporosis. The RDA of calcium in the U.S. is set at 1,200 milligrams. Compare that to the World Health Organization's recommendation of 500 milligrams for children and 800 milligrams for adults. Around the world, some countries have much lower allowances, such as Thailand, for instance, with 400 milligrams daily for people of all ages.

As Charles Attwood, M.D., points out in his book, "Dr. Attwood's Low-Fat Prescription for Kids" (Penguin Books, New York, 1995), among the elderly South African Bantu women, who consume a very low protein diet (50 grams daily, compared with 91 grams for Americans) and only 450 milligrams of calcium daily, there is no osteoporosis despite a calcium drain from nursing an average of 10 children. On the other hand, Eskimos, who eat a very high protein diet (250-400 grams) of fish, and who have a calcium intake of over 2,000 milligrams daily, have the highest rate of osteoporosis in the world!

An interesting study conducted by Yale researchers on women over 50 with hip fractures, a sign of weakened and osteoporotic bones, found that among 16 countries that were investigated, the highest incidence occurred where calcium consumption is the highest.

The bottom line is that you can get your calcium needs from green vegetables. That's right. Green vegetables. One hundred calories of green vegetables will give you much more calcium than dairy. Plus a whole lot more nutrients important for health. Watercress, turnip, mustard and collard greens, spinach and broccoli, just to name a few vegetables, provide more calcium than dairy.

"This calcium stays in the bones, unlike much of that from the high protein-containing dairy products," points out Attwood. "In cultures where the most protein is consumed, the calcium requirement for good bone density and protection against osteoporosis may be UNATTAINABLY high, without supplements — it's a Catch-22. Milk, it now seems clear, is not the solution to the malady of poor bone density. It may be a part of the problem."

Fortunately, osteoporosis can be helped thanks to major advances in nutritional and lifestyle research. Research on specific dietary protocols has consistently shown that a modified vegetarian, high complex fiber diet is of critical importance. And we know from studies conducted here and around the world that good bone density achieved by the age of 18 normally lasts a lifetime for individuals who eat a balanced plant-based diet and who remain physically active

According to "Eat Right, Live Longer," a diet high in meat "is disastrous for bones." Author Neal Barnard points out that the problem is not just the amount of protein in meats but also the type. Protein molecules are made up of tiny string-like beads called amino acids. Meats are loaded with sulfur-containing aminos, "which are especially aggressive at causing calcium to be lost in the urine," says Barnard.

"Grains, beans, vegetables and fruits easily provide enough protein for your body's needs but avoid the excess," he adds. "They are powerful calcium savers that help keep bones strong and calcium dense." He cites a 1994 study in the America Journal of Clinical Nutrition which showed that when people eliminate meats, cheese and eggs, they reduce their calcium losses in the urine in half.

Meats also have high levels of phosphorus — compared to calcium — which also promote calcium loss. Vegetables have an equal amount of the two important minerals.

Other factors that promote calcium and bone-density loss:
- The phosphoric acid content of sodas.
- Caffeine, particularly for women after menopause. Choose herbal teas instead.
- Too much salt, either by itself or in high-salt foods.
- Tobacco.

How we treat osteoporosis

I often recommend Osteocaps, a nutritional osteoporosis formula that contains the nutritional factors essential for this disorder. If you think about it, your bones are not just composed of calcium. If you pulverize and analyze bone you will find a partnership of minerals at work to strengthen your structure. Chief among them are calcium, magnesium, boron, manganese, silica, molybdenum, vanadium, lithium, and potassium.

One of the minerals I mentioned is boron, an unfamiliar name to most people. Boron is critical to bone health. It exerts physiological effects similar to estrogen on bone density. It is commonly deficient as determined by hair analysis studies.

Vitamins, especially A, D, and K, are also critical for this condition. Vitamin K, an under-recognized nutrient also known as phylloquinone, is important for the integrity of proteins found in bone. Older individuals and persons with osteoporotic fractures are known to have lower K levels in the body. A daily supplement of 1 milligram helps to increase the absorption of calcium into the bone and also decreases the excretion of calcium out of the body.

Aging alters the metabolism of vitamin D and calcium. The level of vitamin D, which is normally produced in the skin from exposure to sunlight, declines with age. This is particularly true for individuals who are housebound, institutionalized and physically inactive. They tend to have an insufficient level. Supplementation of 400 to 800 international units of D, along with 1,200 milligrams of calcium, has been found to reduce the incidence of hip fracture by as much as 43 percent.

Phytoestrogens, natural estrogens derived from plants, are safe and effective alternatives to the pharmaceutical versions Premarin and Provera. Osta B3 is the form we use. Since estrogen and progesterone play a major role in bone disease and heart disease, many of my patients opt for these plant-based formulas. They can be taken orally or rubbed on the skin on a daily basis to provide natural hormone replacement therapy.

Regular weight-bearing exercise (walking, aerobics, and weight training) is a must for all women concerned with osteoporosis. Exercise stimulates the cardiovascular system and skeletal structure, which increases the uptake of nutrients and hormones and strengthens bones.

The thyroid connection

Synthroid, a standard hormonal replacement prescription used for low thyroid, can cause or contribute to osteoporosis. This type of medication has been shown to deplete the skeletal sites such as the neck of the femur (hip).

For men and women who do have low thyroid, two other options should be considered.

1) A nutritional evaluation to determine whether or not you have adequate "raw materials" in your body and/or diet to make thyroxine (thyroid hormones).

I often recommend a supplement that combines iodine, vitamin A,

L-tyrosine (an amino acid), and thyroid glandular extract. This preparation, called Thyrosine Complex, provides patients who are slightly hypothyroid with the necessary building blocks to make their own thyroid hormones and avoid the depleting effect of synthetic hormones.

There are probably millions of individuals, especially women, who have nutritionally-induced hypothyroidism, that is, they are deficient in the ingredients the body needs the most to produce thyroid hormones. For the most part, conventional doctors do not look for these factors. As a result, many people are unnecessarily placed onto a lifetime of replacement drug therapy.

2) Those who have true hypothyroidism not due to nutritional deficiencies may want to consider the prescription drug, Armour Thyroid. Although no studies to date have compared synthroid to Armour, the latter contains both T3 and T4 (two types of thyroid hormones) naturally occurring from a bovine (animal) source. Synthroid offers only a synthetic dosage of T4. Thus, Armour may hold the greater promise. Our own thyroid gland produces both T3 and T4.

The chiropractic — osteoporosis connection

Chiropractic adjustments are essential for aging patients because spinal misalignments lead to abnormal wear and tear — arthritis. Realigning the spinal and skeletal structures reduces the effect of gravitational

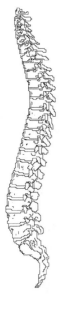

forces on the body by properly distributing this stress across the joint surfaces.

Irene, a women in her sixties, first visited my office 18 years ago and had to be driven by taxi, even though she only lived one block away. Irene had multiple spinal fractures due to osteoporosis. In constant pain, barely able to stand or walk, and facing a lifetime in bed, she opted for chiropractic and nutritional care. Following X-rays and spinal evaluations, I recommended a series of chiropractic adjustments using the activator method. This method utilizes a small spring gauge instrument that delivers 1 to 4 ounces of pressure to misaligned vertebrae. Irene was treated initially in a seated position as I adjusted her multiple misalignments with the instrument.

I also prescribed a modified vegetarian diet and bone-building supplements. Irene gradually progressed to the point where she could walk to the office. In fact, she recovered to the point that within a year she was able to travel with her husband to Europe.

Along with the activator method, the sacral-occipital (SOT) technique is also frequently helpful in these cases. It is a light- touch chiropractic procedure that optimizes structural balance, relieves pain, increases joint motion, enhances flexibility and improves balance.

In addition, chiropractic orthotics are often prescribed at our office for heel spurs, foot pain, and knee problems. They are excellent "shock absorbers" that help reduce overall skeletal stress. This is helpful for osteoporosis sufferers by reducing foot stress that is absorbed into the spine.

Natural Remedies for Osteoporosis

- *The Gallagher Wellness Program*
- *Chiropractic manipulation: Activator or Sacral-occipital (SOT) method*
- *Vegetarian diet high in soy*
- *Phytoestrogen/progesterone* .... .45 to .625 milligrams daily (women only)
- *Thyrosine Complex* ..... 1 or 2 capsules daily (if slight hypothyroid condition exists)
- *Osteocaps* .... 2 capsules, 3 times daily
    If Osteocaps unavailable subtitute with the following supplements:
    - *Calcium* .... 800-1,5000 milligrams daily
    - *Magnesium* .... 500-1,000 milligrams daily
    - *Manganese* .... 5 milligrams daily
    - *Boron* .... 3 milligrams daily
    - *Silica* .... 1 milligram daily
    - *Vitamin K* .... 1 milligram daily
    - *Vitamin D (with folate)* .... 1-3 milligrams daily
    - *Betaine HCL* .... 1 capsule, 3 times daily

PREMENSTRUAL SYNDROME (PMS)

The Jekyl and Hyde PMS personality

Q "*My husband says I have a Jekyl and Hyde personality. I seem to do real well until one week before my period. Then I become extremely irritated, angry and depressed. I have always had painful, heavy menstrual cycles but it has gotten worse the past five years. My gynecologist suggested Prozac (anti-depressant) but I am afraid of drugs.*"

About premenstrual syndrome

Premenstrual tension syndrome affects 33 percent of American women between the ages of 30 and 40. It is typically associated with fatigue, mood swings, depression, irritability, low sex drive, breast swelling and tenderness, headaches, anxiety, and craving for food, especially sweets. For some women (about 10 percent), the condition is actually debilitating.

Common conventional medical treatments include the use of hormones, tranquilizers, mood elevators, water pills and other relatively ineffective and symptomatic treatments.

PMS has a strong nutritional connection. Hypoglycemia (low blood sugar) is often involved. Most patients have a dietary history brimming with refined carbohydrates (that means lots of processed food, "junk food" and sugar) that contribute to all sorts of deficiencies and problems.

Our typical eating habits are a major contributing factor to PMS, fibrocystic breast disease and reproductive diseases. The high consumption of animal protein and dairy products increase the levels of estrogen in women, provoking difficult menstrual cycles and hormonal imbalances. Asian women, whose diets are high in fiber and lower in protein and fat, experience far less debilitating symptoms.

Many PMS sufferers have a history of antibiotics, birth control pills and sometimes steroids. Combined with poor diet, the use of these drugs can create up to two weeks of living hell for many women.

How we treat PMS

At our clinic we recommend vitamin B-6. This vitamin is a natural mood elevator and diuretic. Many individuals are deficient in B complex, particularly if they eat a sugary diet.

Magnesium, a pivotal mineral, works synergistically with B6. We usually suggest 500 milligrams twice day, or a bowel tolerance level. It is particularly helpful for irritability and breast tenderness. A deficiency of magnesium is a sure-fire way to promote PMS and, according to government nutritional surveys, most Americans are indeed deficient, and substantially so. According to Mildred Seelig, Ph. D., of Emory University, who is one of the world's leading magnesium researchers, a deficiency intensifies the body's reactions to stress. Lower magnesium levels have been associated with PMS in research and such a deficiency has been hypothesized as a causal factor for this condition. Magnesium is involved in hundreds of important functions in the body, including the relaxation of muscle tissue.

The combination of magnesium, B-6 and chromium, another mineral, is useful for stabilizing blood sugar to help prevent the roller coaster effects of blood sugar that occurs in hypoglycemia (see the chapter on hypoglycemia).

Vitamin D, along with calcium, has been recently shown in studies to help severe PMS and menstrual migraines. The dosage of vitamin D found effective was 1,600 international units daily, and 1,200 milligrams of calcium.

We have long used Primrose and Flaxseed oil supplements for their ability to ease tension, irritability, nervousness and depressed libido. These beneficial oils contain important omega 3 and 6 fatty acids that are often lacking in women with PMS and migraines. Deficiencies can play a role in the development of pain and inflammation.

Topical creams containing extracts of Mexican wild yams can be effective anti-PMS agents. These popular products contain a natural progesterone-like hormone. They are rubbed onto the forearm from mid-cycle to menses. They can also be effective against menstrual migraine, especially when applied directly over the site of head pain or placed under the tongue.

Herbal remedies include Unicorn root, especially if there is depression associated with PMS. The amino acids tyrosine and DL-phenylalanine are also helpful in relieving PMS-related depression.

Chasteberry, a tree native to the Mediterranean region, has long been used for female complaints. The plant is thought to contain a compound that produces effects almost identical to progesterone.

The European bilberry is another useful herb, particularly for cramping. It relaxes smooth muscles in the body, including those in the uterus wall that tighten with cramps.

I have found these herbals particularly helpful for menstrual cramping, anxiety and mood changes.

Glandular therapy has been a gold standard at our clinic. For PMS, I recommend a raw tissue supplement containing concentrated pituitary, adrenal and ovary extract. I often find that PMS patients have weak adrenal and ovary glands.

Finally, it is best to remember that PMS is not a psychological state but rather an abnormal physiological response to nutritional, hormonal and mechanical stress over a period of time. It takes a comprehensive approach to get good results. And the results, according to our patients, are indeed very good.

Menstrual bleeding

Q *"I have been having heavy periods for the past 5 years. My cycle usually lasts 6-7 days with heavy bleeding and clots. My gyne cologist said that I had 2 choices, either hormones or a hysterec tomy. I tried the hormones for 3 months but they didn't help and I started getting varicose veins. The hysterectomy is out of the questions since I am only 32 and I want to have children. I am hoping you have a third option."*

There are multiple alternative medicine options for women who suffer from menorrhagia (heavy periods).

The Japanese angelica root (Dong quai), which has traditionally been used for hot flashes and depression in menopause, is equally effective for uterine disturbances.

Bromelain, a mixture of sulfur-containing enzymes obtained from the stem of the pineapple plant, is particularly effective in strengthening the blood vessels and decreasing pain and inflammation.

Perhaps the most common nutritional deficiency in this condition is vitamin A. Vitamin A is linked to hormone production and women with heavy menses have lower blood levels of vitamin A, compared to those with normal cycles. I recommend vitamin A in the form of beta carotene, which is also a good anti-oxidant.

Strengthening the blood vessels is crucial. For that purpose, bioflavonoids (derived from the white pulpy part of the citrus fruits) and grape seed extract are recommended supplements.

In extremely resistant cases with prolonged bleeding, or for those who have frequent menstrual cycles, natural progesterone from Mexican wild yams is an excellent option. Skin creams or tablets containing this plant hormone may help to normalize blood flow or regularity without toxic side effects.

The chiropractic — PMS connection

Chiropractic manipulation is an extremely useful — and vastly underused — asset in dealing with most gynecological problems including painful periods, pelvic pain, excessive bleeding, sexual dysfunction and bladder problems. I strongly believe that gynecologists and chiropractors can work together for the benefit of many patients.

Specific chiropractic techniques, especially Applied Kinesiology (AK), can quickly and non-invasively assess the status of the organs and nervous system, and help direct chiropractic and nutritional approaches to aid in recovery. Subluxations or spinal misalignments can cause interference with the nerve and blood supply to the reproductive organs. Hormonal imbalances, among other problems, may be the result.

Manipulation corrects the misalignment. This, in turn, has the potential to normalize the nervous system/hormonal relationship and re-establish menstrual health.

I have successfully used chiropractic adjustments to treat thousands of women with severe PMS, irregular menses, continuous menstrual bleeding, menstrual migraines, and vaginal pain.

A number of studies have demonstrated the benefits of chiropractic care for these types of problems:

• One randomized pilot study, involving 45 women aged 20 to 49, found that immediately after spinal manipulation, women reported a significant reduction in their perception of pain and level of menstrual distress. The symptom improvement among women receiving chiropractic treatment was twice as great as improvements among a comparative non-chiropractic treatment group. The researchers suggested that manipulation may be an effective, safe, drug-free, alternative for relieving the pain of menstruation (dysmenorrhea). They called for further research to substantiate their findings of reduced blood levels of certain prostaglandins, chemicals produced by the body which are believed to be responsible for menstrual pain (Journal of Manipulative and Physiological Therapeutics, 1992).

• Eleven women with histories of PMS reported improvement in all measured symptoms including variation in "sexual drive/habits," "social impairment" and depression, following chiropractic treatment (Journal of Chiropractic Research and Clinical Investigation, 1992).

• An interesting case was reported in 1990 involving a patient suffering from an average of eight days of painful menstrual cramps each month.

This condition had begun with the onset of menses and intensified after the birth of her child four years before. Evaluation determined the presence of subluxations. She was adjusted in the sacroiliac, upper and mid-back, upper neck, and skull. Following the treatment, she experienced cramping an average of 2.25 days. Her pain had diminished by a third (Journal of Manipulative and Physiological Therapeutics, 1990).

   • Earlier, in a 1979 study, 88 percent of women who received chiropractic adjustments reported reduced pain during their periods. In this original study, women were divided into three groups. One received chiropractic adjustments. Another group received "sham" adjustments, that is, ineffective maneuvers meant to give the impression of actual adjustments. The third (control) group was merely monitored. Only the women in the chiropractic care group reported improvements. The researchers concluded that "in primary dysmenorrhea, spinal manipulative therapy should be seriously considered" (Journal of Manipulative and Physiological Therapeutics, 1979).

   • A 1973 European medical publication reported the successful chiropractic treatment of 357 women with gynecological problems (inflammation, dysmenorrhea, and low back pain). The study, conducted at Charles University in Prague, found that a variety of gynecological disorders were associated with spinal misalignments. (Manuelle Medizin, 1973).

Natural Remedies for PMS

• **Gallagher Wellness Program**
• **Chiropractic cervical and lumbar manipulation**
• **High fiber, low fat, low protein, soy-based diet**
• **Chasteberry (standardized extract)** .... 2 capsules, twice daily
between ovulation and menses
• **Magnesium aspartate** .... 500-1,000 milligrams daily
• **Vitamin B-6** .... 50-200 milligrams daily
• **Glandular extracts of ovary and adrenal** .... 2 tablets daily
• **Progesterone cream** .... 1/4 teaspoon between ovulation and menses

Natural Remedies for Menstrual Bleeding

• **Gallagher Wellness Program**
• **Chiropractic lumbar manipulation**
• **Dong quai** .... 2 capsules, twice daily
• **Bromelain/Papain** .... 2 capsules, 3 times daily between meals
• **Beta Carotene** .... 100,000-200,000 IU
• **Vitamin C (with bioflavonoids)** .... 2,000-6000 milligrams daily

PROSTATE ENLARGEMENT

Q *"I am 68 years old and I am up every night urinating three to five times. I sometimes have low back pain and occasional testicle pain. I have been to a urologist who said I need prostate surgery. What about natural alternatives for me?"*

The incidence of what is known medically as benign prostatic hyperplasia (BPH) increases with age. In plain English, the term means a non-malignant enlargement of the prostate.

The walnut-sized prostate gland lies just below a man's bladder, surrounding the narrow urethra tube that carries urine down into the penis and out of the body. The prostate is responsible for secreting a milky fluid that lubricates the urethra, prevents infection and increases sperm motility.

Enlargement can lead to progressive symptoms including frequent night-time urination (nocturia), hesitancy and urgency to urinate, and, in severe cases, obstruction of the urethra. The prostate is the major cancer spot among men — it occurs in about one-fifth of BPH cases, and is rising at an alarming rate. The American Cancer Society predicted that prostate cancer deaths would reach 41,400 in 1996, a number fast approaching the annual breast-cancer toll of 44,300.

About 50 percent of males over 60 in the United States are affected by BPH and by the age of 80 almost all of them. However, only in half the cases is enlargement significant and only a quarter experience urinary symptoms. Nevertheless, it is the No. 1 problem treated by urologists.

Several factors contribute to this male problem. They include aging, hormonal changes, nutrition, spinal dysfunction and lifestyle. The typical American diet is a major risk factor. Sugar, excessive protein, and alcohol all promote prostate enlargement, prostatitis and depressed libido.

Standard medical treatment emphasizes the surgical and drug approach.

TURP, which stands for trans urethral resection of the prostate, is the most common surgery performed on males over the age of 65 — 400,000 operations annually! The swollen prostate is surgically reduced to take pressure off the urethra.

Although the surgical approach claims a 90 percent success rate, there are significant complications involved. They include impotence (5 percent), a need to be re-hospitalized within three months (8 percent), a need for another surgery (20 percent), temporary incontinence, mental confusion, nausea, vomiting, high blood pressure, heart failure and seizures.

More recently, the pharmaceutical industry has touted the prescription drug Proscar, which acts by blocking male hormones responsible for production of prostate cells. However, the drug is so toxic that the FDA has recommended that pregnant women not be exposed to the semen of men who are on Proscar due to the risk of birth defects. Among the side effects are impotence and lowered libido.

Research has shown that mild symptoms sometimes improve with absolutely no treatment at all. In one study, subjects with mild enlargement were followed over a five year period. A quarter of them improved without treatment. One-half of them remained unchanged. The condition of the rest grew worse.

How we treat enlarged prostate
Saw palmetto extract

Exciting natural options include herbal supplements such as saw palmetto berry extract, which has now been proven to be more effective than Proscar, and Pygeum africonum, which has a similar action as saw palmetto. I have had excellent results with the saw palmetto extract in reducing symptoms of enlarged prostate. This herbal is derived from a small palm tree growing along the southeastern coastline, particularly in south Florida.

Although saw palmetto is "made in the U.S.A.," we lag far behind Europe in putting it to use. Extensive research has been done there showing its effectiveness and it is widely used to treat enlarged prostate or benign prostatic hyperplasia.

Germany's Commission E, a division of that country's Federal Health Agency (Bundesgesundheitsamt), evaluates the safety and effectiveness of herbal medicines and publishes its findings. Regarding saw palmetto extract, Commission E notes that this natural medication relieves the difficulties (pain and frequent urination) associated with an enlarged prostate without reducing the enlargement.

One major European study was conducted in 1992 and 1993 by Johan Braeckman, of the department of urology at the University of Brussels. The study looked at the efficacy of a standardized saw palmetto extract on 305 patients with BPH. More than a hundred urologists participated in the multicenter trial.

Braeckman reported the following findings:

• The effects of saw palmetto begin after 30 to 45 days. Most common drugs, such as Proscar, may not kick in until 6 to 12 months.

• Subjectively, most patients said it helped. Eighty-three percent said it was effective after 45 days, and 88 percent after 90 days.

• Objectively, doctors agreed at a similar rate.

• No serious side effects were reported. Twenty-five patients reported side effects, half of which were limited to minor gastrointestinal symptoms. Only two percent of the patients had to prematurely discontinue taking saw palmetto.

• Saw palmetto extract does not change the PSA concentration. PSA (prostate-specific antigen) is a widely used diagnostic test to determine the presence of cancer. The use of Proscar for BPH carries the risk of masking the development of prostate cancer because it significantly decreases PSA levels.

Diet and nutrition

As I mentioned above, the typical American diet probably plays a major role in the development of BHP.

"Your prostate would rather have you be a vegetarian," says Neal Barnard, M.D., president of the Physicians' Committee for Responsible Medicine and a leading advocate for using the power of foods for health.

A meat-based diet encourages many hormone-related conditions and "prostate enlargement is no exception," he says in his 1995 book "Eat Right, Live Longer" (Harmony Books, New York).

In prostate tissue, the male hormone testosterone is modified into dihydrostesterone (DHT), and it is this altered hormone that fuels the enlargement process. Both Proscar and saw palmetto block this conversion.

Barnard notes that foods can "strongly influence sex hormones, including testosterone." He points to research showing that "daily meat consumption triples the risk of prostate enlargement. Regular milk consumption doubles the risk and failing to consume vegetables regularly nearly quadruples the risk."

The condition, he adds, is reportedly on the rise in Asian countries where diets are increasingly becoming Westernized.

Raw flax seed oil, as well as unprocessed raw pumpkin seeds, provide essential fatty acids that are critical for natural shrinkage.

In "Super Nutrition For Men," Ann Louise Gittleman, M.S., a well-known nutritionist and former director of nutrition for the Pritikin Institutes, writes that "by increasing the right fats (from nuts, seeds and therapeutic oils) you can significantly support and nourish this vital gland

and thereby decrease the chances of developing problems with it."

The best "initial medicine," she says, may be the essential fats, and avoidance of the non-essential fats "from margarine, vegetable shortenings, fried foods, and processed vegetable oils."

Zinc is critical in any nutritional program to fend off prostate enlargement. A normal prostate contains more of this important mineral than any other organ in the body. Zinc deficiency among Americans is widespread today, due mainly to its removal in processed foods and the deficient state of agricultural soil in 32 states. Smoking, alcohol, coffee, infections and medications cause a further loss of zinc in the body. In our clinic, we use zinc picolinate supplements to raise prostate tissue levels.

Amino acid therapy, utilizing glycine, alanine, and glutamic acid, has been shown to be beneficial. In one study, this combination reduced or relieved nocturia, urgency, and frequency in a majority of cases.

Scandinavian doctors have long recommended flower pollen extract (Cernilton) as a method of shrinking the prostate, decreasing infection (prostatitis), and increasing libido. I have found this supplement particularly helpful for younger men with chronic prostate infections who were literally living on antibiotics and sulfa drugs.

Glandular therapy

Glandular therapy, based on the concept that "like cures like," has been an important part of natural medicine since the time of Hippocrates. In fact, before the discovery of insulin, whole liver was prescribed as a treatment for diabetes. Scientific studies have demonstrated that glandular extracts, taken as concentrates in capsule form, can be quite effective against a variety of illnesses. Extracts of liver, prostate, thymus, thyroid, and spleen contain small protein molecules which exert hormone or hormone-like action. Taken orally, glandulars are selectively used by the body to repair or assist "target organs."

I have personally used glandulars for many years, in fact since my clinical rounds in chiropractic school. I have found them to be major nutritional factors in recovery from chronic illness.

The use of prostate extract in conjunction with amino acids, herbals, and vitamins, represents another important natural remedy for all prostate problems.

I often use Applied Kinesiology (AK) as a type of "natural cat scan" to test the body for organ weaknesses. Often placing a capsule of a glandular extract under the tongue will neutralize the weakness, thereby providing an important and effective method of restoring organ health. This holds true for prostate conditions.

The chiropractic — prostate connection

Chiropractic manipulation, known for its beneficial effect on female genitourinary problems, can yield significant results for men as well. Over the years I have had good results with BPH, prostatitis, testicular pain, erectile dysfunction of all types, and general male menopausal symptoms.

The nerve and blood supply to the prostate, penis, bladder and urethra are controlled by spinal nerve centers in the lower back. As I have said throughout the book, nerve and blood flow are often impaired by spinal misalignments. As a result you can experience pain or organ dysfunction or both. If the misalignment is located in the lower back area, you may have any number of symptoms, such as sexual difficulties, incontinence or prostate disorders.

Chiropractic manipulation of the lumbar (low back) vertebra and adjustment of the sacroiliac joint that connects the hips to the spine, will frequently improve or reverse these additional conditions.

Ralph, a patient in his late 50s, came to me two years ago for constant neck and arm pain. After a few weeks of chiropractic treatment his pain started to resolve. He also mentioned that he was up four to six times every night urinating due to a prostate problem. Although he had no low back pain, I preceded to examine his low back. I discovered a misalignment in his lumbar spine. After I adjusted it four times, he was sleeping through the night.

Natural Remedies for Prostate

- Gallagher Wellness Program
- Chiropractic lumbar manipulation
- Saw palmetto (standardized extract) .... 250-350 milligrams daily
- Zinc Picolinate .... 50 milligrams, twice daily
- Flax seed oil .... 3 capsules, twice daily

RHEUMATOID ARTHRITIS

About rheumatoid arthritis

Unlike osteoarthritis that primarily affects the back and is more commonly associated with "wear and tear," rheumatoid arthritis is a systemic auto-immune disease. It mostly strikes the extremity joints — the elbows, wrists, knees, feet, and hands. It is sometimes associated with low grade fever, joint stiffness, and fatigue, and affects more women than men, especially those between the ages of 20-40.

In most cases, there is no single cause of the disease. Wholistic doctors believe that a combination of nutritional deficiencies, food allergy, the environment and genetics all play a role.

Conventional medicine offers no effective treatment protocol. In fact, it doesn't even have very safe treatments. This is truly a case where "the cure is worse than the disease."

Medicine focuses on a three-tier approach in an attempt to obliterate the symptoms. In doing so, patients can become severely harmed. Standard treatments involve the use of aspirin, NSAIDs (non steroidal anti-inflammatory drugs), steroids (such as Prednisone) and chemotherapeutic agents (methotrexate).

Initially hailed by pharmaceutical companies as a non-toxic alternative to steroids, NSAIDs have now been linked to thousands of hospitalizations and 2,600 deaths annually in the treatment of rheumatoid arthritis alone. One-quarter of patients placed on these "safe drugs" develop ulcers within four weeks of taking them. Recent studies have confirmed that NSAIDs not only do not cure any type of arthritis, but that they damage the chondrocyte (specialized joint cells) and accelerate arthritis.

Cortisone or "steroid therapy" is another popular medical magic bullet that decreases inflammation. However, it suppresses the immune system in the process. Long term use is problematic. Side effects include ulcers, blood clots, spinal fractures, diabetes, and depression.

The final assault on the immune system is the chemotherapeutic approach that includes the use of the cancer drug methotrexate and other disease-modifying pharmaceuticals. Although the short-term effect may reduce symptoms, if used over time the results can be disastrous and even fatal. A study of 112 patients on aggressive drug therapies for 20 years found that this strategy can increase the rate of disability and shorten lifespan. The study was published in the leading British medical journal Lancet in 1989.

Jessica Malarik's case

Jessica Malarik, from Saltsburg, Pennsylvania, was 13-years-old in the spring of 1994 when her mother first brought the girl to see me. Her problems started in 1988,

> **Rheumatoid arthritis, joint pain, seizures**

when Jessica was seven. Her mother explained her daughter's medical history this way:

"Jessica had two seizures that year and was diagnosed with epilepsy. She was placed on Tegretol, an anti-seizure medication. She never had another seizure, but because her EEGs were abnormal, she continued taking Tegretol for the next six years.

"When she was 11, she began having problems with swollen joints in her hands and began taking Tolectin for rheumatoid arthritis. During the next two years her dosages of Tolectin increased as her hands continued to bother her.

"Jessica also seemed to catch every cold, sore throat or flu that came around. She missed a lot of school and started to become depressed about always being sick."

After starting to treat Jessica with a program of adjustments, diet and supplements, she began to improve.

"By the summer of 1994," her mother said, "her hands no longer bothered her and, with her pediatrician's approval, she gradually stopped taking Tolectin. She was so happy with the improvement she wanted to stop taking Tegretol, too. Again, we checked with her specialist before weaning her from the Tegretol."

In early 1997, Jessica had been off her medicines for more than two years without a seizure.

Always a good student, Jessica seemed to become more alert, self-confident, and ambitious after stopping the medication, according to her mother.

The youngster did suffer some recurrences of joint pain. We attributed that to food factors. For instance, green peppers seem to trigger a reaction, as well as too much wheat.

Jessica also developed menstrual problems and, as I later learned, was too embarrassed to discuss them with me. Her mother took her to a female gynecologist who recommended a short dosage of birth control pills. In a matter of two weeks, Jessica experienced severe joint pain in her feet and hips as well as in her hands. We were later able to control her problem with a herbal supplement, Fem-H.

"Overall," says her mother, "her health is much improved."

Here is a case of a youngster who, if her mother had not discovered alternative medicine, might otherwise have faced a lifetime on the medical treadmill.

A blessing in disguise

Many patients who have a serious diagnosis such as epilepsy or rheumatoid arthritis often accept the medical verdict and live with their problems for the rest of their lives. Untold suffering accompanies these patients who find themselves taking unnecessary drugs, undergoing numerous medical procedures and even operations, and living in fear and despair.

Jessica and her mother decided to reach out and try a new way. We discovered that she had intolerances to certain foods that are linked to rheumatoid arthritis.

Chiropractic manipulation boosted her immune system and contributed to a gradual improvement and ultimate recovery.

Jessica, like many of our young patients, now has the potential to achieve and maintain optimum health throughout life. She has at her disposal natural methods to keep her body well.

Many patients with this problem are young. They are often depressed because they cannot do many of the things their friends do. "My friends can go out, go to restaurants, go drinking, and they don't have any problems," one young woman told me.

Once a patient's health improves, I tell them that their condition is really a blessing in disguise. They have learned how to take care of their bodies. They have knowledge to serve them the rest of their life. On the other hand, I say, you will find that your friends, when they reach 40 or 50 or so, will often be undergoing the same kind of medical procedures that most Americans are going through. That means taking medication, having premature hysterectomies, unnecessary operations, and being on the illness treadmill.

I wonder how many millions of people with rheumatoid arthritis and other serious health problems could become well again if they became aware of natural prescriptions and their ability to heal themselves.

Carol Kirlin's case

One such person who unfortunately went through a horrendous treadmill experience but finally got off and became well again was Carol Kirlin, 55, of Charleroi, Pennsylvania.

> **"I prayed to die...I was so sick of operations."**

Carol was at her "wits end," she said, when she heard one of my radio programs and made an appointment in 1990. She was in extreme pain.

Carol had previously been diagnosed with severe rheumatoid arthritis and had undergone many years of treatment. She had been on heavy steroid therapy and gold shots. She said she had been "in and out of hospitals, had eight foot operations, two surgeries to replace finger joints, had an elbow transplant, and been on 32 pills a day.

"The medication hasn't helped me get better and in fact is making me worse, I believe. The doctors practically destroyed everything in my bones as well as the way I was feeling and my mental outlook. At one point, I prayed to die. I was so sick and so weary of operations."

When I examined Carol I found misalignments in her neck that were affecting her shoulders, arms, and hands. She also had sacro-iliac misalignments that impaired her knees and feet. Tests showed she had food allergies and severe nutritional deficiencies.

Once we started her on a program of detoxification, chiropractic adjustments, removal of food allergies, and nutritional supplements, Carol's medical nightmare came to an abrupt halt.

"After the first couple of months," Carol said, "I experienced a total transformation in me, in my mental outlook and physical health. I felt 100 percent better.

Today, she is another woman. "I feel better mentally and physically," she says. "I follow the diet that Dr. Gallagher gave me, and if I go off it, believe me, my rheumatoid arthritis flares up."

How we treat rheumatoid arthritis

Individuals with rheumatoid arthritis have a hyperfunctioning or overly-vigilant immune system that can, if left unchecked, create joint damage and disability. Our goal, therefore, is to identify the reasons why this is happening and then develop a restorative health strategy.

Digestion and absorption difficulties are common among rheumatoid arthritis patients. Thus we often utilize a functional digestive analysis to determine the right course of treatment. This analysis often shows poor pancreatic enzyme production and deficiency of hydrochloric acid. By supplementing these substances that are in short supply, we can minimize allergic reactions.

A common starting point is our ten-day detoxification program, which combines raw fruits and vegetables, herbal teas and fasting (please refer to chapter six).

398 Dr. Gallagher's Guide To 21st Century Medicine

This unique approach is both diagnostic and therapeutic. Removal of common food allergens (such as dairy, wheat, beef, and eggs) along with fasting (1-5 days) will often eliminate potentially offending foods that can stir up and overload the immune system.

Additionally, we recommend colon hydrotherapy to reduce bowel toxins which have now been proven to be triggering agents for rheumatoid arthritis. Researchers are not sure yet why the toxins move from the gut to joints in the body. It is known, however that patients with inflammatory bowel disease suffer attacks of joint inflammation especially in the major limb joints and that the severity of the problem in the joints often parallels the degree of disease in the bowel.

Parasites, candida (yeast), enzyme deficiencies, and chemical toxins are factors often associated with rheumatoid arthritis. We recommend blood antibody studies to assess their involvement.

MFP Herbal, a formula that contains artemesia (Chinese wormwood) and grapefruit seed extract, has potent anti-bacterial, anti-fungal and anti-parasitic activity. I have found it to provide critical help in many rheumatoid cases.

Indian turmeric, Panax Ginseng, Devil's Claw, and the enzymes extracted from pineapples and papayas (Brom/Pap) can be taken in capsule form individually or in combination to generate anti-inflammatory and analgesic effects. Their anti-inflammatory effect is similar to drugs, but without side effects. Instead of capsules, you can do juice fasts emphasizing pineapples and papayas.

Glucosamine sulfate helps reduce infection and promote cartilage repair. Glucosamine has been proven to be more effective than non-steroidal anti-inflammatory drugs (NSAIDs) in the treatment of arthritis, but for the right reason: it helps repair damaged cartilage cells.

Desert plants such as aloe vera and yucca help ease inflammation and joint pain. Years ago, Dale Alexander, affectionately known as the "Cod Father," popularized the use of cod liver oil. Scorned as a quack by the arthritis establishment, his therapy has now been proven by scientific research to be beneficial in reducing inflammation and decreasing pain. Cod liver oil, as well as flax seed oil, are rich in omega 3 fatty acids that enhance the body's own natural pharmacy to produce anti-inflammatory compounds.

One interesting study was conducted recently using 66 rheumatoid patients who were taking diclofenac (Voltaren), a non-steroidal anti-inflammatory drug. The subjects were divided into two groups by researcher Joel M. Kremer, M.D., of the Albany Medical College in New York. Along with their regular medication, one group was given a fish oil supplement and the other a placebo for the 30 week duration of the experiment. For the last 8 weeks, the medication was discontinued in both groups and replaced with a placebo. This meant that during the final stage of the study, one group was taking two placebos and the other taking the fish oil and a placebo.

Results:

• for the fish oil takers, significant decreases in the number of tender joints, pain, duration of morning stiffness, and both patient and physician assessments of arthritic activity.

• for the placebo group, no similar improvements.

Supplementation with fish oil enabled a number of patients to stop their medication without a disease flare-up. This is a most desirable outcome in as much as NSAIDs often cause peptic ulcers, and liver and kidney damage.

During the past decade, 15 scientific articles have been published demonstrating improvement of rheumatoid arthritis symptoms in patients taking fish oil supplements.

Fish oil supplements have also been found to lower cholesterol levels and reduce platelet clumping, thus reducing the risk of blood clots, and reduce some of the symptoms of bowel dysfunction and premenstrual syndrome.

Antioxidants such as vitamins C and E, selenium, and the enzyme superoxide dismutase help prevent free radical damage which is involved in the rheumatoid arthritis process. (See the discussion on free radicals in chapter 11)

Pantothenic acid, an important B complex vitamin, is commonly deficient in rheumatoid patients. Supplementation helps reduce the severity of symptoms.

The chiropractic-rheumatoid arthritis connection

Just as in the cases of Jessica Malarik and Carol Kirlin, we are routinely able to help rheumatoid arthritis patients and accelerate their recovery with chiropractic care.

Manipulations can enhance the immune system and stimulate the body's natural painkillers.

Many patients don't realize there is a chiropractic connection because they may not have back pain. Back pain is just one symptom of spinal misalignment. A more frequent consequence is interference with the nervous system. You need to remember that the nervous system controls and coordinates all systems of the body, including the immune system.

Chiropractic manipulation, well documented for its effectiveness in treating chronic pain, should not be overlooked. If your structure is misaligned, your body cannot function correctly.

Natural Remedies for Rheumatoid Arthritis

• *General Chiropractic manipulation*
• *Juice fasting, especially papaya and pineapples*
• *Eliminate food allergens*
• *Glucoflex Forte (glucosamine sulfate,*
        chondroiten sulfate) .... 2 capsules, 3 times daily
• *MFP Herbal* .... 2 capsules, 3 times daily
• *Flax seed oil* .... 3 capsules, twice daily
• *Pantothenic acid* .... 500 milligrams twice daily
• *Vitamin C and hydrochloric acid (HCL) intravenous infusions*

SINUS INFECTIONS

Q **"I have been on antibiotics for 52 consecutive days for sinus infections. I have constant pain in my head, my ears ring,my neck is stiff, and my nose bleeds. I have been to my family doctor who keeps switching antibiotics but I keep going downhill. He told me my next step is sinus surgery. I own my own computer business but I am having a hard time keeping up. Do you think nutrition or chiropractic could help?"**

This call, from a listener of one of my radio shows, is a good example of how the medical system fails to deal with the cause of problems. Here is a person on long-term antibiotics, prescribed by a doctor who is undoubtedly concerned about his patient's health. The medication isn't working, so now the doctor recommends surgery! For sure, that won't solve the underlying problem of an originally weakened immune system that must now be devastated from repeated antibiotics.

How many people are trapped in a similar medical treadmill?

Sinusitis, or inflammation of the sinuses, is one of the most common health problems in the country. It affects more than 2 million people annually.

The sinus cavities are believed to be a sort of "air control system" of the lungs. Air is drawn into these tiny cavities, cleaned and filtered, and then passed along into the lungs. Because the cavities are extremely tiny they can become easily clogged with mucous.

Foreign substances such as bacteria, viruses, drugs, allergens, and chemicals can irritate the mucous membranes in the eyes, ears, nose, and throat, leading to excessive mucous, draining, pressure, itching, inflammation, infection and pain. The body's natural response to irritants is to produce histamine, water and mucous. In the case of the sinus membranes, repetitive irritation promotes thick mucous production that does not drain readily from the cavities, setting the stage for problems.

Many chronic cases of sinus infections are allergic in nature. Food, dust, molds, pollen and chemicals inflame the sinus tissue. The swelling decreases circulation in the area, permitting the spread of germs.

The conventional medical treatment includes antibiotics, decongestants, antihistamines, allergy shots, and then, if necessary, surgery.

The use of antibiotics for chronic infections is questionable. In one experiment, researchers divided subjects into two groups. One group was were given an antibiotic (amoxicillin, amoxiciloin clavlanate potassium, or trimethoprim-sulfamethoxazole). The other group received no treatment. The results — a similar response in each group!

One problem with antibiotics, notes environmental allergy expert Doris Rapp, M.D., is that some individuals can "develop an allergic reaction to the major components of an antibiotic itself, or to the dye, flavor, sweetener, or corn (dextrose) that it contains."

A major problem with antibiotics, as I have explained elsewhere in this book, is that this type of medication often destroys the beneficial bacteria in the body and promotes the development of yeast infections (see the chapter on yeast infections).

Judy Tusky's case

Judy Tusky, 50, a Pittsburgh court reporter, looks back on her life as one series of illnesses after another. Her problems began as a child with a continual sense of "just not feeling quite right." She was prescribed antibiotics "for everything from a tooth problem or infection in the mouth, to a virus, flu or cold," she recalls.

> "I don't feel like I have one foot in the grave now."

In high school, she was plagued with a bad sinus condition. She began using three pillows at night in order to facilitate breathing. Doctors used cotton probes into the sinus cavities and steroids to alleviate the blockage but these methods caused pain or side effects and no enduring relief.

Later, during the 1980s, she developed bronchitis, pneumonia, bad congestion, sinus infections and upper respiratory illness almost every year. Bronchitis would affect her at least several times a year.

"My family doctor prescribed at least seven different antibiotics for me," she recalls. "After a few weeks I would feel better and then the bronchitis and infections would come back and I would get another antibiotic. This would go on winter after winter, a vicious cycle of illness, an inability to breath, and antibiotics until my immune system was almost destroyed. I began to dread winter. I even wondered if I would make it through the winters. One November I woke up at four in the morning and I just couldn't move."

It was around this time that Judy decided to try the natural approach.

"I started on a program of chiropractic adjustments, pulsed diathermy (electromagnetic heat) and supplements," she says. "I was skeptical for a long while. I thought, can these supplements and treatments really break the chain of constant illness? I waited to get sick again, but instead I started to feel better. I had a bad cold in February the following year and treatment helped my lungs feel a lot better. I waited for another bout of bronchitis and sinus or pneumonia and I'm still waiting. That was two years ago.

"When I began to experience the results of chiropractic neck adjustments, supplements, eliminating food allergies and excess sugar from my diet, along with other natural methods, I went though a period of anger directed at the doctors and hospitals, who, for over 50 years never gave me real choices. What they gave me seems to have worked to destroy my immune system.

"My energy level has increased and enables me to endure busy 18 hour days sometimes. I don't feel like I have one foot in the grave now. It took a while to get used to the idea that I wouldn't be sick like before. I can breathe properly now. I threw away two pillows and now sleep with one like any other person. After two years, I am still in awe that we have all these alternatives available and still angry most people aren't given the choices."

By switching to natural healing, Judy made a major health transaction — trading in minimal health for optimal health. She no longer regards infections as inevitable suffering in her life. Chiropractic thoracic (mid-back) adjustments helped relax her bronchial tubes and neck adjustments aided sinus drainage. With the help of chiropractic and nutrition, Judy has discovered the healer within.

Had she been exposed to alternative medicine as a child, she could have been saved much needless misery. I am reminded of the popular Steven Stills song from the 1960s — "Teach Your Children Well." In this case, it behooves us all to teach our children about the benefits of chiropractic and natural healing.

Linda Cozza's case

Linda Cozza, a 40-year-old Pittsburgh clerk, sought my help in 1996 for a chronic sinus problem. She suffered from headaches all her life, she told me, and over the previous five years her sinus condition had been getting worse. She had overall congestion, runny eyes, headaches, and voluminous drainage requiring a box of tissues a day. She experienced lack of energy and depression and had been taking Prozac for about a year.

> **A box of tissues a day....no more**

Two different doctors had prescribed antibiotics, Seldane, Entex LA, Claritin, and Beconase, a nasal spray. She had some relief but the year before the condition came back "with a vengeance much worse that it ever was," she said.

We put Linda on a detoxification program and advised her to avoid tomatoes, mushrooms, refined carbohydrates, white flour products and foods containing yeast. Among other things, she had a yeast infection, a likely result of her numerous antibiotic prescriptions.

We also put her on a program of supplements to help strengthen her immune system. Chiropractic manipulations, originally four times a week, were later reduced to once a week.

Linda told us that her sinuses improved "at least 50 percent" during the 10-day detoxification program. In July of 1996, some three months after she started treatments in our clinic, she reported she was "100 percent better."

In Linda's words: "I adhere to the nutrition regime which excludes sugar, white flour and all processed foods. I basically eat all fresh meats, much brown rice, steamed vegetables, fruit with occasional consumption of 100 percent natural wheat flour or corn meal products.

"I have found that by keeping a diet record of only the 'bad' food items I consume (rarely), I can predict a sinus drainage/congestion episode to occur within three days. This has helped me to understand the connection of the highly refined carbohydrate food products to the adverse reaction it causes in my body.

"I also continue my nutritional supplement regime which includes a multiple vitamin and a few other specific vitamins and herbs. Above all I have learned what it takes to keep myself healthy.'"

Linda is no longer a Prozac queen. Her problem wasn't depression. Rather it was her uncorrected health condition contributing to feelings of fatigue and hopelessness.

Linda is a classic case of a patient on the medical treadmill. You start with one problem. You take medication. You then develop other problems as a result of the ripple effect of drug side effects. You become chronically fatigued and settle into a way of life that can only be described as a half-life. Then you receive the diagnosis of depression and the pharmaceutical coup de gras: Prozac. Unfortunately, this is a pattern that describes the way millions of Americans live. Don't let it happen to you!

How we treat sinus infections

Applied kinesiology (AK) is an effective method I use to identify allergenic substances contributing to sinusitis. It works this way:

We place extracts of potential allergens (wheat, dairy, sugar, food dyes, etc) under the tongue to be "challenged." If a normally strong muscle becomes weak while the substance being tested is in the mouth, this indicates that the body is incompatible with that particular substance.

We then proceed to find out why. Often there is an associated spinal misalignment that will lower the immune response and trigger allergic reactions. Chiropractic adjustments raise and stimulate the immune system and help to counteract allergic reactions.

Patients tell me routinely that after a series of adjustments they can eat foods they haven't been able to eat for years. Likewise, many patients report that seasonal allergies are reduced or eliminated.

Digestive impairment, especially low hydrochloric acid (HCL) and pancreatic enzyme production, will often trigger allergic sinusitis and cause your immune system to work overtime. Improper digestion permits incompletely digested food proteins to enter the bloodstream. There, they are perceived by your body as "foreign invaders" and become the targets of antibody "counterattacks." Betaine Plus, a time-released formula of HCL, along with a pancreatic supplement called Allerzyme, can help eliminate this problem and promote optimum digestion and absorption of food.

The mucous membranes of our sinuses and throat are composed of specialized cells called epithelial cells. The nutritional therapy that protects and repairs these cells are crucial for our well being. Antioxidant vitamins A, E, and C, along with the flavonoids (pycogenol, grape seed extract), protect cell membranes against damaging free radical activity and can help prevent sinus infections (for details on free radicals, see chapter 11).

For over 20 years, I have recommended Antronex to sinus patients. This product contains a natural antihistamine called yakitron, derived from liver. Unlike medical antihistamines, it does not cause side effects.

In some cases where the sinuses are so congested that drainage seems impossible, alternating applications of moist heat and ice helps provide relief.

The Chinese botanical ephedra, if used prudently, has natural decongestant activity, as well as a beneficial effect in asthmatic cases.

Herbal supplements such as echinacea and goldenseal have been long used to combat infections, including those caused by funguses, parasites, and even the tuberculosis bacterium. They are also available in the form of nasal sprays to treat sudden sinus flare-ups and infections.

I also recommend bromelain and papain, the well-known enzymes found in pineapples and papayas. They exert an anti-inflammatory effect on swollen sinus tissue. These enzymes are most effective taken between meals on an empty stomach.

A series of three to six intravenous Vitamin C infusions will often reverse the problems encountered in chronic sinus infections. Taken as a drip over two hours, this nutritional "cocktail" is a standard therapy in our clinic.

Pulsed diathermy, ultrasound and lymphatic drainage techniques are often employed with good results.

The chiropractic — sinus connection

As I mentioned above, chiropractic offers potential relief for allergy-related sinus conditions, and when allergies are not involved, it may provide the missing element to otherwise unsuccessful treatments

Gillespie and Barnes, writing in the Journal of Craniomandibular Practice, found that mechanical misalignment of the cranium (skull) and injury to soft tissues (muscles, ligaments, tendons, fascia) in the head act as "primary" causes of headaches, neck pain, throat infections, ear infections, sinus congestion, and asthma.

Such medical research helps explain my clinical observations involving thousands of sinus patients over 20 years. During this time I have consistently found spinal misalignments in the upper neck, especially at "the axis," or second cervical vertebrae. My interpretation has been that such misalignments can cause inadequate nerve and blood supply which adversely affects the sinuses. Countless cases of both acute and chronic sinus conditions have completely resolved following a series of chiropractic adjustments, and in some cases even after a single adjustment.

Acupressure treatments over the sinus reflexes in the forehead and around the nose are excellent "points" that can be manually stimulated to promote sinus drainage.

Like Judy Tusky and Linda Cozza, your days of being a sinus sufferer or antibiotic junkie may be numbered once you enter the chiropractic-nutritional zone.

Natural Remedies for Sinus Infections

- The Gallagher Wellness Program
- Chiropractic manipulation
- Lymphatic drainage and acupressure
- Pulsed diathermy/ultrasound
- Identify/remove allergens
- DL Winter (herbal combination with echinacea, goldenseal and red clover) .... 2 capsules, 3 times daily
- Botanical nasal drops (echinacea, goldenseal) .... 3 drops as needed
- Bromelain/papain .... 2 capsules, four times daily between meals
- Beta carotene .... 100-200,000 IU daily
- C1000 (with bioflavonoids) .... 1,000 milligrams every hour
- IV vitamin "cocktails" in resistant cases

Barbara's psoriasis case

Barbara Olson-Douglas, 44, a store manager from Monongahela, Pennsylvania, suffered from eczema and psoriasis. In 1994, she experienced a severe outbreak requiring hospitalization for two days. The following year she developed a severe reaction to poison ivy. Then more eczema and psoriasis. Her treatments included Medrol, Benadryl, Zantac and steroid medications, both oral and injected.

> **No more psoriasis**

When Barbara expressed her concern about the side effects of the many drugs her dermatologist and general practitioner assured her there was no problem.

"I also complained about poor digestive function and weight gain and was told these were due to my age!" Barbara said when she came to see me.

In May of 1996 we started Barbara on a detoxification program and restricted diet after we found evidence of yeast infection. We recommended the herb silymarin, which is helpful to detoxify the liver.

Three months later, Barbara reported that she had made considerable progress. Her skin has cleared considerably. She lost 25 pounds. Her digestion was returning to normal and her energy level had dramatically increased.

Along with her improved health, Barbara said the experience of natural health care taught her an important lesson. During an office visit, she told me this: "It's really up to you, the patient, to understand, to listen to your body, and seek out a good health care professional interested in your feelings, not just in their reputations. Doctors mean well, but too often they refuse to believe that vitamins and herbs are a beneficial source of healing and maintaining good health. But we, as patients can and must have a say in this, in our treatment, and help change those views. I have now learned to follow natural therapies and they work."

Psoriasis is conventionally treated with cortisone creams, oral steroids, shots and other drugs. Unfortunately for Barbara and many other people, standard treatment is frequently unsuccessful. Complications are common.

Psoriasis can be debilitating, both physically and psychologically, to people, especially women. But like most skin diseases, it begins inside the body. Although topical treatments such as cortisone creams or oatmeal baths are helpful for the symptoms, they cannot get at the root of the problem.

In Barbara's case, I prescribed a wholistic treatment program in which we detoxified her digestive tract and her liver. This was the foundation. A special diet was created that eliminated food allergens, especially dairy and grain products, as well as all yeast-containing foods. She also received a series of chiropractic adjustments to improve her immune system, energy and digestive function.

Barbara no longer suffers from the heartbreak of psoriasis. Her condition has totally cleared up and she is receiving maintenance care.

Dolores Leopardi's psoriasis case

Dolores, now 70, of Tarentum, Pennsylvania, came to see me more than 20 years ago. She had psoriasis all over.

> "My feet and hands are so bad that people turn away when they see them."

I will never forget the sight of this poor, suffering woman. It was summer, yet she was wearing gloves to cover her hands. Bright, white gloves.

"My feet and hands are so bad that people turn away when they see them," she told me. "I looked like a corpse."

Dolores said she had gone to many skin doctors in the Pittsburgh area, but none of them could help her. All of them had given her creams, medicines and put her hands under ultraviolet light that didn't help.

I asked her to remove the gloves. It was a painful and embarrassing process for her. As she peeled the gloves away, I saw hands that were split, cracked and bleeding, that had the appearance of raw meat.

Dolores had come to see me after I had helped her priest who also had had a psoriasis problem. I told her I could help her but she had to follow a strict program. She said she was willing.

We did a blood test, hair analysis and diet questionnaire. Based on the results and my examination, we placed her on a natural food diet with no citrus, dairy or sugar. She started to take supplements of zinc, B complex and liver extract.

"In two weeks, I felt good and did not itch anymore and took off the gloves forever. People did not turn away from me anymore," Dolores reminisced during a recent checkup. "It has been over 20 years and the psoriasis has not come back. What's more, I feel and look 20 years younger."

Dolores indeed remains psoriasis-free to this day. She follows a nutritional program and receives maintenance chiropractic adjustments.

Albert Tringhese's eczema case

Albert, a retired truck dealer from Uniontown, Pennsylvania, was also among my first patients more than 20

> **Cured — a food allergy-related condition**

years ago. Over the years he had received regular chiropractic maintenance, followed a good diet and taken nutritional supplements, and enjoyed good health.

In 1996, however, he developed a troublesome case of eczema on both of his legs. Albert was perplexed. He couldn't understand how he could have severe eczema with the kind of lifestyle he was following.

"I went to several doctors and got no results," he told me.

After analyzing his case, we tested him for food and environmental sensitivities and determined he had developed allergies to wheat and several other grains. I recommended he remove these items from his diet. Along with that I suggested he take milk thistle to help with liver detoxification, flax seed oil to improve immune function and decrease inflammation.

In a short period of time, Albert's eczema completely cleared up. No drugs. No creams.

SORE THROATS

Herlinde Yugar's case

Ever since she was a child, Herlinde Yugar has had throat problems. In 1992, when she first consulted with me, she described a 35-year history of chronic recurring throat and sinus infections.

Resolved — a 35-year history of sore throats that baffled doctors

Most of that time, she said, "I have been taking antibiotics on a regular basis, and every three weeks or so for the last 10 years."

Despite the long-term medication, her problems persisted. In addition, she was constantly tired, had muscle aches and pains, and generally felt poorly.

Herlinde, a real estate agent in Canonsburg, Pennsylvania, told me that "doctors were baffled and continued to prescribe different antibiotics to see which one would work."

Examination showed her to have spinal subluxation complexes which were likely causing her immune system and other organs to malfunction. This made her susceptible to repeated infections. Years of taking antibiotics had also decimated the beneficial bacterial colonies in her digestive tract, contributing to intestinal toxicity, imbalances and a yeast infection.

There was no one single treatment for her chronic condition. It would take a multiple, natural approach, including modification of her diet, embarking on a nutritional program, and undergoing comprehensive chiropractic care. I felt confident we could help her overcome decades of unwellness if she was willing to follow the program.

She said she would try anything. She was tired of not feeling good.

Q *"Do you have any natural remedies for sore throats? I don't smoke and I exercise often but I seem to catch everything that comes along."*

A I treat many people with chronic infections, such as Herlinde Yugar and this particular caller. "Catching everything that comes along" has less to do with the strength of germs and more to do with poor resistance. When you take better care of your body your resistance is better. Recurrent infections reflect a weakened system.

As a method of treatment, antibiotics have little to offer. They are neither preventive nor curative. Quite to the contrary, incising evidence indicates they actually contribute to repeat infections or trigger disturbances in the body that cause a variety of problems. Such was the case with Herlinde.

Applied kinesiology evaluation (see chapter 13) determined weaknesses of her lymphatic system, sinuses, spleen and liver. These weaknesses and malfunctions were connected to the misalignments in her spine and accompanying interference in the nervous system.

A key to regaining health was a series of chiropractic manipulations. Chiropractic manipulations often provide astonishing relief of ear, nose and throat infections by restoring nervous system function. In Herlinde's case, many organs and systems were beneficiaries, including the sinuses, throat, thymus gland, the spleen and the immune system. Glandular extracts of thymus and spleen were also used as part of her treatment program to help strengthen those weakened organs.

We started her on a 10-day detoxification diet, part of our general wellness program (see chapter 6), to eliminate intestinal toxicity. After the fourth day on the diet, she called to tell us she had started to feel better.

Herlinde also began taking a herbal combination that acts as a "natural antibiotic." It consists of echinacea, goldenseal and red clover. This formula helps activate the specialized cells in the immune system that recognize bacteria, viruses and other foreign substances and then destroy them naturally without harming the host.

An anti-yeast nutritional plan was also prescribed. She avoided yeast-containing foods such as bread and pastry, and took a supplement called ADP (timed-release oregano), which has a strong anti-fungal (yeast) property. The reason for these measures is that people who have taken many antibiotics often have an overgrowth of yeast in the body, which contributes to many other health problems.

Part if Herlinde's recovery program was taking a good probiotic supplement that restores friendly bacteria in the body.

Sambuchol, a popular Israeli remedy whose active ingredient is elderberry, is an effective lozenge. Studies have shown it to have strong anti-viral and anti-bacterial activity.

Zinc lozenges are also beneficial. They inhibit the growth of harmful bacteria.

If you have chronic sore throats, or any other recurrent infections, and have taken many antibiotic prescriptions over the years, you may, like

Herlinde Yugar, required a multi-faceted natural program to restore order to your body.

Herlinde has stayed with the program and hasn't had to take a single antibiotic in more than five years. She feels great, she says.

"I have become an avid believer in the combination of diet, vitamins, and chiropractic care," she told me during a recent checkup. "I tell my story to everyone whether they want to hear it or not."

Gargle away your sore throats

You may be able to stop a developing sore throat in its tracks by gargling with the either of the following preparations:

• A simple time-honored folk remedy is apple cider vinegar. I recommend taking one ounce undiluted and gargle with it every hour. Then spit it out.

• Vitamin C (ascorbic acid) powder is nothing short of remarkable. Mix a half teaspoon (two grams) of powder in four ounces of cold water and gargle every hour. Swallow the mixture after gargling.

Natural Remedies for Sore Throats

• *Gallagher Wellness Program*
• *Chiropractic cervical manipulation*
• *Lymphatic Drainage*
• *Sambuchol or zinc lozenges as needed*
• *Vitamin C (ascorbic acid) powder* .... one-half teaspoon in 4 oz. of water; gargle every 1-2 hours. Drink mixture after gargling according to bowel tolerance.
• *DL Winter (echinacea, goldenseal, red clover)* ...... 2 capsules, 3 times daily
• *Zinc picolinate* .... 50 milligrams daily
• *Thymoglan (Thymus extract)* .... 2 capsules, 3 times daily

---

STRESS
AND YOUR ADRENAL GLANDS

The importance of being "adrenally healthy"

The adrenal glands — there are two in your body, each one sitting atop your kidneys — are major hormone manufacturers. Among their output are hormones that allow your body to respond to stress. However, if the stress is strong enough or long enough (chronic), your adrenals can become overworked and incapable of meeting all the demands your body puts upon them. Poor diet and structural misalignments in the body can also affect the adrenal glands negatively.

The medical name for exhausted adrenals is functional hypoadrenia. The term means underfunctioning adrenals, just like hypothyroid refers to an underfunctioning thyroid gland. It is unlikely you have heard about this condition, but it is very prevalent and in fact underlies many illnesses, particularly those that are stress-related.

According to research, this condition can contribute to many symptoms including the following:

- fatigue
- dizziness and fainting
- light-headedness
- low stress tolerance
- nervousness
- anxiety
- mental confusion
- sensitivity to bright light
- asthma
- skin rash
- joint pain
- headaches
- back pain
- arthritis
- ulcers
- digestive upsets
- heart palpitations
- impotence
- crave salty foods
- crave sweets

Weak adrenals can also underlie many auto-immune disorders including rheumatoid arthritis, colitis and psoriasis.

Conventional doctors don't generally recognize functional hypoadrenia until it becomes a clear case of Addison's disease, that is, a total breakdown in the function of the adrenal glands. Probably the most famous Addison's patient was the late President John F. Kennedy.

Because the contemporary medical system tends to treat symptoms and not deal with underlying causes, the presence of exhausted adrenal glands may never be determined. More likely, patients will simply receive prescriptions for relief of symptoms such as anxiety, depression or pain. The adrenals, meanwhile, continue to wilt away while a new chemical stress is introduced in the body. Patients may be described as hypochondriacs, or as having nervous conditions.

Standard lab tests can determine Addison's disease but may not pick up the signs of adrenal exhaustion and functional hypoadrenia. Clues can be more readily picked up with a thorough medical history, clinical examination and applied kinesiology. All of these are primary diagnostic tools of chiropractic care.

Applied kinesiology, a muscle testing method, is extremely useful. I use it daily in my clinic to help determine adrenal function (see the section on chiropractic diagnostics in chapter 13).

Other diagnostic techniques include the following:

1. Check your blood pressure. You can do this at home, too. Do it first when seated. Now stand up and check it again. If the systolic blood pressure (the first number) does not rise at least eight points higher than your resting blood pressure, it is a sign of hypoadrenia.

What's happening is this: The adrenals produce the hormone adrenaline, which elevates blood pressure, quickens the pulse and heart rate, and prepares the body for "fight or flight." The mere physical effort involved in rising from a sitting to a standing position represents a minor stress on your body. If your adrenals are overworked, they may not be capable of producing the adrenaline necessary to even create the elevated blood pressure and pulse rate for optimum blood flow into the brain. Thus, it's a sign of adrenal exhaustion if your pressure doesn't rise like it should.

2. Look in the mirror at a fixed point. Now shine a light (a small pen light) into your eye. Your pupil should quickly get smaller (constrict). If it remains dilated (open) or fluctuates rapidly back and forth, you may have weak adrenals.

The adrenal glands play an important role in the regulation of the autonomic nervous system. This is the part of the nervous system that functions "automatically," without our active involvement. The autonomic system controls our organs, including constricting and dilating the pupils.

3. ASI Test (Adrenal Stress Index). This is a new saliva test done in the clinic that helps determine normal or abnormal production of adrenal hormones, including DHEA. I prefer the salivary hormone test over standard blood testing because it more accurately determines shifting hormone levels at different stages of the day and night.

Whether I use the AK test, the ASI, or the functional adrenal tests I have just described, the key to the correct treatment is the interpretation. Your adrenal glands can overfunction as well as underfunction and must be viewed in the proper context. Also you may have abnormal test results for other reasons, such as the presence of another disease.

Once this condition is determined, repair of the adrenals is vital to restore energy and normal bodily functions.

The adrenal hormone factory

Your adrenals are tiny, waxy-looking glands that are big-time producers of important hormones.

Among them are:

• Glucocorticoids — Hormones that convert fats and protein for use as sugar and energy and also act as anti-inflammatory agents.

• Sex corticoids — Small amounts of testosterone, the male hormone, and estrogen, the female hormone, are made here. Estrogen from the adrenal glands is believed to have an important balancing role in menopause.

• Mineralocorticoids — Help to keep the body's minerals and fluids in balance and also contribute anti-inflammatory activities.

• Adrenaline (also known as epinephrine) is the so-called "fight or flight hormone" and gives us the ability to combat stress. It also helps in the body's utilization of sugar and the control of the autonomic nervous system which governs organs and glands.

• DHEA, short for dehydroepiandrosterone (pronounced dee-hi-dro-epp-ee-ann-dro-stehr-own), is a prohormone, or, in more popular terms, the "mother of all hormones." The body uses DHEA as a raw material to make other important hormones. DHEA itself has no known function.

The case of a mother and daughter with fatigued adrenals

"I'm a mess and have been for 15 years," the patient told me at her first appointment. "I am chronically fatigued. It takes all the determination I can muster to get up off the couch. Some days I never make if off the couch. I watch life pass me by like a spectator sport."

> "I watch life pass me by like a spectator sport."

The patient was Gail Sorace, 47, a Ph.D. candidate from Sarver, Pennsylvania, who first came to see me in 1996.

Her story was a litany of imbalance and ill health.

• Bulemia and anorexia since the time she was a teenager. She had an extreme craving for chocolate and sweets. She would binge to satisfy her cravings and later control her weight by not eating.

• Menstrual cycles every two weeks. A gynecologist had insisted on a hysterectomy. Gail refused and switched doctors. The second specialist put her on progesterone which helped extend the cycle to three weeks.

• Digestive disorders since elementary school. Her stomach always ached. She was constantly constipated. Many tests over the years showed nothing abnormal.

• Confusion much of the time. "My family thought that I was a case of early dementia," she said.

• Severe depression from lack of energy. "When I became suicidal, I checked myself into a residential psychiatric treatment center," she said. "No one there seemed to understand that I was basically a very 'up' person who was suffering from severe physical fatigue and an eating disorder."

Gail received a prescription from a psychiatrist for the anti-depressant Prozac, along with a regimen of therapy.

"I kept saying I didn't really feel depressed, that there was something out-of-whack with my body. But the psychiatrist just dished out more Prozac," she said.

"I went to another doctor who diagnosed me with attention deficit disorder (ADD). All the tests and history indicated that was my problem. A lot of people with eating disorder and alcoholism are diagnosed with ADD.

"I spent two years on Ritalin and during that time my brain did seem to function better. I had energy and the depression went away. When I decided to get off all the drugs due to severe mood swings, all the old problems returned two-fold."

• A doctor in California treated her for hypothyroidism. "I made some progress," she said. "My depression eased with a return of some energy and the regulation of my menstrual cycle, but I was still tired, mentally confused, and exhibiting severe hypoglycemic (low blood sugar) reactions."

Gail had a full-blown case of functional hypoadrenia, that had never been diagnosed, along with hypoglycemia. We were able to stabilize her with chiropractic manipulation, a very high protein/low carbohydrate diet, and nutritional supplements, including 12 to 14 adrenal extract tablets a day. For most adrenal patients, I usually prescribe 2 to 6 tablets a day, but her case was so advanced that it required 2 capsules virtually every couple of hours. This type of glandular supplementation helps to provide the nutritional repair elements necessary for overcoming "adrenal wipeout."

"Now I am back to feeling as I did when I was a kid and I have been able, in fact, to enter a doctorate program," Gail says. "As long as I stay on my diet, my cycle is regular. I have minimal clotting. I don't have any digestive upsets or constipation."

Gail's daughter Stacy, aged 17, was also having health problems. She had gone from being an energetic and active teenager to being "lethargic, a couch potato and seriously overweight," in the words of her mother.

She also developed narcolepsy, a condition where a person can fall asleep at any time. Stacey did so, in school, in a car, anyplace, anytime. "In the middle of a sentence," her mother said.

Gail took her daughter to several specialists. "The doctors always had the same answer," she told me. "They said nothing was wrong that a weight-loss diet wouldn't fix, even though I had told them we had tried different diets and portion control and all that. I had given up hope that Stacey would be her same old self again. She seemed doomed."

Although Gail and Stacey differed greatly in age and symptoms, they both had spinal stress and functional hypoadrenia. Gail received chiropractic manipulation to the twelfth thoracic vertebra (T12) which is often misaligned in adrenal exhaustion cases. Stacey, in addition to being narcoleptic, was considered to have ADD (attention deficit disorder). Chiropractic evaluation revealed that she had misalignments in the neck and thoracic area.

With chiropractic manipulation we corrected the mechanical stresses affecting both mother and daughter. The nutritional support provided the raw materials to repair their adrenals.

Neither of them — Gail or Stacey — had psychiatric, neurological or psychosomatic problems. They had chiropractic and nutritional problems that were not addressed in the conventional medical system.

How we treat weak adrenals

Our program is designed to help give overworked adrenal glands an opportunity to rest, rejuvenate and resume their normal role as the "military defense system" of our body, protecting us against stress.

Experience has shown that chiropractic manipulation and nutritional supplements offer effective means of achieving this goal. We also recommend small, frequent and nutritious meals and snacks

For more than 20 years I have used Adrenoglan Chelate, an excellent glandular supplement that contains important nutritional factors to rebuild the adrenals. It contains potassium, pantothenic acid (vitamin B-5), the amino acid tyrosine, which research has shown to be a powerful anti-stress nutrient, and raw adrenal extract. Adrenal extract is one of many "glandular" therapies I have pre-scribed to patients for more than 20 years. These substances provide the "nucleoproteins" necessary for cell regeneration.

Adrenoglan also contains sodium. Many patients ask me about that. Isn't sodium what salt is all about, they want to know. Yes, they are right. Sodium is a major component of salt. Although many people are wary of salt, individuals tend to dump salt (and therefore sodium) during stressful events. Studies have now pointed to an association between weak adrenals and chronic fatigue syn-drome, with increased salt intake being recommended as a remedy.

For this reason, I recommend that individuals with weak adrenals and chronic fatigue use extra salt. One teaspoon daily is sufficient. Simply add it to food. The form I recommend is either sea salt or "Real Salt," a product mined in Utah from an ancient sea bed that contains multiple trace minerals. The problem with regular table salt is that it contains sugar (dextrose), aluminum (a toxic substance), and has no additional trace minerals.

Most of us are familiar with the unique and pleasing taste of licorice candy. Did you know that the flavor comes from the root of the licorice plant (glycyrrhiza glabra)? Medicinally, licorice root has a long history of use. Throughout the world it has been widely applied to help with coughs and bronchial complaints. In addition it has been shown to be helpful for cases of adrenal insufficiency, inflammation and mild Addison's disease. It has also been suggested that licorice may help address the chronic fatigue syndrome as well as the tiredness often affecting individuals with weak adrenal function.   Licorice, it turns out, is a "phyto-hormone," or plant hormone, that offers natural pharmacological activity to boost the adrenal glands. It specifically contains a chemical called glycyrrhizin that has a similar structure and activity as certain adrenal steroids. I use this regularly in my treatment of hypoadrenia. The best form is standardized deglycyrrhizinated licorice. Other forms may have a slight blood pressure elevating effect.

Vitamin C, along with vitamin B-5 (pantothenic acid) and cholesterol — yes, cholesterol — are critical factors for the production of adrenal hormones. Did you know that only 10 percent of your total cholesterol comes from your diet. Ninety percent is manufactured by your body, and particularly in the brain, liver and intestines. Cholesterol is a necessary fat for the production of hormones, and especially adrenal and sex hormones.

I frequently prescribe the homeopathic remedy kalium phosphoricum, especially when low adrenal activity is associated with depression.

A word on fainting

Q *"My daughter is 16 and she has frequent fainting spells and fatigue. She was checked by the family doctor for anemia and thyroid and everything was okay. We have been to a neurologist and had a brain scan and an MRI. So far all the tests are normal but my daughter is going downhill. My husband and I are willing to try anything to help her."*

A In my experience, there are two consistent findings in individuals who have a sudden loss of consciousness but who have been found to be normal medically:
   1) The "atlas syndrome"
   2) Functional hypoadrenia

"Atlas syndrome" refers to the misalignment of the first cervical vertebra, that is the uppermost neck bone upon which the skull rests. This vertebra is known as the atlas.

When it is misaligned, excessive and abnormal nerve input can be generated into the brain. Over time, this can cause dizziness, loss of balance and fainting spells. Cervical manipulation will often correct this structural distortion, and allow the nervous system and brain to achieve balance.

When adrenal depletion is involved, we use the comprehensive approach I have mentioned above.

Natural Remedies for Hypoadrenia

- *Chiropractic manipulation*
- *Cranial manipulation*
- *Adrenoglan Chelate* .... 2 capsules, 3 times daily
- *Ultrapreventive III (high dosage multiple vitamin)* 2 capsules, 3 times daily
- *Licorice root (standardized extract)* .... 2 capsules, 3 times daily
- *American Ginseng* .... 1 capsule, twice daily
- *Kali phosphoricum (30X)* .... 2 pellets, 4 times daily
- *Sea salt or "Real Salt" (available in health food stores)*

SWALLOWING DISORDERS (ESOPHAGEAL SPASMS)

Q "*I am 32 and work as a computer software programmer. In the past two years, I have been in the emergency room six times because I can't swallow. The doctors at the hospital give me a shot and send me home. An internist ran every test in the book and said I was too tense and I should change jobs. He has also given me different tranquilizers but I quit them because they make me drowsy. I always feel like there is something stuck in the back of my throat. Is there anything you know of that might help?*"

I have seen many cases like these. Although conventional medicine often views swallowing problems as a "nervous disorder," I look at them much differently.

The esophagus is the tube leading from your mouth to your stomach and is a muscular structure. I have found that it can become contracted due to misalignments in the adjacent cervical or thoracic spine.

One dramatic case involved a three-year-old girl who was progressively losing weight because she was unable to swallow properly. The pediatrician sent the child to an ear, nose, and throat specialist. The specialist dilated her throat, evaluated her condition, and then referred the girl to a hospital for "exploratory throat surgery."

Out of desperation, the mother brought her to me. We took a history and examined the girl's spine. The examination revealed the presence of a vertebral subluxation at C5 (the fifth neck vertebra). After the first pediatric chiropractic manipulation, the child was able to eat again. She quickly regained her lost weight and was able to avoid surgery.

Another dramatic case involved a woman in her mid-forties who spontaneously vomited with any slight backward movement of her head. She had gone through exhaustive medical examinations and treatments without relief. She had a drawerful of pills that caused undesirable side effects.

Chiropractic examination revealed restricted motion at the site of the "axis" vertebra — the second vertebra in the neck. Following six chiropractic manipulations, the condition was completely resolved.

This type of condition, known in the chiropractic profession as "esophageal spasms," is usually caused by mechanical distortion in the neck.

My recommendation is that patients with swallowing or esophageal conditions consult a chiropractic physician. Determining and correcting spinal misalignments may be the missing link to restored function.

TINNITUS

See also:
• *chapter on dizziness / vertigo*

About tinnitus

Tinnitus is a Latin word meaning "ringing." The medical condition refers to a ringing in the ear. However, many people also experience buzzing, roaring, clicking, hissing, crickets, chirping, music, static and other acoustic sensations that can become increasingly disturbing.

Tinnitus is believed to affect some 50 million Americans. It may be constant and unrelenting, or intermittent, and change in frequency and intensity. It may be experienced in both or one ear. There is no consensus as to cause nor is there a consensus for treatment to cure the condition.

Music to the ears — not in this case

For Mary Barrett, 80, of Lower Burrell, Pennsylvania, the tinnitus she developed included not only the customary ringing but music as well, and specifically church and Christmas melodies.

> **"I hear church music. And it doesn't stop."**

Mary came to see me in March of 1995, some seven years after she began experiencing ringing in the ears. Since late 1994, she began hearing the music also. She also had hearing loss and had been fitted for a hearing aid. She heard the music whether she wore the hearing aid or not.

She had been treated by a neurologist and had undergone a battery of tests — MRI, Cat Scan, X-rays, EEGs — to determine the possibility of mini strokes. Her neurological evaluation: all was normal.

I will never forget Mary's words at the time of her first appointment. "I hear 'Silent Night,'" she said. "I hear church music. And it doesn't stop."

Mary had other complaints: a pulse beating in her right ear, occasional loss of balance, sharp pains in the upper neck and back of the skull, daily headaches, and heaviness in the back of the head. She was taking Tylenol and Naprosyn, an anti-inflammatory drug. She was unable to sleep more than two hours a night since she suffered a fall in 1992. Mary's neurologist suggested a psychiatrist, which often happens in cases like this when medical tests come out normal. Instead, she came to see me.

After analyzing her cervical spine, we began a series of adjustments. Her problems began to diminish gradually. There was a reduction in the volume of the music. The headaches and skull pressure lessened. She began sleeping longer each night. Her memory and concentration improved. And, after a dozen adjustments, her problem was gone.

After the twelfth adjustment, she told me she hadn't heard any music for a week. The last song she was able to discern, she said, was "How great Thou art."

Think of your nervous system like a compact disk or stereo record. Did you ever have a stereo malfunction and the same song keeps playing over and over again? When the spine misaligns, as in Mary's case, the nervous system malfunctions and the part of the brain responsible for recorded sound literally gets "stuck."

This scenario, in fact, is the basis of many diseases. Isn't depression usually associated with the same repetitive thought pattern? Isn't anxiety characterized by uncontrollable and repetitive anxious thoughts?

When the spine or skull is misaligned, unhealthy "grooves" are created in the nervous system. You can try to talk your way out of them or think your way out of them, or drug yourself out of them. Fortunately, Mary and many of my other patients turned to the chiropractic connection and were able to break the vicious cycle of illness and turn down the volume.

Nancy Ireland's case

Nancy Ireland, 56, a homemaker from North Versailles, Pennsylvania, suffered for years from Meniere's syndrome, an ear disorder that involves dizziness, nausea, tinnitus, and loss of hearing.

> **After 35 years of treatments, she was told to learn to live with it...but she refused comply!**

"It started at age 19, with dizzy spells so violent I couldn't stand up and couldn't keep food down," she told me. "After 35 years of seeing six different specialists and being tested, drugged, retested and having more drugs, with little results, they said I have to live with it. There was nothing more they could do."

When Nancy first came to see me almost all her hearing was gone in her left ear. Her hearing in the right ear was deteriorating. She still had unexpected dizzy spells, nausea, and a growing problem with chronic diarrhea.

Nancy was a prime candidate for our comprehensive program. Her hearing has been restored in her right ear and is coming back in her left. The noise level has been reduced considerably as well. "I have relief from my symptoms at last," she told me during a recent visit.

In her words: "The treatments have done wonders not just for my hearing, but for my vision as well. I wear no glasses or contacts anymore. No more sinus headaches. I'm free of fibrocystic breast disease. My on-and-off diarrhea of the past 5 years is now under control. And I lost the 20 pounds that I've been trying to lose for 10 years. All this in 2 years of treatments."

Nancy was typical of many patients I see. They suffer from multiple health problems and have multiple reasons why they become ill. Similarly it takes multiple treatments or therapies to help them get well.

Nancy had significant subluxations of the upper part of her neck. Her TMJ (jaw) was also out of alignment. We corrected that. Following a series of chiropractic manipulations she experienced a marked improvement of her vertigo, nausea, ringing in the ears, and her vision.

We discovered through laboratory antibody tests that Nancy also had a parasite infection. She was placed on an anti-parasitic diet, received colonic hydrotherapy (colon irrigation), and started a special nutritional program. This relieved her daily diarrhea problem. She really required our entire wellness program to bring her back into balance. Now, two years later, she is another person.

The health of people supposedly declines with age. Aging is synonymous with illness, so they say. It doesn't have to be that way. I have literally treated thousands of middle aged and elderly patients who are able to regain lost health, stay out of hospitals, avoid drugs, and maintain an optimum level of vigor and well-being by following a nutritional and chiropractic program. They may not be stopping the clock, but they are sure slowing it down.

The chiropractic — tinnitus connection

Mary Barrett and Nancy Ireland represent two good examples of the vast healing potential that chiropractic adjustments offers for what most people and conventional doctors regard as "medical problems." Such problems typically take patients through a maze of specialists, high tech tests, varying diagnoses, and often bizarre drug treatments. When nothing can be done for you, you get categorized as having "mental problems."

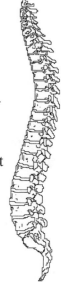

Remember the concept of "brain hibernation," which we spoke about in chapter 13? This refers to spinal misalignments that cause a reduction in the brain's ability to receive oxygen. Nancy Ireland, at age 56, no longer has to wear contacts or glasses for the first time in over 30 years. Mary Barrett, at age 80, didn't have a psychiatric problem; rather, she had spinal misalignments that caused her to hear religious hymns at rock concert volume.

What does this say for our children who start out life and

progress throughout the course of their lives misaligned, constantly malfunctioning, disconnected to chiropractic because of ignorance, fear and misinformation, and become the walking wounded forever stuck on the medical treadmill?

Break through the bonds of medical disinformation and experience the chiropractic optimum health model. Although not a panacea, chiropractic should be at the core of everyone's health and wellness program.

The TMJ connection

Temporomandibular joint misalignment (TMJ) is an often overlooked cause of tinnitus, hearing loss and headaches. This joint, which is formed by the mandible (jaw bone) and the temporal bone (the skull bone just above the ear), can misalign due to dental problems, trauma, abnormal sleeping positions, neck misalignment and spinal scoliosis.

Here's how to tell if you have a TMJ problem:

• Look in the mirror. Keep your mouth open but relaxed. See if your two front teeth line up with your two bottom front teeth. When you open and close your mouth does it pop, click or shift to the side?

• Put your little fingers in your ears and slowly open your mouth as wide as possible. Do you feel your little finger being pushed more on one side?

• Open your mouth as wide as possible. See how many fingers you can put in your mouth vertically. You should be able to put in at least three and usually four.

These simple tests may indicate you have TMJ syndrome. Not only can tinnitus and hearing loss result from the abnormal joint stress, but a whole constellation of symptoms including facial numbness, headaches, dizziness, and neck pain.

I have treated thousands of TMJ sufferers. Many have been on the medical treadmill of pain pills, braces, TMJ splints, and surgery. Fortunately, for TMJ patients there are specific chiropractic manipulations that are either helpful or corrective.

Raymond Nimmo, D.C., a prominent chiropractic researcher from Texas, developed a method that treats specific trigger points in the muscles along the jaw and inside the mouth. The Nimmo method can effectively relieve TMJ stress.

Although the TMJ splint — a type of mouth guard used for jaw stress — is a common and sometimes successful treatment, it has serious limitations. It does not address the spinal and cranial misalignments which are the usual causes of the problem. In my clinical experience most TMJ sufferers resolve following a course of chiropractic spinal and TMJ manipulations. A small percentage may need a skilled dental TMJ specialist.

Help from China

Ginkgo biloba is one of the world's oldest living tree species — believed to have survived for 200 million years. Ginkgo is considered a sacred tree by the Chinese" writes Rebecca Flynn in "Your Guide to Standardized Herbal Products," and has been "used in oriental medicine since ancient times for respiratory ailments and for brain function."

Ginkgo's active ingredients have antioxidant properties and help cerebral blood flow, vertigo, headaches and tinnitus.

In a study reported in 1988 in Germany, 103 patients with recent onset tinnitus experienced significant reduction in symptoms with Ginkgo.

I have also found bioflavonoids, especially rutin, hesperidin and the flavonoids in grape seed extract to be beneficial, probably due to their ability to strengthen blood vessels and therefore promote optimum brain flow and oxygen uptake. Deficiencies of niacin (vitamin B-3) is also sometimes linked to ringing in the ears. Niacinate, the non-flushing form of niacin, promotes blood flow and lowers cholesterol and triglycerides.

Food allergies, which we can often identify with applied kinesiology (AK) or through specialized blood tests (IgG4) that pinpoint delayed food allergies, are sometimes a culprit in tinnitus. Although any food or chemical can act as an allergen, some of the most common are milk, wheat, eggs and citrus.

Chelation therapy, an intravenous nutritional therapy used by our medical staff, can be of great benefit to those whose tinnitus is vascular in origin.

Natural Remedies for Tinnitus

- *Gallagher Wellness Program*
- *Cranial manipulation*
- *Spinal manipulation*
- *TMJ manipulation*
- *Ginkgo Biloba Extract (standardized 24% extract)* 40 milligrams, 3 times daily
- *Flav 1,000 (bioflavonoid complex)* .... 2 capsules, 3 times daily
- *Niacinate (non-flush vitamin B-3)* .... 500 milligrams, twice daily
- *Grape seed extract (standardized)* .... 100 to 200 milligrams daily
- *Identify food allergens*
- *Intravenous chelation therapy, if vascular disease is present*

VISION PROBLEMS

Many times over the years people have called in to my weekly radio program and asked how they can improve their vision.

Whether it is blurred vision, night vision problems, painful eyes, difficulty focusing, sensitivity to bright light, seeing spots in front of your eyes, or diseases such as cataracts, glaucoma, or macular degeneration, many callers and patients want to know if there are any natural remedies to help their sight.

I can assure you there are. Very often problems with the eyes are secondary symptoms of problems elsewhere in the body. When you correct the underlying problems with natural means you are often able to improve the vision, as well as other symptoms.

Among the major conditions of the eyes are:

• Chronic glaucoma — essentially, hypertension of the eyeball, a progressive disorder causing tunnel vision, extreme pain, blurred vision, and reddened eyes. It affects about two million Americans.

• Cataracts refer to a degeneration of the lens tissue and the gradual inability to permit light from being transmitted into our eyes. Over time, this leads to loss of vision and ultimately blindness.

• Macular degeneration, currently the leading cause of vision loss for persons over the age of 50, is a moderately dense scar found in the macula of the eye. This disorder is usually associated with aging, hardening of the arteries and high blood pressure.

• Retinopathy, an illness of the retina, affects many diabetics and causes loss of vision. It involves deterioration of the tiny blood vessels supplying the retina, the thin layer of light receptor cells at the back of the eyes that produce the sensation of vision.

While topical medication for chronic glaucoma sufferers is helpful, and cataract surgery essential in advanced cases, conventional medical care has no effective treatment for macular degeneration. Additionally, millions of people suffer from functional vision disorders which are often worrisome and interfere with daily activities.

Consider if you will the following varied cases of patients who benefited from a natural approach of nutrition and chiropractic.

The Grazulis' case

Anthony and Lillian Grazulis, an elderly couple from Coraopolis, Pennsylvania, both had eye problems.

> **Cataract surgery averted...nutritionally**

In October 1993, Anthony was informed by an optometrist that he had cataracts and would probably need surgery within a year.

A short time later, Anthony shared the news with me. He was a patient of mine. I suggested several nutritional supplements — selenium, vitamin E, and a special formula for the eyes called Opthalplex Plus. He started taking the supplements at once.

In August 1994, Anthony consulted with an ophthalmologist, thinking he would need surgery by then.

"When the examination was over I realized the doctor hadn't mentioned cataracts," Anthony told me later. "I asked him about this. He replied that my condition was so minimal that I would not have a problem for 'years and years and years.'

"In December 1996 I had an eye examination by another optometrist who told me that I didn't have a problem."

Meanwhile, wife Lillian's health problems were improving with a comprehensive program of chiropractic, diet, nutrition, prayer and meditation, and exercise. After 20 years she was able to quit her high blood pressure medication. Her sinus problems resolved. And, she told me recently, "I have more energy than I could hope for." This is a woman of 73.

She also told me that during a recent eye exam her doctor was amazed at the improvement of her vision and said it was "like a different person taking the exam." Lillian followed the same nutritional supplement program for the eyes as did her husband.

Margie Fulton's case

This 42-year-old patient from Jeannette, Pennsylvania, was disabled as a result of diabetes. She was an insulin-dependent diabetic and had started to develop

> **Reversing diabetic retinopathy**

many of the serious vascular complications common to the disease around the age of 25. She experienced kidney failure in 1986, underwent a kidney transplant in 1995, and also suffered from neuropathy and poor circulation in the lower extremities.

Diabetic retinopathy had also adversely affected her vision. Despite laser treatments and surgery in both eyes, she lost the sight in her left eye.

When she came to see me in December of 1996, the vision in her right eye was deteriorating. She had developed a corneal abrasion with decreased circulation to the retina. In addition, the pressure had begun to increase and measured 33 in spite of medication. That is considered a high and dangerous level for glaucoma.

Margie came to see us for chiropractic and nutritional care. She received specific adjustments to her upper neck as well as a supplement prescription for her diabetes and vision problems.

Margie said she never dreamed that her vision would improve, but within two weeks it did just that. During one follow-up treatment she said her vision had improved to the level she was at a year before. An examination by her ophthalmologist showed that the pressure had dropped to 18.

The adjustments had helped restore better nerve and blood supply to the eyes. The nutritional supplements, namely Opthalplex Plus and bilberry, delivered raw materials essential for repair.

Sister Vera's case

Sister Vera Stanchec, OSBM, of Uniontown, Pennsylvania, is an 80-year-old nun who was diagnosed with retinopathy in 1987. She was losing her vision.

> **"You have no retinopathy!"**

For 2 1/2 years she returned every three months to her ophthalmologist for an examination. No treatment was prescribed.

"You are holding your own," he commented. But Sister Vera felt her vision was deteriorating. She had "bloody eyes," meaning that tiny blood vessels in her eyes were becoming fragile and hemorrhaging.

She decided to try a different approach — the natural approach. That's when she made an appointment at our clinic.

We recommended she take a simple prescription of selenium (200 micrograms daily) and vitamin E (800 international units).

Here's the rest of her story: "I took this faithfully for another 2 1/2 years and then decided to change eye doctors. After the new doctor examined me, he said, 'Everything is just fine, Sister.'

"I then asked how my retinopathy was doing. He double checked and then triple checked. 'What retinopathy?' he said.

"At that point I related my selenium and vitamin E story. He just nodded and said, 'That must have been what cured you.'"

That was five years ago.

"I'm still doing great," she told me during a checkup in early 1997.

Sister Vera discovered the power of two very important anti-oxidants for the eyes — vitamin E and selenium. These important nutrients protect the cells in our bodies, including the eyes, from undergoing premature degeneration. In Sister Vera's case, the effect was more than preventive; it was curative.

The case of Anthony Christofano, Jr.

> **Distorted vision from a corneal abrasion...reversed by chiropractic care**

In the summer of 1995, Anthony Christofano, Jr., 24, of Jeannette, Pennsylvania, scratched his left eye on the corner of a paper bag. He went immediately to the hospital emergency room where he received a diagnosis of corneal abrasion and a patch to wear for several days. The eye should be back to normal by then, he was told.

Usually, corneal abrasions resolve in a few days, but not in this case. When the patch came off, his vision out of the left eye was blurry and with his right eye he saw one image on top of another.

Anthony went from one doctor to another seeking medical help. His odyssey took him to the top eye specialists in Pittsburgh and to Johns Hopkins Medical School. A total of 15 different doctors.

"Their diagnosis," Anthony said, was 'we don't know what caused it.' Time will heal it.'"

In the meantime, his vision was not getting better. He was unable to drive a car and was becoming depressed at the prospect of a lifetime of vision problems.

Anthony's quest for answers brought him to my clinic. My impression was that the trauma to his eye caused a reflex reaction to his brain and spinal cord, resulting in cranial and cervical misalignments. I initiated a series of cranial, neck and back adjustments, along with a nutritional therapy program.

Within four to six weeks, Anthony's vision began improving. The wholistic approach worked. His condition reversed. Today, he drives his car without a problem and can see normally.

"I regained my normal sight," Anthony says. "It was truly a miracle."

How we treat vision problems

Many people suffer from visual disorders because of lack of exercise, improper nutrition and spinal subluxation. For these reasons, exercise, chiropractic adjustments, and nutritional prescriptions are a major part of our strategy.

Over the years we have had excellent results from two particular nutritional formulas: Opthalplex Plus and Ora Key. Both contain important antioxidants which can counteract the activity of free-radical destruction in the eyes (see discussion of free radicals in chapter 11) and promote optimum circulation.

Since many visual problems are due to damage from free radical activity and impaired circulation, antioxidants and natural blood vessel dilators are essential. One such natural agent is European bilberry, a type of blueberry that has beneficial chemical components that aid night vision and naturally opens constricted blood vessels.

During World War II, British air force pilots ate jelly made from bilberry and experienced improved vision at night. During the 1960s, studies on bilberry confirmed that it produced improvements in night vision among both healthy subjects and individuals with visual disorders. One study demonstrated its benefits to air traffic controllers, pilots and truck drivers. Bilberry also helps bleeding gums, hemorrhages, phlebitis, varicose veins, and high blood pressure.

Vitamin C with rutin, a member of the bioflavonoid family, helps to strengthen blood vessels and prevent collagen (cell cement) breakdown.

Supplemental vitamin E is extremely beneficial for individuals with diabetes (see information on vitamin E in the diabetes chapter) and diabetic retinopathy.

Butcher's Broom, a herb used by ancient Greek physicians for swelling and varicose veins, also has been found helpful for diabetic retinopathy and eye hemorrhages.

Since hardening of the arteries and hypertension are common features of advanced eye problems, oral chelation and intravenous chelation should be strongly considered (see the chelation therapy section in chapter 11).

For localized eye inflammation from allergies or viral conjunctivitis, not associated with eye disease, homeopathic eye drops such as Similasan can be used with a good deal of success. Natural eye washes that use distilled water with goldenseal tea can work effectively to relieve eye strain and reddened irritated eyes.

Eye fitness

We are supposedly a nation obsessed with exercise, or at least we talk a lot about exercise.

We do all kinds of exercise for our muscles. Even our tongue gets a good daily workout. But the eyes? Regular eye exercise can do wonders for many visual problems.

At our clinic we have developed a program of visual exercises designed to strengthen your eye muscles and improve visual acuity. We have used the program for years to help patients.

These exercises are not a replacement for proper eye care or examination by a trained physician.

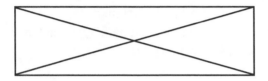

Exercise # 1 ("The box")

Hold your index finger out in front of you.
Without moving your head, follow your finger as it makes a rectangular box.
Next, make and follow an "X" inside the box.

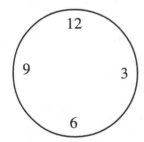

Now, go backwards. Repeat several times.

Exercise # 2 ("The clock")

Sit comfortably and gaze outward, imagining a large clock.
Follow the clock, stopping at each hour and seeing each number.
Do it slowly for 12 through 1 and then back.
Stretch your eyes and reverse the procedure.
Repeat several times.

Exercise # 3
Blink your eyes rapidly. Rest. Repeat several times.

Exercise # 4
Hold your thumb up in front of you and focus directly on it.
Next, focus on the tip of your nose.
Now, look at a distant object, such as a tree or a sign.
Go back and forth now several times from the tip of your nose to the distant object.

Exercise # 5 ("Cupped breathing")
Vigorously rub the palms of your hands together.
Now breathe in deeply while cupping each hand over each eye.
Hold for 10 seconds. Repeat several times.

Not all light is created equal

Natural light and lighting is extremely important to your general well-being and particularly your eyes. Consider full-spectrum glasses or contact lenses when purchasing eye care products. Overhead lighting should utilize full-spectrum lights such as the Ott light or the Vita light.

The chiropractic — vision connection

Cranial manipulation and upper cervical manipulation may often be helpful for visual problems. By correcting misalignments, manipulation can increase blood blow to the brain and also eliminate interference with nerve impulses essential to vision.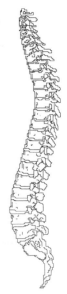

The ability of the pupil to constrict and relax and allow light into the eyes, for instance, is dependent upon the autonomic nervous system, which is influenced by the cervical spine. If your neck is misaligned, nerve signals that control the operation of the pupil could be impaired.

A number of published reports indicate vision improvements, even very dramatic ones, after manipulation:

• One described the case of a 75-year-old man who injured his head in a fall. Afterward, he experienced headaches and dizziness, and the next morning he woke up completely blind. Three months later the patient was referred to a chiropractor who found subluxations in the neck. A series of 11 manipulations over a three-month period gradually restored the man's vision (Journal of Behavioral Optometry, 1990).

    • An interesting observation on the benefits of chiropractic for vision problems comes from an Australian ophthalmologist, R. F. Gorman, M.D. Gorman, and three other eye specialists evaluated 16 patients before and after spinal manipulation. In all cases their visual field and/or visual acuity improved.

The eye doctors also commented that the chiropractic adjustments resulted in additional benefits for their patients, such as less fatigue, elevated mood, more happiness, better arm range of motion, and improved spinal posture/alignment.

Gorman has theorized that spinal misalignments can block blood flow to the brain and affect various sensory and mental functions, including vision. Allen Terrett, D.C., an Australian chiropractor and educator, has expanded on this theory, which he calls "brain hibernation." The theory says that misalignments can cause interference in blood flow and nerve impulses in the brain, resulting in some areas of the brain to "hibernate," that is, function at reduced capacity.

"I'm sure that this is exactly what happens to many people every day, and that this is why they suffer problems such as tiredness, headache, depression, irritability, difficulty concentrating, visual difficulty, etc.," wrote Terrett in a 1994 issue of Chiropractic Technique.

In my practice I encounter many patients who do not have clearly-defined eye disease but rather an array of functional disturbances that they may, or may not, mention among their health complaints. These disturbances include reduced vision, blurred vision, tunnel vision, and focusing difficulties.

The observation of Gorman, the Australian ophthalmologist, regarding additional benefits to patients from chiropractic manipulation is something I experience routinely on a daily basis. By utilizing chiropractic and nutritional care, we are able to correct deficiencies or impairments in the body's natural intelligence and order. The benefits can be both systemic and localized. By manipulating the neck, for instance, we may be able to reduce or eliminate a patient's headaches and clear up a visual difficulty as well.

I have patients everyday in my practice who, following adjustments, spontaneously comment that they "can see better," or that "the room is much brighter," or "my vision isn't as blurry."

I treated Nancy Ireland, one of my patients, for Meniere's disease, a disorder of the ear. She also had vision problems and had used glasses for 35 years. Chiropractic treatment restored much of her lost hearing, eliminated most of the tinnitus, and, as an added benefit, improved her vision.

"The treatments have done wonders," she said. "I don't have to wear glasses or contacts anymore."

Another interesting case involved a 59-year-old woman I was treating for low energy. She reported that one of the "surprising side benefits" of chiropractic adjustments was improved vision. "I no longer have to wear my bifocals when shopping in the supermarket," she said. "I can now read both the distant aisle signs and the small print on package labels without my glasses. If my vision blurs up a bit, I just get another manipulation of my neck, and that immediately puts me back in focus."

One of the great joys in alternative medicine are the "side benefits" that occur as a result of treatment. For me, as a chiropractor, it's just common sense. When you correct structure, you affect function, and correcting the function of the nervous system brings a multitude of gratifying and even unexpected results. You get beneficial effects rather than side ones.

Natural Remedies for Vision

- Gallagher Wellness Program
- Cranial and chiropractic manipulation
- Opthalplex Plus ....2 capsules, twice daily
- Ora Key (magnesium,
         vitamin C, hawthorn, CoQ10, carnitine) .... 2 capsules, twice daily
- Anti Oxidants (including vitamin E and selenium) .... 2 capsules daily
- Vitamin C (with bioflavonoids) .... 3,000-6,000 milligrams daily
- Intravenous chelation therapy, if eye conditions are associated with
         hypertension, atherosclerosis, diabetes.

YEAST SYNDROME (CANDIDIASIS)

Q *"I am 35 and always sick and tired. I have non-stop yeast infec tions, sore throats, bladder trouble, allergies, depression and anxiety. I catch everything that comes around. I have been to eight medical specialists and have had every test in the book. I have tried at least 15 prescription drugs. I need help. I am at the end of my rope."*

This caller to one of my radio broadcasts was suffering from candidiasis, better known as the yeast syndrome, a complex condition that can cause symptoms throughout the body. In today's overmedicated society, the yeast syndrome is virtually an epidemic.

Yeasts are single-cell micro-organisms belonging to the plant kingdom. They are cousins of molds and they live all around us — and inside us as well. The family of yeasts include organisms that have served mankind well since time immemorial. Yeast is what causes bread to rise, fruits to ferment into wine, and hops into beer.

One common family of yeast — Candida albicans, as it is known in scientific terms — is normally present in the mouth, skin, bowels and vagina. However, when the body's normal defenses have been weakened, colonies of yeast can multiply rapidly and produce toxins that further debilitate the immune system. They then become an aggressive force causing many chronic ailments that are often misdiagnosed and never traced to yeast.

One way to picture this overgrowth is to think of a yeast problem as you would a yard that is overrun with weeds.

"Yeasts are mild-manner creatures incapable of producing infec-tion in the normal healthy individual," writes the University of Chicago's John W. Rippon, Ph.D., an authority of yeast, in his 1982 book, "Medical Mycology." "They only cause trouble in the person with weakened defenses. The severity of the disease will depend on how weak a person's resistance is, rather than on any disease-producing properties" of the yeast.

Candida is perhaps most notorious for its tendency to overgrow in the vagina and cause itching, burning and inflammation. It is also in-volved in "jock itch" and the fungal annoyance between the toes known as "athlete's foot." Many babies, with immune systems not fully developed, contract a condition in the mouth called "thrush" that is yeast-related. So, too, many AIDS patients, who suffer from immune dysfunction, become plagued with yeast infections in many organ systems.

Yeast may also be involved in so-called "incurable" conditions such as psoriasis, multiple sclerosis, autism and arthritis. According to William G. Crook, M.D., author of "The Yeast Connection: A Medical Break-through," the most frequent symptoms linked to yeast include:

- fatigue
- irritability
- hyperactivity
- depression
- short attention span and memory loss
- menstrual problems
- digestive and intestinal disorders
- muscle pain
- headache
- vaginitis
- skin problems
- impotence
- urinary disorders

In many, many cases, yeast infections affect more than just localized parts of the body. When they become systemic in nature, they can cause any of the above conditions, in any combination, plus trigger other reactions.

Why yeast rises in your body

By far the major cause of yeast infections is the over-prescribing of broad-spectrum antibiotics by physicians. As I mentioned at the end of chapter eight, these medications can devastate the colonies of beneficial bacteria that reside in your body and open the door for the overgrowth of other micro-organisms, including yeast.

The medical literature "clearly supports the theory that antibiotics can lead to candida overgrowth which suppresses immune function thereby predisposing one to recurrent infections," says James Brodsky, M.D., of Georgetown University School of Medicine. "We must help our patients overcome this illness, which is probably, for most, iatrogenic in origin." Iatrogenic refers to complications caused by medical treatment.

Other causes of yeast infections that have been suggested are diets high in sugar and other simple carbohydrates (yeasts thrive on sugar!), environmental toxins that may impair the immune system, food allergies, oral contraceptives, smoking, and stress.

According to William Crook, "ingestion of sugar causes a 200-fold increase in the growth of candida."

Mainstream medicine, for the most part, does not recognize systemic yeast infections but only localized vaginal, mouth, toenail or skin infections. This is a great disservice to patients. Many go from doctor to doctor, are treated for individual symptoms, receive prescriptions (including more antibiotics!) that further suppress the immune system and promote yeast activity, and never get better.

Often, at the end of this medical treadmill, patients wind up in a psychiatrist's office, convinced that their problem is "mental." I can assure you, that if a systemic infection is present, the problem is very, very real.

As a rare exception, conventional doctors will acknowledge the general condition in cases of severe immune deficiency, such as in AIDS. It is largely in the wholistic healing community where you will find the necessary recognition and good treatment programs. Diagnosis can be elusive but patient history, physical examination, a special candida questionnaire and blood candida antibody levels, are helpful in pinpointing the problem. Sometimes the best way of confirming a suspected diagnosis is to do a trial anti-yeast program. If the patients feels better on the program, then the suspicion of yeast was correct.

Mary Jo Sweeney's case

Pittsburgh housewife Mary Jo Sweeney was very sick when she made an appointment to see me.

> **Pain, lethargy, nervousness...
> "I am dying
> at age 45."**

"I have pain throughout my whole body," she said. "Some days I can hardly walk. It is painful just to bend over. I am fatigued to the point of lethargy. I have to rest after taking a shower. I can't think straight and I am very nervous."

Mary Jo didn't know that she had a systemic yeast infection. "I am dying at age 45," she said, desperately.

She had consulted a long list of medical specialists. A year before she had seen a nutritionist. No blood tests were done. The nutritionist told her to avoid fruit, fruit juice, and dairy products.

"But I just kept getting sicker and sicker," she said. "I could not breath and my chest felt tight. My stomach was bloated. I blamed all my symptoms on stress. I had no idea that candida could be so widespread in my body and destroy my immune system and eventually kill me if not treated correctly."

I first saw Mary Jo in April of 1996. We did a thorough medical history, blood tests, and hair analysis. We started her first on a detoxification program followed by a strict, high-protein, low carbohydrate diet.

"The diet is hard to stay on," she complained, "but I know I have to do it to get better."

We also recommended colonics. At first she was reluctant. It was an uncomfortable prospect and too unconventional for her. But now she's glad she did it. She benefited immensely from colonic hydrotherapy (see chapter six on detoxification). This treatment helps to rapidly flush out toxins and yeast byproducts from the colon that contribute to problems in other parts of the body. Colonics is often a missing link among patients whose attempts to overcome candidiasis reach a standstill.

Mary Jo's determination paid off. Slowly and surely, her energy and strength returned. She realized her problems were not psychological nor was she dying from some dreaded disease. She lost more than 20 pounds. Her bloated abdomen vanished. Several months after starting on the healing path, Mary Jo had come a long way. She still had a ways to go but she was confident that she would reach her goal of optimum health.

Jalaire Craver's case

Jalaire Craver, of Mt. Lebanon, Pennsylvania, a 45-year-old homemaker, developed problems over a period of nine months. Her symptoms included a sore tongue, nausea, anxiety attacks, and tingling in all her limbs. Ringing in her ears kept her awake at night. When she laid

> **Nausea, anxiety, ringing in the ear, muscle weakness... all resolved**

down her back was "alive" with what she felt were "waves of electrical sensations running up and down" her spine. Then she experienced muscle weakness that made even walking a difficult proposition.

Her doctor first prescribed an anti-viral drug. A neurologist said there was nothing serious and to come back in three months. He prescribed anti-anxiety drugs.

Jalaire felt that although her physicians were very caring individuals, they were unable to help her. Through word of mouth she came to us.

On her first visit she said she was particularly concerned about her condition because of a family history of multiple sclerosis. Moreover, she had difficult breathing fully and thought she might have a lung disease.

Our evaluation pointed to none of these. Her symptoms, which had defied medical specialists, were due to the yeast syndrome coupled with spinal misalignments.

We recommended a strict diet of vegetables and brown rice along with relevant supplements. The diet suppressed yeast growth. The vitamins rejuvenated her weakened organs. A series of twice-a-week chiropractic adjustments turned on her immune system. Following manipulation of her thoracic spine (mid-back), her "lung disease" was gone.

Looking back, Jalaire recently said that "improvement was noticeable within two weeks. I began to sleep better, and every week more of my numerous symptoms disappeared. It probably took eight months for the last tingle to fade away. But overall, my health had never been better."

How we treat yeast infections

Our approach to the problem often includes the following:

• First a 10-day detoxification program to rid the body of yeast-generated poisons.

• Colon hydrotherapy.

• Because their immune system has been ravaged, many people with yeast problems are sensitive to a wide variety of foods, chemicals and environmental substances. We test patients to help determine their sensitivities so they can as best as possible avoid exposure (see chapter nine).

• A diet plan emphasizing high-protein, soluble fiber, vegetables, and avoidance of typically allergenic foods.

A patient's menu should strictly exclude yeast-containing foods, such as bread, crackers, and other bakery items.

Avoid junk or processed foods, as well as fermented and pickled food. No fruit juices.

According to yeast expert, John Rippon of the University of Chicago, "yeasts thrive on the simple carbohydrates, including cane sugar, beet sugar, honey, corn syrup, maple syrup and molasses."

Eating fruits promotes yeast growth because they are rich in fructose (a simple sugar), he points out.

Avoid milk and dairy, Rippon says, until a patient improves. These foods contain lactose, a naturally-occurring sugar. In the intestines, the lactose is broken down into simple sugar, providing more food for yeast.

Although some individuals may tolerate sugar-free, fruit-free yogurt preparations, many people are intolerant to yogurt. In addition, many commercial yogurt cultures taken to reintroduce beneficial bacteria (such as lactobacillus acidophilus) are ineffective for that purpose.

I have long used a supplement in my clinic called "Yeast Defenders." It is a useful source of soluble fiber combined with caprylic acid and acidophilus. These substances inhibit yeast, and re-introduce healthy bacteria into the intestinal tract.

Yeast-free B complex, vitamin C, zinc picolinate, along with thymus and adrenal extracts, are important nutrient support factors to increase resistance, inhibit yeast and raise energy levels.

Certain herbal supplements are excellent strategies in overcoming yeast infections and boosting the integrity of the immune system.

Among them are:

• Echinacea and goldenseal. These well-known herbals are potent anti-microbial agents that increase white blood cells, the immune system "soldiers" that surround and destroy bacterial and viral invaders in the blood.

• MFP (grapefruit seed extract) and Pau D'Arco tea are potent inhibitors of yeast.

• Japanese research has demonstrated that licorice root contains anti-bacterial, anti-viral and anti-inflammatory agents. It was found to be effective against strains of Staphylococcus arureus bacteria that were resistant to penicillin and streptomycin.

• Studies now indicate that essential oils found in plants such as clove, thyme and oregano exert a powerful anti-yeast effect. We recommend patients use liberal amounts of these culinary herbs in their cooking. Garlic, ginger, curry, and lemon balm can also be helpful .

• ADP (time-released oregano) is a gold standard at our clinic. Oil of oregano has a 21 times greater anti-septic potency than the phenol substances found in Lysol, Pine Sol, and Chloraseptic throat spray.

• Although the prescription drug Nystatin may be part of a yeast recovery program, the common garlic we use in cooking, has been found to be more effective. Garlic is famous for its natural antibiotic qualities.

Super Oxy Plus is a unique supplement that combines 35 percent food grade hydrogen peroxide with aloe vera juice and different herbal factors. Both oral and intravenous hydrogen peroxide offer potent anti-fungal and anti-viral effects. I usually recommend one tablespoon between meals on an empty stomach. It is important to use only the 35 percent food grade level because other types of hydrogen peroxide can be toxic.

The chiropractic — yeast connection

In our clinic, chiropractic manipulation is a core element of the yeast recovery program. You would never think chiropractic has a role,

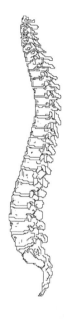

but as in many other disease processes, it can indeed play a major and surprising healing role.

The reason is simple — misalignments in the head, neck, and back can be primary or secondary causes for malfunctioning systems in the body. Remember: structure affects function.

Most wholistic experts focus their attention on the immune system as the primary factor in combating yeast and do all they can to strengthen the system. However, most don't take into account the possibility of a malfunctioning nervous system that may prevent the immune system from waging the strongest possible fight. Such malfunction may stem from subluxations in the cranium or spine.

Using applied kinesiology (AK) and other chiropractic techniques, we can quickly perform a "natural cat scan" to determine structural abnormalities and their connections to malfunctioning organs and glands.

Over the years I have often found yeast patients with misaligned bones that are "short-circuiting" the communication network between the brain and the vital glands and organs involved in immune system function, such as the pineal, thymus, spleen, liver, adrenals and lymph.

No matter how many vitamins, minerals, herbs, or homeopathics you take, uncorrected misalignments can stand in the way of effective immune system function and the goal of beating a systemic yeast infection. It often takes chiropractic care to re-open blocked pathways between your brain and cells and permit the immune system to fight back effectively.

Natural Remedies for Yeast Infections

- *The Gallagher Wellness Program*
- *Chiropractic manipulation*
- *High protein, low carbohydrate diet*
- *Avoid yeast-containing foods*
- *Super Oxy* .... *1 tbsp. between meals*
- *ADP* .... *2 capsules, 3 times daily*
- *MFP* .... *4 drops, 3 times daily in 6 ounces of water*
- *Yeast Defenders* .... *2 capsules, 3 times daily*

ABOUT MEDICAL WELLNESS ASSOCIATES

91 Lincoln Highway East,
Jeannette, PA 15644
(724) 523-5505 • Fax (724) 523-6875
(800) 834-4325 (toll-free in western Pennsylvania)

Medical Wellness Associates is a multi disciplinary healthcare facility located in Jeannette, Pennsylvania, 20 miles southeast of Pittsburgh, that incorporates the latest alternative medicine therapies.

Our emphasis is on addressing the root causes of health problems and eliminating them through detoxification techniques, chiropractic manipulations, elimination of food allergies, improving the diet and digestion, and enhancing mental and physical function through nutritional supplementation, exercise and stress reduction.

Our comprehensive program is designed to educate the patient, inspire them to become involved in process of regaining health, to wean them away as much as is medically safe from dependence on medications. In short, to awaken the healer within.

This unique clinic was founded in 1977 by Martin Gallagher, D.C., and Charlotte Ciotti, D.C., and brings together Doctors of Chiropractic (D.C.) and Doctors of Medicine (M.D.) to provide a balanced and state-of-the-art approach to acute and chronic health problems. The physician staff currently includes five D.C.s and three M.D.s.   Services are also provided by 65 health professionals, including registered nurses, licensed practical nurses, exercise and massage therapists, colon therapists, radiology technicians, and medical and chiropractic assistants.

The clinic is self-contained in a modern 20,000 square foot building that serves patients throughout the U.S. and Canada.

Clinical services

- Lifestyle Evaluation: includes current history, work status, exercise, stress factors, nutrition, and vitamins.

- Physical Examination: traditional medical exam that also incorporates nutritional characteristics.

- Chiropractic Examination: evaluation of spinal and cranial motion to assess the nervous system.

- Applied kinesiology (AK) exam is used to determine muscle, organ and nutritional imbalances.

- EKG to evaluate cardiac function at rest.

- 24 Hour Holter test to monitor changes in blood pressure over 24 hours.

- Vascular evaluation using a Doppler ultrasound (non invasive) to assess arterial blockages and circulatory problems

- X-rays to determine bone disease, fractures, and structural patterns

- Nerve Conduction Tests to evaluate the presence of nerve injury or damage.

- Spirometry, a test to determine lung capacity, an important diagnostic tool for allergies and respiratory disorders.

- Nutritional Diagnostics:

Many people are thoroughly confused about which vitamins to take and how much. In our practice, we see two distinct types of nutritional patients.

The first has extensive health problems even though often taking a large number and variety of vitamins, based on what he or she hears, reads or tries.

The second type usually takes minimal or no vitamins and is more health conscious, prevention-oriented and would like to have regular nutritional evaluations to find out about metabolic status and changing nutritional requirements.

Nutritional evaluation: includes the medical history and lifestyle assessment with computerized diet analysis, trace mineral and toxic metal screening, and specialized blood tests for vitamin and mineral deficiencies.

Additional individual testing may include food sensitivity tests, chemical antibody studies, parasite and candida evaluation or digestive analysis.

The collected information is correlated and incorporated into an individualized program to help overcome specific conditions or prevent disease. It will include a consultation to discuss the findings, outline a nutritional program and prescribe the necessary vitamins, minerals, homeopathics, enzymes or herbal therapies.

The specific tests include:

Trace Minerals and Toxic Metal Analysis: utilizing hair to assess the balance of minerals and screen for toxic metals (such as lead and aluminum) in the body.

EMA: a blood test used to determine the levels of vitamins and minerals in the body.

Elisa Test: evaluates immune responses to foods, chemicals and the environment through simple blood testing.

Food Sensitivity Test: utilizes blood testing to determine immediate and delayed responses to food up to four days after exposure.

CDSA: evaluates the stool to determine digestive capabilities. Screens for parasites and yeast.

GI Antibody Studies: blood test to determine the state of the digestive system.

Candida Testing: uses specific blood antibody tests to determine immune response to yeast.

Parasite Testing: blood antibody tests for specific parasitic organisms.

Hormone Evaluation: blood and saliva testing for levels of DHEA, testosterone, estrogen, progesterone, thyroid, and other hormones.

Executive Profile: Blood test to evaluate blood fats and major organs. Functional Liver Test: utilizes a caffeine tablet and urine test to determine liver detoxification.

• Our physical medicine programs include:

Chiropractic Manipulation: specific manipulative procedures to enhance joint function, decrease pain and improve the nervous system. Several different methods are employed for all age groups including Applied Kinesiology, Leander, Sacro/occipital technique, Activator, diversified and extremity manipulation.

Cranial Manipulation: a specific evaluation and treatment using pressure point therapy to enhance brain, jaw, and whole body function.

Myotherapy: incorporates massage, trigger point therapy, lymphatic drainage and myofascial release techniques to reduce pain and induce relaxation.

Electro Acupuncture: analysis and treatment of meridians (energy pathways) using acupuncture points on the hands, feet and ears to create energy balance.

Laser Therapy: non-surgical cold laser therapy for pain control.

Pulsed Diathermy: electromagnetic heat, helpful for arthritis, bursitis and organic disorders.

Ultrasound: micro massage using sound waves to reduce pain and soft tissue inflammation.

Interferential Therapy: a type of electrical stimulation, developed in Germany, to help reduce pain and inflammation.

Intersegmental Traction: a therapy designed to create increased spinal motion and relaxation.

Russian Muscle Stimulation: a type of electric therapy that helps muscle atrophy and increases muscle strength.

T.E.N.S.: a portable unit for pain control.

Biofeedback: a technique that facilitates relaxation and stress management.

• Exercise rehabilitation

Cybex: a state of the art computerized isokinetic testing and rehab facility supervised by staff sports medicine doctors and exercise therapists.

• Nutritional programs

Detoxification: specific foods, juices and supplements to remove toxic substances from the body.

Colon Hydrotherapy: certified colon therapists administer water infusions to enhance digestive and whole body rejuvenation. Specific implants complement this procedure.

Homeopathy: both oral and injectible remedies.

Herbal Medicines: single and combination formulas used to enhance immune function and create balance.

Oral vitamins and minerals: both pediatric and adult formulas for supporting nutritional deficiencies.

Vitamin and mineral injectables: including B-12, B Complex, and magnesium, for specific health problems.

Chelation Therapy: utilizes a man made amino acid (EDTA) in an intravenous solution. Helpful for heart disease, diabetes, toxic metal syndrome and much more.
See chelation section in chapter 11 for more details.

IV Vitamin Infusions: Intravenous vitamin treatments that deliver direct nutrition including vitamin C, magnesium, B Complex, and trace minerals. Often used for flu, energy loss and chronic health problems.

Insurance

Insurance Information: MWA is a participating Medicare facility. Our doctors participate with Blue Shield. Over 700 insurance carriers cover our services. For those who are underinsured, individual payment plans are available at our office.

The office is open six days a week. Monday through Friday from 8:00 AM until 9:00 PM and Saturday from 8:00 AM until 12:00 PM.

Nutritional and educational supplies

Dr. Gallagher's video tapes, cassettes, books, and nutritional supplements used in our clinic can be obtained by calling our office at 724-523-5505 or faxing in your order at 724-523-6875. See appendix B for a list of available tapes.

APPENDIX B

EDUCATIONAL TAPES FROM DR. GALLAGHER

The following video cassettes and audio tapes by Dr. Gallagher are available through Medical Wellness Associates. To obtain these, or any additional tapes completed since the printing of this book, please call (724) 523-5505.

Video cassettes from Dr. Gallagher's NATURAL HEALTH television show (including interviews with patients). All cassettes are 30 minutes in length. Cost: $7 each.

1. Allergies/migraines
2. Arthritis
3. Ulcerative colitis/Crohn's Disease
4. Multiple sclerosis
5. Back surgery
6. Candida (yeast infections)
7. Irritable bowel syndrome
8. Reversing heart disease
9. Chronic fatigue syndrome
10. Depression/anxiety
11. Reversing visual disorders
12. Hypoglycemia
13. Fibromyalgia
14. Chronic infections
15. Diabetes
16. Ear infections
17. Sinus infections
18. Psoriasis/eczema
19. Premenstrual syndrome
20. Bladder infections
21. Gall bladder disease
22. Attention deficit disorder/hyperactivity
23. Rheumatoid arthritis
24. Lupus
25. Meniere's disease and tinnitus
26. Vertigo

27. Chronic sore throat
28. Seizures
29. Anorexia
30. Weight control
31. Anemia
32. Asthma
33. Carpal tunnel syndrome
34. Cold sores
35. Colic
36. Fibromyalgia
37. Heartburn and hiatal hernia
38. High blood pressure
39. Hypoglycemia
40. Hypothyroidism
41. Memory loss
42. Menopause
43. Osteoporosis
44. Prostate
45. Stress and your adrenal glands

Video cassettes of Dr. Gallagher lectures. Cassettes range from one to three hours in length. Cost: $25 each.
1. "How to increase your energy and maximize your health."
2. "Wellness."
3. Martin Gallagher, interviewing alternative medicine and natural health pioneers.
4. "Natural health prescriptions," practical advice from A to Z on how to combat health problems.
5. "Surviving and preventing health crises."
6. Chronic fatigue syndrome.
7. "Health steps to high energy."
8. "Wholistic Health."

The following are audio tapes of Dr. Gallagher lectures. Cost: $5 each.
1. "Natural Health Prescriptions."
2. "Surviving and Preventing Health Crises."
3. Food Allergies.

RESOURCES

American Academy of Environmental Medicine
4510 W. 89th Street
Prarie Village, KS 66207
(913) 642-6062
Referrals for specialists in food, chemical and environmental allergies.

American Association of Acupuncture and Oriental Medicine
4101 Lake Boon Trail
Suite 201
Raleigh, NC 27607
(919) 787-5181
 The AAOM is a national professional organization of acupuncturists.

American Association of Naturopathic Physicians
2366 East Lake Avenue, Suite 322
Seattle, WA 98102
(206) 323-7610
Provides directory of naturopathic physicians and offers referrals to nationwide
network of accredited or licensed practitioners.

American Chiropractic Association (ACA)
1701 Clarendon Boulevard
Arlington, VA 22209
(703) 276-8800
Major source for chiropractic information. Monthly publication and
newsletter. Clinical counsels with specialization in sports injuries and
physical fitness, mental health, neurology, diagnosis, internal disorders,
nutrition, orthopedics, physiological therapeutics, diagnostic imaging, and
occupational health.

Foundation for Chiropractic Education and Research (FCER)
66 Washington Avenue
Des Moines, Iowa 50314
(800) 622-6309
This organization funds chiropractic research and provides scientific
updates, newsletters and literature on alternative medicine.

Great Lakes Association of Clinical Medicine, Inc.
70 West Uhrin Street
Chicago, IL 60610
(312) 266-7246
Members are MDs and DOs who practice preventive nutritional medicine
and offer chelation therapy.

International Association for Colonic Therapy I/ACT
2204 NW Loop 410
San Antonio, TX 78230
(210) 366-2888
Referrals to a nationwide network of colon therapists. Funds a national
certification panel for colon therapists.

International Association of Professional Natural Hygienists
Regency Health Resort and Spa
2000 South Ocean Drive
Hallandale, FL 33009
(305) 454-2220
Professional organization of doctors who specialize in therapeutic fasting.

International Chiropractic Association (ICA)
1110 North Glebe Road
Suite 1000
Arlington, VA 22201
(703) 528-5000
The original Chiropractic Association founded by B.J. Palmer, the son of
the founder of chiropractic, Daniel David Palmer. Concerned with
legislation, healthcare policy, public relations, continuing education, skills
development, publications, and interprofessional relations.

International College of Applied Kinesiology (ICAK)
PO Box 905
Lawrence, KS 66044-0905
(913) 542-1801
Referral service for those seeking an applied kinesiologist. Founded by
George Goodheart, D.C.

Koren Publications, Inc.
2026 Chestnut Street
Philadelphia, PA 19103
(800) 537-3001
A resource for consumer and professional information on chiropractic.

National Center for Homeopathy
801 North Fairfax
Suite 306
Alexandria, VA 22314
(703) 548-7790
Provides information on homeopathy and referral list of practicing homeopaths.

National Health Federation
212 West Foothill Boulevard
Monrovia, CA 91016
(818) 357-2181
Consumer advocacy group that monitors health care legislation, provides national workshops, and distributes a monthly health magazine.

Neurological Fitness
PO Box 1634
Vienna, VA 22183
(703) 938-6441
A quarterly newsletter focusing on research on spinal manipulation and somato-visceral/neurological conditions.

Practice Makers Products, Inc.
PO Box 213
Palmerton, PA 18071
(800) 345-3099
A resource for professional and consumer information on chiropractic.

Rheumatoid Disease Foundation
5106 Old Harding Road
Franklin, TN   37064
(615) 646-1030
This non-profit charitable organization provides a listing of physicians who perform nutritional and chelation therapy.

SORSI
PO Box 8245
Prairie Village, KS 66208
(913) 649-3475
Teaches post graduate courses and certifies chiropractors (D.C.s) in the
sacral occipital technique as taught by Dr. Major D. DeJarnette.

The Chiropractic Report
3080 Yonge Street
Suite 3002
Toronto, Ontario, Canada
(416) 484-9601
A professional newsletter on global chiropractic research.

APPENDIX D

BIBLIOGRAPHY

The following books are useful sources of additional information. They can be obtained through regular commercial bookstores or ordered directly through the publishers listed.

- Attwood, Charles, "Dr. Attwood's Low-Fat Prescription for Kids," Penguin Books, New York, 1995.
- Barnard, Neal, "Eat Right, Live Longer," Harmony Books, New York, 1995.
- Beasley, Joseph, and Swift, Jerry, "The Kellogg Report: The Impact of Nutrition, Environment & Lifestyle on the Health of Americans," The Institute of Health Policy and Practice, Bard College Center, 1989, Annandale-on-Hudson, NY 12504.
- Braly, James, "Dr. Braly's Food Allergy & Nutrition Revolution," Keats Publishing, 1992, New Canaan, CT 06684.
- Brecher, Harold and Arline, "Forty Something Forever: A Consumer's Guide to Chelation Therapy and other Heart-Savers," Heart Savers Press, 1994, POBox 683, Herndon, VA 22070. Phone: (714) 471-4734.
- Casdorph, H. Richard, and Walker, Morton, "Toxic Metal Syndrome: How Metal Poisoning Can Affect Your Brain," Avery Publishing, Garden City Park, NY, 1995..
- Colgan, Michael, "Your Personal Vitamin Profile," Quill Publishing, New York, 1982.
- Janson, Michael, "The Vitamin Revolution in Health Care," Arcadia Press, 1996, POBox 205, Greenville, NH 03048. Phone: (800) 398-8851.
- Klatz, Ronald and Goldman, Robert, "Stopping the Clock: Dramatic breakthroughs in anti-aging and rejuvenation techniques," Keats Publishing, 1996, New Canaan, CT 06684.
- Koren, Tedd, "Chiropractic and Spinal Research," Spring 1995 edition, available through Koren Publications, 2026 Chestnut Street, Philadelphia, PA 19103. Phone: (800) 537-3001.
- Lisa, Joseph P, "The Assault on Medical Freedom," Hampton Roads Publishing Co.,1994, 891 Norfolk Square, Norfolk, VA 23502. Phone: (804) 459-2453.

- Lonsdorf, Nancy and Butler, Veronica, "A Woman's Best Medicine: Health, Happiness and Long Life Through Ayur-Veda," Tarcher/Putnam (G.P. Putnam's Sons Publishers), New York, 1993.
- Mandell, Marshall, and Scanlon, Lynne, "Dr. Mandell's 5-Day Allergy Relief System," Thomas Y. Crowell Publishers, New York, 1979.
- Moss, Ralph, "Cancer Therapy: The Independent Consumer's Guide to Non-Toxic Treatment & Prevention," Equinox Press, 1996, Brooklyn NY 11217. Phone: (718) 636-1679.
- Ornish, Dean, "Dean Ornish's Program for Reversing Heart Disease," Random House, New York, 1990.
- Rapp, Doris, "Is This Your Child's World: How You Can Fix the Schools and Homes that are Making Your Children Sick," Bantam Books, New York, NY, 1996.
- Sahley, Billie Jay, "The Anxiety Epidemic," Pain and Stress Center, 5282 Medical Drive, Suite 160, San Antonio, TX 78229-6043. Phone: 1-800-669-CALM.
- Selye, Hans, " The Stress of Life," McGraw-Hill, New York, 1956.
- Sorvino, Paul, "How to become a former asthmatic: Easy twice-a-day breathing exercises to prevent asthma, spasms, and reduce reliance on drugs," Wm Morrow & Co., New York, 1985).
- Wolinsky, Howard, and Brune, Tom, "The Serpent on the Staff: The Unhealthy Politics of the American Medical Association," Tarcher/Putnam (G.P. Putnam's Sons Publishers), New York, 1994.

APPENDIX E

CHAPTER REFERENCES

The Treadmill — How Bad Is It?

Hoffman, Catherine, Rice, Dorothy, Sung, Hai-Yen, "Persons with chronic conditions," The Journal of the American Medical Association, November 13, 1996, 276: 1473-1479.

U.S. National Center for Health Statistics, "Vital Statistics of the United States," Volumes for 1970-1980 (Rockville, MD: 1975), as quoted in Colgan, Michael, "Your Personal Vitamin Profile," Quill Books, New York, 1982, 24.

"America's vast sick-care economy," Alternative Medicine Digest, Issue 17, 1997, 94.

Office of Technology Assessment (Library of Congress), "Assessing the Efficacy and Safety of Medical Technology," 1978.

Leape, Lucian L., "Error in medicine," special communication, Journal of the American Medical Association, December 21, 1994, 272 (23): 1851.

Waddell, G., "A new clinical model for the treatment of low back pain," Spine, 1987, 12 (7): 632-644

Bailar III, John D., MD,Ph.D., and Smith, Elaine M., "Progress against cancer," New England Journal of Medicine, Special Articles, May 8, 1986, 314:1226-1232.

Bailar III, John D., Gornick, Heather L., "Cancer undefeated," New England Journal of Medicine, Special Articles, May 29, 1997, 336: 1569-1574..

Johnson, Jeffrey A., and Bootman, Lyle, "Drug-related morbidity and mortality: a cost-of-illness model," Archives of Internal Medicine, October 9, 1995, 155: 1949-1964.

Bates, David W., et al, "Incidence of adverse drug events and potential adverse drug events," Journal of the American Medical Association, July 5, 1995, 274 (1): 29.

"High doses of heart medicine raise risk of death, study find," Associated Press report of study on calcium channel blockers published in Circulation, September 1, 1995. (AP article appeared in Los Angeles Times, September 1, 1995, 30).

Fries, J.F., Miller, S.R., et al, "Toward an epidemiology of gastropathy associated with nonsteroidal anti-inflammatory drug use," Gastroenterology, 1989, 96: 647-655.

Perneger, Thomas, et al, "Risk of kidney failure associated with the use of acetaminophen, aspirin, and non-steroidal anti-inflammatory drugs," New England Journal of Medicine, December 22, 1994, 331 (25):1675.

Dhawan, Anil, and Sorrell, Michael, "Acetaminophen overdose: Need to consider intravenous preparation of N-Acetylcysteine in the United States," American Journal of Gastroenterology, 1996, 91 (7): 1476.

Norrby, S. R., "Antiobiotic resistance: a self-inflicted problem," Journal of Internal Medicine, 1996, 293: 373-375.

Hauser, W.E., and Remington, J.S., "Effect of antibiotics on the immune response," American Journal of Medicine, 1982, 72: 711-716.

Kogan, Michael D., et al, "Over-the-counter medication use among U.S. preschool-age children," Journal of the American Medical Association, Oct 5, 1994, 272 (13): 1025-1030. See also in same issue, JAMA editorial on OTC medications.

Weber, Tracy, "Tarnishing the golden years with addiction," Los Angeles Times, December 20, 1996, 1.

Wolfe, Sidney, "Worst Pills, Best Pills II," Public Citizen Health Research Group, Washington D.C., 1993, as quoted in "There's peril in mixing prescriptions," by Pamela Warrick, Los Angeles Times, October 12, 1993, p. e-1.

Coles, L. Stephen, & Harris, Steven B., "Coenzyme Q-10 and Lifespan Extension," in "Advances in Anti-Aging Medicine," vol. 1., edited by Ronald M. Klatz, Mary Ann Liebert, Inc., publishers, Larchmont, N.Y., 1996, 214-215.

The Shifting System — From Disease Care to Health Care

Eisenberg, D.M., et al, "Unconventional medicine in the United States," New England Journal of Medicine, January 28, 1993, 238: 246-252.

Wolinsky, Howard & Brune, Tom, "The Serpent on the Staff: The Unhealthy Politics of the American Medical Association," Tarcher/Putnam, New York, 1994, 12-13.

Goodwin, Jan, "A Health Insurance Revolution," New Age Journal, March/April 1997, 95.

Alternative Medicine Gaining Credibility, USA Today, October 11, 1996.

Goldberg, Burton, "Insuring the future of your health — Why alternative medicine is the way," Townsend Letter for Doctors and Patients, August/September,1996, 130.

Zucker, Martin, "Dean Ornish's Program for Reversing Heart Disease: Lifestyle changes to unblock clogged arteries," Let's Live Magazine, February 1996, 24-26.

Ebrall, P.S., "Mechanical low-back pain: A comparison of medical and chiropractic management within the Victorian WorkCare Scheme," Chiropractic Journal of Australia, June 1992, 22 (2): 47-53.

Jarvis, K.B., et al, "Cost per case comparison of back injury claims of chiropractic versus medical management for conditions with identical diagnostic codes," Journal of Occupational Medicine, August 1991, 33 (8): 847-852.

Colt, George, "The Healing Revolution," Life Magazine, September 1996, 35-50.

Coulter, Anne H., "Second Annual International Congress stimulates discussion among alternative medicine luminaries," July/August 1996, 2 (4): 264-265.

"Ten Leading Causes of Death in the United States," Update, Centers for Disease Control and Prevention, Atlanta, 1994.

Beasley, Joseph D., & Swift, Jerry J., "The Kellogg Report: The Impact of Nutrition, Environment & Lifestyle on the Health of Americans," The Institute of Health Policy and Practice, The Bard College Center, Annandale-on-Hudson, New York, 12504, 1989, 454.

Remaking Yourself Healthier — The Basics of 21st Century Medicine

"Diet related to killer diseases," Hearing before the Select Committee on Nutrition and Human Needs of the U.S. Senate, 95th congress, July 22-26, 1977. U.S. Government Printing Office, Washington D.C.

Allen, Scott, "Study: Air pollution killing thousand," Des Moines Register, May 9, 1996, p. 1. Also: 1996 study on pollution in the U.S., National Resources Defense Council, Washington D.C.

Moyers, Bill, "Healing and the Mind," Doubleday & Co., New York, 1993. The molecules of emotion modulate all cellular activity through intercellular communication and provide a plausible mechanism for the role of the mind and emotions in health. See also: Interview with Candace Pert, Alternative Therapies, July 1995, 1 (3): 71-76.

Detoxification

Lonsdorf, Nancy, Butler, Veronica, Brown, Melanie, "A Woman's Best Medicine: Health, Happiness, and Long Life through Ayur-Veda," Tarcher/Putnam, New York, 1993, 149.

Mandell, Marshall & Scanlon, Lynne, "Dr. Mandell's 5-day Allergy Relief System," Thomas Y. Crowell Publishers, New York, 1979, 11.

Zucker, Martin, "Environmentally sick schools: Sick children who can't learn, sick teachers who can't teach," Let's Live Magazine, September 1995, 43-46.

Beasley, Joseph D., & Swift, Jerry J., "The Kellogg Report: The Impact of Nutrition, Environment & Lifestyle on the Health of Americans," The Institute of Health Policy and Practice, The Bard College Center, Annandale-on-Hudson, New York, 12504, 1989, 172.

"The Biotype Diet"

Barnard, Neal, "Eat Right, Live Longer," Harmony Books, New York, 1995.

Ames, Bruce N., et al, "Oxidants, antioxidants, and the degenerative diseases of aging," Proceedings of the National Academyof Science, 1993, 90: 7915-7922.

Continuing Survey of Food Intakes by Individuals, U.S. Department of Agriculture, 1989-91.

Price, Weston, "Nutrition and Physical Degeneration: A Comparison of Primitive and Modern Diets and Their Effects," Price-Pottenger Nutrition Foundation, PO Box 2614, La Mesa, CA 92041, 1945.

Optimizing Your Digestion

Lanza, E., et al, "Dietary fiber intake in the U.S. population," American Journal of Clinical Nutrition, 1987, 46 (5): 790-797.

Burkitt, Denis, and Trowell, H., " Western Diseases: Their Emergence and Prevention," Harvard University Press, Cambridge, MA, 1981.

Hoffer, Abram, "Orthomolecular Medicine for Physicians," Keats Publishing, New Canaan, CT, 1989, 17.

Burkitt, Denis, and Trowell, H., editors, "Refined Carbohydrate Foods and Disease," Academic Press, New York, 1975.

Zucker, Martin, "Chewing Well: Megabites of information to digest," Let's Live Magazine, July 1989, 38.

Pixley, F., et al, "Effect of vegetarianism on development of gallstones in women," British Medical Journal, 1985, 291: 11-12.

Breneman, J.C., "Allergy elimination diet as the most effective gallbladder diet," Annals of Allergy, 1968, 26: 83-87.

Food, Chemical and Environmental Sensitivity Identification

Braly, James, "Dr. Braly's Food Allergy & Nutrition Revolution," Keats Publishing Co., New Canaan, CT, 1994.

Rapp, Doris, "Is This Your Child's World: How You Can Fix the Schools and Homes that are Making Your Children Sick," Bantam Books, New York, 1996.

Exercise and Conditioning

Klatz, Ronald, and Goldman, Robert, "Stopping the Clock: Why Many of Us Will Live Past 100 — And Enjoy Every Minute," Keats Publishing Co., New Canaan, CT, 1996, 182-187.

Elmer-DeWitt, Philip, "Extra Years for Extra Effort," Time Magazine, March 17, 1986, 66.

Powell, K.E., Pratt, Michael, "Physical activity and health," British Medical Journal, July 20, 1996, 313: 126-127.

Nutritional Rehabilitation

National Research Council: Diet and Health. Implications for Reducing Chronic Disease Risk. National Academy Press, Washington D.C., 1989.

Seelig, Mildred, "Consequences of magnesium deficiency on the enhancement of stress reactions; preventive and therapeutic implications (a review)," Journal of the American College of Nutrition, 1994, 13 (5): 429-446.

Colgan, Michael, "Your Personal Vitamin Profile," Quill Books, New York, 1982, 26-44.

Janson, Michael, "The Vitamin Revolution in Health Care," Arcadia Press, Greenville, NH, 1996, 21.

For a comprehensive understanding of nutritional deficiency in the United States, see Beasley, Joseph D., & Swift, Jerry J., "The Kellogg Report: The Impact of Nutrition, Environment & Lifestyle on the Health of Americans," The Institute of Health Policy and Practice, The Bard College Center, Annandale-on-Hudson, New York, 12504, 1989, 155-169.

P.J. Skerrett, "Vitamins: Emerging as disease fighters, not just supplements," Medical World News, January 1993, 34 (1): 24-32.

Gey, K.F., et al, "Poor plasma status of carotene and vitamin C is associated with higher mortality from ischemic heart disease and stroke: Basel Prospective Study," Clinical Investigator, January 1993, 71 (1): 3-6.

"Scientists link low B vitamin levels with heart disease risk," Council for Responsible Nutrition news release, April 24, 1995.

Joosten Etienne, et al, "Metabolic evidence that deficiencies of vitamin B-12 (cobalamin), Folate, and vitamin B-6 occur commonly in elderly people," American Journal of Clinical Nutrition, October 1993, 58 (4): 468-476.

Enstrom, James E., et al, "Vitamin C intake and mortality among a sample of the United States population," Epidemiology 1992, 3 (3): 194-202.

Stampfer, Meir J., et al, "Vitamin E consumption and the risk of coronary disease in women," New England Journal of Medicine, May 20, 1993, 328 (20): 1444-1449.

Rimm, Eric B., "Vitamin E consumption and the risk of coronary disease in men," New England Journal of Medicine, May 20, 1993, 328 (20): 1450-1456.

Geoffrey Cowley," Vitamin E for a healthy heart," Newsweek Magazine, May 31, 1993.

Mortensen, S.A., et al, "Co-enzyme Q10: Clinical benefits with biochemical correlates suggesting a scientific breakthrough in the management of chronic heart failure," International Journal of Tissue Reactions, 1990, 12 (3): 155-162.

Langsjoen, Per, et al, "Pronounced increase of survival of patients with cardiomyopathy when treated with Co-enzyme Q10 and conventional therapy," International Journal of Tissue Reactions, 1990, 12 (3): 163-168.

Langsjoen, Per, et al, "Long-term efficacy and safety of Co-enzyme Q10 therapy for idiopathic dilated cardiomyopathy," American Journal of Cardiology, February 15, 1990. 65: 521-523.

Sharma, Hari, "Freedom From Disease: How to Control Free Radicals, A Major Cause of Aging and Disease," Veda Publishing, Toronto, 1993, 23-25.

Brecher, Harold & Arline, "Forty Something Forever: A Consumer's Guide to Chelation Therapy," Health Savers Press, Herndon, VA 22070, 1994.

Relaxation and Stress Management

U.S. Department of Health and Human Services, "Healthy People 2000: National Health Promotion and Disease Prevention Objections." DHHS Publication No. (PHS) 91-50212, Government Printing Office, Washington D.C., 1991.

"Drowsy America," cover story, Time Magazine, December 17, 1990.

Klinkenborg, Verlyn, "Awakening to sleep," New York Times Magazine, January 5, 1997, 6, 26.

The healing power of prayer, quoted in Well Being Journal, North Bend, Washington, January/February 1997, 1 (1): 1.

Rees, Brian, "Heal Your Self, Heal Your World," Manu Publishing, PO Box 561, Pacific Palisades, California, 90272, 1997, 320.

Chiropractic — Much more than just treating back pain

Stary, O., "The concept of research of vertebrogenic disease in Czechoslovakia," Acta Universitatis Carolinae (Med), supplement, 1965.

Koren, Tedd, "Chiropractic and Spinal Research," Koren Publications, 2026 Chestnut Street, Philadelphia PA 19103, spring 1995, 6.

Palmer, D.D., "The Science, Art and Philosophy of Chiropractic," Portland Printing House, Portland, OR, 1910.

John Bourdillon, M.D., a medical manipulator who recorded his experiences in "Spinal Manipulation," Wm. Heinemann Medical Books, London, 1982 (third edition); 205-206, 218-219. (These pages refer to his work on organic illness).

Wolinsky, Howard, and Brune, Tom, "The Serpent on the Staff: The Unhealthy Politics of the American Medical Association," Tarcher/Putnam (G.P. Putnam's Sons), New York, 1994. For a detailed account of the chiropractic-AMA litigation and other AMA activity against alternative medicine, see chapter six: "Medical Monopoly."

Manga, P., Angus, D., et al, "The effectiveness and cost effectiveness of chiropractic management of low back pain," The Ontario Ministry of Health, Ottawa, Canada, August 1993.

Chapman-Smith, David, "The Chiropractic profession," The Chiropractic Report, March 1997, 11 (2): 2.

Demographic characteristics of users of chiropractic services," The Gallop Organization, Princeton, N.J., 1991.

Patel, Christopher, "Family physicians and chiropractors: A need for better communication and cooperation," Faculty of Medicine, University of Toronto, 1990 thesis, unpublished.

Cherkin, D., et al., "Patient evaluations of low back pain care from family physicians and chiropractors," Western Journal of Medicine, March 1989, 150: 351-355.

Gonyea, M.A., "The role of the doctor of chiropractic in the health care system in comparison with doctors of allopathic medicine and doctors of osteopathic medicine," The Center for Studies in Health Policy, Inc., Washington D.C., September 1993.

Eisenberg, D.M., et al, "Unconventional medicine in the United States," New England Journal of Medicine, January 28, 1993, 238: 246-252.

Miller, W.D., cited in "Research Status of Spinal Manipulative Therapy," edited by M. Goldstein, U.S. Department of Health, Education and Welfare, Bethesda, MD, 1975, 295-301.

Senstad, O., et al, "Frequency and characteristics of spinal manipulative therapy," Spine, 1997, 22 (4): 435-440.

Terrett, A.G.J., and Leynhans, A.M., "Complications from manipulations of the low back," Journal of the Australian Chiropractors Association, December 1992, 4: 129-140.

Goldberg, Burton, "Alternative Medicine: The Definitive Guide," Future Medicine Publishing, Tiburon, CA, 1993; 149-155

Terrett, A.G.J., "The cerebral dysfunction theory," chapter in "Foundations of Chiropractic Subluxations," edited by Meridel Gatterman, Mosby, St. Louis, 1995, 341-352.

Zhang, C., et al, "Study on cervical visual disturbance and its manipulative treatment," Journal of Traditional Chinese Medicine, 1984, 4: 205-210.

Gorman, R.F., "Chiropractic Medicine for Rejuvenation of the Mind," Academy of Chiropractic Medicine, 1983. Published privately: Available ($30) from R.F. Gorman, 7-324, Marrickville Road, Marrickville, Australia 2204.

Terrett, A.G.J., "Cerebral dysfunction: A therapy to explain some of the effects of chiropractic manipulation," Journal of Chiropractic Technique, December 1992, 5(4): 168-73.

Thomas, M.D., and Wood, J., "Upper cervical adjustments may improve mental function," Journal of Manual Medicine, 1992, 6: 215-216.

Coulter, I.D., et al, "Chiropractic patients in a comprehensive home-based geriatric assessment, follow-up and helth promotion program," Topics in Clinical Chiropractic, 1996, 3 (2): 46-55.

Yates, R.G., et al. "Effects of chiropractic treatment on blood pressure and anxiety: A randomized, controlled trial," Journal of Manipulation and Physiological Therapeutics, December 1988, 11 (6): 484-488.

"Chiropractic treatment vs. Tylenol," Family Practice News, June 1, 1996.

Kokjohn, J., Schmid, D. M., et al, "The effect of spinal manipulation on pain and prostaglandin levels in women with primary dysmenorrhea," Journal of Manipulative and Physiological Therapeutics, June 1992, 15 (5): 279-285.

Thomason, P. R., Fisher, B.L., "Effectiveness of spinal manipulative therapy in treatment of primary dysmenor-rhea: A pilot study," Journal of Manipulative and Physiological Therapeutics, 1979, 2: 140-145.

Davydov, O.V., "Spinal syndrome of abdominal pain pathogenesis and treatment," Klin. Med, 1991, 69: 90-91.

Svatko, L.G., et. al., "Manual treatment of impaired hearing associated with cervical spine pathology," Vestn Otolaringol, 1987, 2: 28-31.

Browning, J.E., "Mechanically induced pelvic pain and organ dysfunction in a patient without low back pain," Journal of Manipulative and Physiological Therapeutics, 1990, 13: 406-411

Browning, J.E., "Chiropractic distractive decompression in the treatment of pelvic pain and organic dysfunction in patients with evidence of lower sacral nerve root compression," Journal of Manipulative and Physiological Therapeutics, 1988, 11 (5): 426-432.

Chapman-Smith, David., "The Chiropractic Profession: Myths and Facts," commentary in The Chiropractic Report, July 1992, 6 (5).

Koren, op. cit., 46.

Seifert, J., "Die kopfgelenksblockierung des neugeborenen," Rehabilitacia (edited by Lewit & Guttman), Prague/Bratislava, 1975, 8: 53.

Lewit, Karel, "Manuelle Therapie," J.A. Barth, Leipzig, 1973, chapter 2, 50-54.

Guttman, G., "The atlas fixation syndrome in the baby and infant," Manuelle Medizin, 1987,25: 5-10.

Vanbreda, Wendy M., and Juan M., "A Comparative Study of the Health Status of Children Raised under the healthcare models of chiropractic and allopathic Medicine," Journal of Chiropractic Research, Summer 1989.

Baughman, T.R., et. al, "Management of pediatric asthma and enuresis with probable traumatic etiology," Proceedings of the National Conference on Chiropractic and Pediatrics, ICA, 1991: 14-22.

Gillman, G., Bergstrand, J., "Visual recovery following chiropractic intervention," Journal of Behavioral Optometry, 1990, 1: 73-74.

Fallon, J., "The effect of chiropractic treatment on pregnancy and labor: A comprehensive study," Proceedings of the World Federation of Chiropractic, 1991; 24-31.

Goodman, R., "Cessation of seizure disorder: Correction of the Atlas Subluxation Complex," Proceedings of the National Conference on Chiropractic and Pediatrics, ICA, 1991: 46-56.

Hospers, L.A., "EEG and CEEG studies before and after upper cervical or SOT category 11 adjustment in children after head trauma, in epilepsy, and in hyperactivity," Proceedings of the National Conference on Chiropractic and Pediatrics, 1992; 84-139.

Woo, C.C., "Post traumatic myelopathy following high jump: A pilot case of spinal manipulation," Journal of Manipulative and Physiological Therapeutics, June 1993, 16 (5): 336-341.

Woo, C.C., "Traumatic spinal myoclonus," Journal of Manipulative and Physiological Therapeutics, 1989, 12: 478-481.

Stude, D.E., et al., "Clinical presentation of the patient with multiple sclerosis and response to manual chiropractic adjustive therapies," Journal of Manipulative and Physiological Therapeutics, 1993, 16: 595-600.

Selano, J.L., et al, "The effects of specific upper cervical adjustments on the CD4 counts of HIV positive patients," Chiropractic Research Journal, 1994, 3: 32-39.

Allergies and Chemical Sensitivities

Mandell, Marshall & Scanlon, Lynne, "Dr. Mandell's 5-day Allergy Relief System," Thomas Y. Crowell Publishers, New York, 1979, 11.

Braly, James, "Dr. Braly's Food Allergy & Nutrition Revolution," Keats Publishing, 1992, 38.

King, D.S., "Can allergic exposure provoke psychological symptoms? A double-blind test," Biol. Psychiatry, 1981, 16 (1): 3-19.

Eaton, K.K., et al, "Gut permeability measured by polyethylene glycol absorption in abnormal gut fermentation as compared with food intolerance," Journal of the Royal Society of Medicine, February 1995, 88: 63-66.

Clemetson, C.A., "Histamine and ascorbic acid in human blood," Journal of Nutrition,1980, 110 (4): 662-668.

Bucca, C., "Effect of vitamin C on histamine bronchial responsiveness of patients with allergic rhinitis," Annals of Allergy, 1990, 65: 311-314.

Rogers, S.A., "Zinc deficiency as model for developing chemical sensitivity," International Clinical Nutrition Reviews, 1990, 10 (1): 253-259.

Osgasawara, H., et al, "Effect of selected flavonoids on histamine release (HR) and hydrogen peroxide (H202) generation by human leukocytes," Journal of Allergy Clin Immunol, 1985, 75: 184.

Galland, L., "Increased requirements for essential fatty acids in atopic individuals: A review with clinical descriptions," Journal of the American College of Nutrition, 1986, 5 (2): 213-228.

Lee, T.H., Arm, J.P., "Modulation of the allergic response by fish oil lipids and eicosapentaenoic acid," Prog Clin Biol Res, 1989, 297: 57-69.

Van Breda, Wendy M, and Juan M., "A comparative study of the health status of children raised under the health care models of chiropractic and allopathic medicine," Journal of Chiropractic Research, Summer 1989.

Anemia

Jacobs, A., et al, "Gastric acidity and iron absorption," British Journal of Haematology, 1966, 12: 728-736.

Lane, M., et al, "The anemia of human riboflavin deficiency," Blood, 1965, 25 (4): 432-442.

Rogers, L.E., et al. "Thiamine-responsive megaloblastic anemia," Journal of Pediatrics, 1969, 74 (4): 494-504.

Hines, J.D., Harris, J.W., "Pyridoxine-responsive anemia: Description of three patients with megaloblastic erythropoiesis," American Journal of Clinical Nutrition, 1964, 14: 137-146.

Berk, L., et al, "Effectiveness of vitamin B12 in combined system disease," New England Journal of Medicine, 1948, 239: 328.

Hoffman, H.N., et al, "Zinc induced copper deficiency," Gastroenterology, 1988, 94: 508-512.

Anxiety and panic disorders

King, D.S., "Can allergic exposure provoke psychological symptoms? A double-blind test," Biol Psychiatry, 1981, 16 (1): 3-19.

Crammer, J.L., "Calcium metabolism and mental disorder," Psychol. Med., 1977, 7 (4): 557-560.

Kinzler, E., et al, "Effect of a special kava extract in patients with anxiety, tension, and excitation states of non psychotic genesis. Double blind study with placebos over 4 weeks," Arzneim Forschung, 1991, 41 (6): 584-588.

Charney, D.S., et al, "Increased angiogenic effects of caffeine in panic disorders," Arch. Gen. Psychiatry, 1985, 42:233-243.

Buist, R.A., "Anxiety neurosis — the lactate connection," International Clinical Nutrition Review, 1985, 5 (1): 1-4.

Potthoff, S., et al, "Panic attacks and the chiropractic adjustment: a case report," Journal of Chiropractic, December 1993, 30: 26-28.

Sullivan, E.C., "The chiropractic management of anxiety: a case report," Journal of Chiropractic, September 1992, 29: 29-34.

Arthritis

Robbins, S.L., Cotran, R.S., and Kumar, V., "Pathological Basis of Disease," W.B. Saunders, Philadelphia, 1984, 1356-61.

Petersdorf, R., et al, "Harrison's Principles of Internal Medicine," McGraw-Hill, New York, 1983, 517-24.

Newman, N.M., and Ling, R.S.M., "Acetabular bond destruction related to non-steroidal anti-inflammatory drugs," Lancet, 1985, ii: 11-13.

Solomon, L., "Drug induced arthropathy and necrosis of the femoral head," Journal of Bone Joint Surgery, 1973, 55B: 246-51.

Hazenberg, M.P., "Intestinal flora, bacteria and arthritis: Why the joint," Scandinavian Journal of Rheumatology, 1995, 24(supplement 101): 207-211.

Zucker, Martin, "Boswellia, an Ancient Herb Combats Arthritis," The Natural Way Magazine, June/July 1995, p. 60.

Deal, C.L., et al, "Treatment of arthritis with topical capsaicin: A double-blind trial," Clinical Therapy, 1991,13 (3): 383-395.

Drovanti, A., et al, "Therapeutic activity of oral glucosamine sulfate in osteoarthrosis: A placebo-controlled double-blind investigation," Clinical Therapy, 1980, 3 (4): 260-272.

Prudden, J.F., Balassa, L.L., "The biological activity of bovine cartilage preparations," Semin Arthritis Rheum, 1974, 3 (4): 287-321.

Annand, J.C., "Pantothenic acid and osteoarthritis," Lancet, 1963, 2: 1168 (letter). Annand, J.C., "Osteoarthrosis and pantothenic acid," Journal of Coll Gen Pract, 1962, 5: 136-137.

Schwartz, E.R., "The modulation of osteoarthritis development by vitamins C and E," International Journal of Vitamin Nutritional Reseach, 1984, 26 (supplement): 141-146.

Walker, W.R. and Keats, D.M., "An investigation of the therapeutic value of the copper bracelet: dermal assimilation of copper in arthritic/rheumatoid conditions," Agents Action, 1976, 6: 454,

Videman, T., "Experimental models of osteoarthritis: the role of immobilization," Clinical Biomechanics, 1987, 2: 223-229.

Lewis, T., "Osteoarthritis in lumbar synovial joints: A morphological study," Acta Orthop Scand, 1964, (supp) 73:1-12.

Ressel, O.J., "Disc regeneration: Reversibility is possible in spinal osteoarthritis," ICA Review, March/April 1989: 39-61.

Woo, S.L., Matthews, J.V., et al, "Connective tissue response to immobility: Correlative study of biomechanical and biochemical measurements of normal and immobilized rabbit knees," Arthritis Rheum, 1975, 18: 257.

St. Pierre, D. and Gardiner, P.R., "The effect of immobilization and exercise on muscle function: A review," Physiotherapy Canada, 1987, 39: 24-36.

Seifert, M., et al, "A 5-year follow-up of 50 cases of idiopathic osteoarthritis of the hip," Ann Rheum Dis, 1969, 28:325.

Asthma

Potterton, D., "The politics of asthma: Out of control," Nursing Times, 1992, 88 (2): 26-31.

Lindahl, O. and L., et al, "Vegan diet regimen with reduced medication in the treatment of bronchial asthma," Journal of Asthma, 1985, 22: 45-55.

Bauer, K., et al, "Pharmacodynamic effects of inhaled dry powder formulations of fenoterol and colforsin in asthma," Clin Pharmacol Ther, 1993, 53 (1): 76-83.

Reynolds, R.D., Natta C.L., "Depressed plasma pyridoxal phosphate concentrations in adult asthmatics," American Journal of Clinical Nutrition, 1985, 41: 684-688.

Simon, R.A., et al, "Sulfite-sensitive asthma," Res Instit Scripps Clin Scientif Rep, 1982-83, 39: 57-58.

Crocket, J.A., "Cyanocobalamin in asthma," Acta Allergologica, 1957, XI: 261-268.

Schwartz, J., Weiss, S.T., "Dietary factors and their relation to respiratory symptoms. The Second National Health and Nutrition Examination Survey," American Journal of Epidemiology, 1990, 132 (1): 67-76.

Haury, V.G., "Blood serum magnesium in bronchial asthma and its treatment by the administration of magnesium sulfate," Journal of Lab Clin Med, 1940, 26: 340-344.

Arm, J., et al, "The effects of dietary supplementation with fish oil on asthmatic responses to antigen," Journal of Clinical Allergy, 1988, 81: 183.

Pelikan, Z., Pelikan-Filipek, M., "Bronchial response to the food ingestion challenge," Annals of Allergy, 1987, 58 (3):164-172.

Bray, G.W., "The hypochlorhydria of asthma of childhood," Quart J Med, 1931, 24: 181-197.

Chilmonczyk, Barbara, et al, "Association between exposure to environmental tobacco smoke and exacerbations of asthma in children," New England Journal of Medicine, June 1993, 328 (23): 1665-1669.

Gillespie, B.R., Barnes, J.F., "Diagnosis and treatment of TMJ, head, neck and asthmatic symptoms in children," Journal of Craniomandibular Practice, October 1990, 8 (4).

Peet, J.B., Marko, S. K., Piekarczyk, W., "Chiropractic response in the pediatric patient with asthma," Chiropractic Pediatrics, 1995, I: 9-12.

Lines, D.H., "A wholistic approach to the treatment of bronchial asthma in a chiropractic practice," Chiropractic Journal of Australia, 1993, 23: 4-8.

Jamison, J.R., et al, "Chiropractic adjustment in the management of visceral conditions: A critical appraisal," Journal of Manipulative and Physiological Therapeutics, 1992, 15:171-180.

Attention Deficit Disorder

Rapp, Doris, "Is This Your Child's World," Bantam Books, New York, 1996, 7.

Hancock, LynNell, "Mother's Little Helper," Newsweek Magazine, March 18, 1996, 51-56.

Batoosingh, Karen A., "Ritalin prescriptions triple over last four years," Family Practice News, June 1, 1995: 4.

Jarrell, Tom, "20/20," ABC-TV, December 8, 1995.

Physicians' Desk Reference, Medical Economics Co., Montvale, N.J., 07645, 1996, 848.

Rapp, op. cit., 211.

"Drug Abuse Alert," USA Today, Lifeline Column, March 28, 1996.

Boris, Marvin et al, "Foods and additives are common causes of the Attention Deficit Hyperactivity Disorder in children," Annals of Allergy, May 1994, 72: 462-468. This and other sources linking hyperactivity disorders to food/environmental sensitivities are cited in Rapp, "Is This Your Child's World," 223.

Menzies, I.C., "Disturbed children: The role of food and chemical sensitivities," Nutri Health, 1984, 3: 39-54.

Prinz, R. J., et al, "Dietary correlates of hyperactive behavior in children," Journal of Consult Clin Psycho, 1980, 48: 760-769.

Kershner, J., Hawke, W., "Megavitamins and learning disorders: A controlled double-blind experiment," Journal of Nutrition, 1979, 109 (5): 819-826.

Colquhoun, I., Bunday, S., "A lack of essential fatty acids as a possible cause of hyperactivity in children," Medical Hypotheses, 1981, 7: 673-679.

Durlach, O.J., "Clinical aspects of chronic magnesium deficiency," in "Magnesium in Health and Disease," edited by Mildred Seelig, Spectrum Publications, New York, 1980.

Hoffer, Abram, "Treatment of hyperkinetic children with nicotinamide and pyridoxine," Journal of the Canadian Medical Association, 1972, 107: 111-112.

Brenner, A., "The effects of megadoses of selected B complex vitamins on children with hyperkinesis: Controlled studies with long-term follow up," Journal of Learning Disabilities, 1982, 15: 258.

Wood, D.R., et al, "Treatment of attention deficit disorder with DL-phenylalanine," Psychiatry Res., 1985, 16: 21-26.

Armstrong, Thomas, CNN broadcast, November 2, 1995

Walton, E.V., "The effects of chiropractic treatment on students with learning and behavioral impairments due to neurological dysfunction," International Review of Chiropractic, 1975, 29: 4-5, 24-26.

Giesen, J.M, et al, "An evaluation of chiropractic manipulation as a treatment of hyperactivity in children," Journal of Manipulative and Physiological Therapeutics, 1989, 12:353-363.

Webster, L., "First report on ADD study," International Chiropractic Pediatric Association Newsletter, January 1994.

Phillips, C.J., "Case study: The effect of utilizing spinal manipulation and craniosacral therapy as the treatment approach for attention deficit hyperactivity disorder," Proceedings on the National Conference in Chiropractic and Pediatrics (ICA), 1991: 57-74.

Barnes, T.A., "A multi-faceted chiropractic approach to attention deficit hyperactivity disorder: A case report," ICA International Review of Chiropractic, January/February 1995, 41-43.

Arme, J., "Effects of biomechanical insult correction on attention deficit disorder," Journal of Chiropractic Case Reports, January 1995, 1 (1).

Block, Mary Ann, "No More Ritalin: Treating ADHD Without Drugs," Kensington Publishing Corp., New York, 1996, 121.

Back Pain

Chapman-Smith, David, "Managing patients with low-back pain," The Chiropractic Report, January 1997, 11 (1): 1.

Burton, A.K., et al, "The natural history of low back pain in adolescents," Spine, October 15, 1996, 21 (20): 2323-2328.

Deyo, R., "Description epidemiology of low back pain and its related medical care in the United States," Spine, 1987, 12 (3): 264-268.

Mierau, D.R., Cassidy, J.D., et al, "Sacroiliac joint dysfunction and low back pain in school-aged children," Journal of Manipulative and Physiological Therapeutics, 1984, 7 (2): 81-84.

Bourne, I.H.J., "Back pain — What can we offer?" British Medical Journal, 1979, I: 1085.

Bernard, T., Kirkaldy-Willis, K.W., "Recognizing specific characteristics of non-specific low back pain," Clinical Orthopedics, April 1987, 217: 266-280.

U.S. Agency for Health Care Policy and Research, "Acute Low Back Problems in Adults," Clinical Practice Guideline No. 14, 1994. Available through AHCPR Publications Clearing House, PO Box 8547, Silver Springs, MD., 20907, or by calling 1-800-358-9295. Single copies of the Quick Reference Guide and Patient Guide are sent free. Inquire for the cost of the Clinical Practice Guideline.

Manga, P., Angus, D., et al, "The effectiveness and cost effectiveness of chiropractic management of low backpain," The Ontario Ministry of Health, Ottawa, Canada, August 1993.

U.S. Agency for Health Care Policy and Research, op. cit.

Meade, T.W., Dyer, S., et al, "Low back pain of mechanical origin: Randomized comparison of chiropractic and hospital outpatient treatment," British Medical Journal, 2 June 1990, 300 (6737): 1431-1437.

Waddell, G., Feder, G., "Low back pain evidence review," Royal College of General Practitioners, London, 1996

Waddell, Gordon, "Modern management of spinal disorders," Journal of Manipulative and Physiological Therapeutics, 1995, 18 (9): 590-596.

Wolk, S., "Chiropractic versus medical care: A cost analysis of disability and treatment for back-related workers' compensation cases," Foundation for Chiropractic Education and Research, Arlington, VA, September 1988.

Jarvis, K.B., Phillips, R.B., et al, "Cost per case comparison of back injury claims of chiropractic versus medical management for conditions with identical diagnostic codes," Journal of Occupational Medicine, August 1991, 33 (8): 847-852.

Cherkin, D.C., "Family physicians and chiropractors: What's best for the patient?" The Journal of Family Practice, November 1992, 35 (5): 505-506.

Ebrall, P.S., "Mechanical low back pain: A comparison of medical and chiropractic management," Chiropractic Journal of Australia, June 1992, 22 (2): 47-53.

Cox, J.M., Shreiner, S., "Chiropractic manipulation in low back pain and sciatica: statistical data on the diagnosis, treatment and response of 576 consecutive cases," Journal of Manipulative and Physiological Therapeutics, 1982, 7: 1-11.

Mathews, J.A., Mills, S.B., et al, "Back pain and sciatica: Controlled trials of manipulation, traction, sclerosant and epidural injections," British Journal of Rheumatology, 1987, 26: 416-423.

Stern, P. J., et. al, "A series of consecutive cases of low-back pain with radiating leg pain treated by chiropractors," Journal of Manipulative and Physiological Therapeutics, 1995, 18 (6): 335-341.

Spengler, et al, "Back injuries in industry: A retrospective study, part 1, Overview and Cost Analysis," Spine, 1987, 11 (3): 241-245

Fries, J.F., et al, "Toward an epidemiology of gastropathy associated with nonsteroidal anti-inflammatory drug use," Gastroenterology, 1989, 96: 647-655.

U.S. Agency for Health Care Policy and Research, op. cit.

Cherkin, D.C., Deyo, R.A., Loeser, J.D., Bush, T., Waddell, G., "An international comparison of back surgery dates," Spine 1994, 19 (11):1201-1206.

Waddell, Gordon, "A new clinical model for the treatment of low back pain," Spine, 1987, 12 (7): 632-644

Wiesel, Sam, editor, "How many spine operations are performed in the U.S.?" The Back Letter, April 1997, 12

(4), Lippincott-Raven Publishers, Philadelphia, 48.

Dommisse, G.F. and R. P. Grahe, "The Failures of Surgery for Lumbar Disc Disorders," Lippincott, New York, 1978, 202.

Mayer, T.G., and Gatchel, R.J., "Functional Restoration for Spinal Disorders: The Sports Medicine Approach," Lea and Febiger, Philadelphia, 1988.

Burton, C.V., and Cassidy, J.David, "Economics, epidemiology and risk Factors," chapter one in "Managing Low-Back Pain," editors Kirkaldy-Willis, William H., and Burton, C.V., third edition, Churchill Livingstone, New York, 1992.

Pang, F.K., and Loh, Z., "Treatment of lumbar intervertebral disc protrusions by manipulation," Clinical Orthopedics and Related Research, February 1987, 215: 47-55.

Delauche-Cavalier, M.C., Budet, C., et al, "Lumbar disc herniation: Computed tomography scan changes after conservative treatment of nerve root compression," Spine, 1992, 17 (8): 927-933.

Koes, B.W., Bouter, L., "Randomized clinical trial of manipulative therapy and physiotherapy for persistent back and neck complaints: Results of one-year follow-up," British Medical Journal, 7 March 1992, 304: 601-605.

Kirkaldy-Willis, William H., Cassidy, J. David, "Spinal manipulation in the treatment of low-back pain," Canadian Family Physician, 1985, 31: 535-540.

Bladder problems

Coronado, Boris E., et al, "Antibiotic-Induced D-lactic acidosis," Annals of Internal Medicine, June 1, 1995, 122 (11): 839-842.

Sobota, A.E., "Inhibition of bacterial adherence by cranberry juice: Potential use for the treatment of urinary tract infections," Journal of Urology, 1984, 121:1013-1016.

Avorn, J., et al, "Reduction of bacteriuria and pyuria after ingestion of cranberry juice," Journal of the American Medical Association, 1994, 271: 751-754.

Saelhof, C.C., "The capillary syndrome in hemorrhagic cystitis: Therapeutic evaluation of bioflavonoids," American Journal of Digestive Disorders, 1955, 22: 204.

Van Duzen, R.E, Mustain, R., "Alpha-tocopherol in treatment of interstitial cystitis: preliminary report," Journal of Urology, 1951, 65: 1033.

Zechner, O., et al, "Nutritional risk factors in urinary stone disease," Journal of Urology, 1981, 125: 51.

Rao, P.N.,et al, "Are stone formers maladapted to refined carbohydrates?" British Journal of Urology, 1982, 54: 575.

Browning, J.E., "Mechanically induced pelvic pain and organ dysfunction in a patient without low back pain," Journal of Manipulative and Physiological Therapeutics, 1990, 13: 406-411

Browning, J.E., "Chiropractic distractive decompression in the treatment of pelvic pain and organic dysfunction in patients with evidence of lower sacral nerve root compression," Journal of Manipulative and Physiological Therapeutics, 1988, 11 (5): 426-432.

Browning, J.E., "Distractive manipulation protocols in treating the mechanically-induced pelvic pain and organic dysfunction patient," Chiropractic Technique, February 1995, 7 (1).

Reed, W.R., Beavers, S., et al, "Chiropractic management of primary nocturnal enuresis," Journal of Manipulative and Physiological Therapeutics, November/December 1994, 17 (9), 596-600.

LeBouf, C., Brown, P., et al, "Chiropractic care of children with nocturnal enuresis: A prospective outcome study," Journal of Manipulative and Physiological Therapeutics, 1991, 14 (2): 110-115.

Carpal Tunnel Syndrome

Ellis, J.M., Kishi T., Azuma, J., Folkers, K., "Vitamin B6 deficiency in patients with a clinical syndrome including the carpal tunnel defect: Biochemical and clinical response to therapy with pyridoxine," Res Comm Chem Pathol Pharmacol, 1976, 43:743.

Driskell, J.A., et al, "Effectiveness of pyridoxine hydrochloride treatment on carpal tunnel patients," Nutrition Reports International, 1986, 34:1031-40.

Folkers, K, et al, "Enzymology of the response of the carpal tunnel syndrome to riboflavin and to combined riboflavin and pyridoxine," Proceedings of the National Academy of Sciences USA, 1984, 81(22):7076-7078.

Upton, A., McComas, A., "The double crush in nerve entrapment syndromes," Lancet, August 18, 1973; 359-61.

Ferezy, J.S., Norlin, W.T., "Carpal tunnel syndrome: a case report," Chiropractic Technique, January/February 1989; 19-22.

Bonebrake, A.R., et al., "A treatment for carpal tunnel syndrome: evaluation of objective and subjective measures," Journal of Manipulative and Physiological Therapeutics, November/December 1990, 13 (9).

Chest Pain

Barker, M., "Manipulation in general medical practice for thoracic pain syndromes," British Osteopathic Journal, 1983, vol. 15 (2): 95-97.

Johnson, Harlen, "Thoracocostal subluxation: An often overlooked cause of chest and arm pain," Journal of Chiropractic Technique, November 1995, 7 (4): 134-138.

Kamikawa, T., et al, "Effects of L-carnitine on exercise tolerance in patients with stable angina pectoris," Japan Heart Journal, 1984, 25: 587.

Ferrari, R., et al, "The metabolical effects of L-carnitine in angina pectoris," International Journal of Cardiology, 1984, 5: 213.

Cranton, Elmer, Frackelton, J.P., "Current status of EDTA chelation therapy in occlusive arterial disease," Journal of Adv Med, 1989, 2: 107-119.

Olszwer, E., Carter, J.P., "EDTA chelation therapy: A retrospective study of 2,870 patients," Journal of Adv Med, 1989, 2: 197-211.

"If you haven't heard about this vitamin, you better get to know it. It could save your life!" (CoQ10) Health/Science Newsletter, May 1996.

Chronic Fatigue Syndrome

Lapp, C.W., "Chronic fatigue syndrome is a real disease," North Carolina Family Physician, 1992, 43 (1): 6-11.

Baschetti, Riccardo, "Chronic fatigue syndrome and licorice," New Zealand Medical Journal, April 26, 1995; 157.

Cox, I.M., et al, "Red blood cell magnesium and chronic fatigue syndrome," Lancet, 1991, 337: 757-760.

Horrobin, D.F., "Post viral fatigue syndrome, viral infections in atopic eczema and essential fatty acids," Medical Hypotheses, 1990, 32 (3): 211-217.

"Chronic fatigue syndrome update. Findings now point to CNS involvement," Postgraduate Medicine, November 1994, 96 (6).

Rowe, Peter, C., et al, "Is neurally-mediated hypotension an unrecognized cause of chronic fatigue?" Lancet, March 11, 1995, 345: 623-624.

Cold Sores

Amsterdam, J.D., et al, "A possible antiviral action of lithium carbonate in herpes simplex virus infections," Biol Psychiatry, 1990, 27 (4): 447-453.

Gordon, Y.J., et al, "Irreversible inhibition of herpes simplex virus replication in BSC-1 cells by zinc ions," Antimicrobial Agents Chemotherapy, 1975, 8 (3): 377-380.

Eby, G., "Use of topical zinc to prevent recurrent herpes simplex infection: Review of literature and suggested protocols," Medical Hypotheses, 1985, 17: 157-165.

Griffith, R.S., et al, "Success of L-Lysine therapy in frequently recurrent herpes simplex infection," Dermatologica, 1987, 175: 183-190.

Gertenrich, R., Hart, R.W, "Treatment of oral ulcerations with Bacid (Lactobacillus acidophilus)," Oral Surgery, 1970, 30 (2):196-200.

Kritz, Fran, "Government taking a closer look at medicinal plants," Medical Tribune, January 19, 1995; 11.

Kahn, Jason, "Vitamin A may help suppress herpes outbreaks," Medical Tribune, May 18, 1995; 10.

Colic

Klougart, N., Nilsson, N., & Jacobsen, J., "Infantile colic treated by chiropractors: A prospective study of 316 cases," Journal of Manipulative and Physiological Therapeutics, 1989, 12: 281-288.

Biedermann, H.J., "Kinematic imbalances due to suboccipital strain in newborns," Manual Medicine, 1992, 6: 151-156.

Pluhar, G. H., Schobert, P.D., "Vertebral subluxation and colic: A case study," Chiropractic: The Journal of Chiropractic Research and Clinical Investigation, 1991, 7: 75-76.

Weber, Marion, Masarsky, Charles, editors, Neurological Fitness, January 1995, 1.

Depression

"What you should know about women and depression," American Psychological Association, Office of Public Affairs, 750 First Street, N.E., Washington, D.C., 20002

Peter Breggin, "Talking Back to Prozac: What Doctors Aren't Telling You About Today's Most Controversial Drug" (St. Martin's Press, New York, 1994).

Breggin, quoted in Gary Null, "The hidden side of psychiatry," Townsend Letter for Doctors and Patients, January 1997, 90.

Christensen, Larry, "Psychological distress and diet — Effects of sucrose and caffeine," Journal of Applied Nutrition. 1988, 40 (1): 44-50.

Christensen, Larry and Somers, Sharla, "Adequacy of dietary intake of depressed individuals," American College of Nutrition, 1994, 13 (6): 597-600.

Christensen, Larry and Burrows, Ross, "Dietary Treatment of Depression," Behavior Therapy, 1990 , 21:183-193.

Reynolds, E.H., et al, "Folate deficiency in depressive illness," British Journal of Psychiatry, 1970, 117:287-292.

Carney, M., et al, "Thiamin and pyridoxine lack in newly-admitted psychiatric patients, British Journal of Psychiatry, 1979, 135:249-254.

Baldessarini, R.J., "Neuropharmacology of S-adenosylmethionine," American Journal of Medicine, 1987, 83 (supplement SA): 95-103.

Murray, Michael, "The Encyclopedia of Nutritional Supplements" (Prima Publishing, Rocklin, CA, 1996, 366 SAM)

Harrer, G., Schulz, V., "Clinical investigation of the antidepressant effectiveness of hypericum," Journal of Geriatric Psychiatry Neurol, 1994, 7 (supplement 1): S6-S8.

Gaby, Alan, "Herbal antidepressant," Townsend Letter for Doctors and Patients, August/September 1996: 26.

Blumenthal, Mark, "St. John's Wort: The leading herb for mild to moderate depression," Natural Pharmacy, February 1997, 1 (2): 8.

Hibbeln, Joseph R., and Salem, Norman, Jr., "Dietary polyunsaturated fatty acids and depression: When cholesterol does not satisfy," American Journal of Clinical Nutrition, 1995, 62: 1-9.

Davis, Donald R., et al, "Omega-3 fatty acids in clinical practice," Journal of the Advancement of Medicine, Spring 1995, 8 (1): 5-35.

Thalen, B.E., et al. "Light treatment in seasonal and nonseasonal depression," Acta Psychiatr Scand., 1995, 91:352-360.

Oren, Dan A., et al, "A controlled trial of cyanocobalamin (vitamin B12) in the treatment of winter seasonal affective disorder," Journal of Affective Disorders, 1994, 32:197-200.

Meesters, Y., et al, "Light therapy for seasonal affective disorder: The effects of timing," British Journal of Psychiatry, 1995, 166: 607-612.

Terrett, A.G.J., "Cerebral dysfunction: A therapy to explain some of the effects of chiropractic manipulation," Journal of Chiropractic Technique, December 1992, 5(4): 168-73.

Gorman, R.F., "Chiropractic Medicine for Rejuvenation of the Mind," Academy of Chiropractic Medicine, 1983. Published privately: Available ($30) from R.F. Gorman, 7-324, Marrickville Road, Marrickville, Australia 2204.

Diabetes

Virtanen, Suvi, and Aro, Antti, "Dietary factors and the etiology of diabetes," Annals of Medicine, 1994, 26: 469-478.

Barnard, R. James, et al, "Diet and exercise in the treatment of non-insulin dependent diabetes mellitus," Diabetes Care, December 1994, 17(12): 1469-1472.

Brun, Jean-Frederic, et al, "Effects of oral zinc gluconate on glucose effectiveness and insulin sensitivity in humans," Biological Trace Element Research, 1995, 47: 385-391.

Anderson, J.W., "Recent advances in carbohydrate nutrition and metabolism in diabetes mellitus," Journal of the American College of Nutrition, 1989, 8 (suppl): 61S-67S.

Anderson, R., Kozlovsky, A.S., "Chromium intake, absorption and excretion of subjects consuming self-selected diets," American Journal of Clinical Nutrition, 1985, 41: 1177-1183.

Anderson, R., "Beneficial effect of chromium for people with type II diabetes," Diabetes, 1996, 45 (supplement 2): 454.

Martinez, O.B., et al., "Dietary chromium and effect of chromium supplementation on glucose tolerance of elderly Canadian women," Nutrition Research, 1985, 5: 609-620.

Mertz, W., "Effects and metabolism of glucose tolerance factor," Nutrition Reviews, 1975, 33 (5):129-135.

White, J.R., and Campbell, R.K., "Magnesium and diabetes: A review," Annals of Pharmacotherapy, 1993, 27: 775-80.

Arslanoglu, I., et al, "Hypomagnesemia in childhood insulin-dependent diabetes mellitus and risk of nephropathy," Diabetologia, 1995, 38:629-634.

Harland, B.F., Harden-Williams, B.A., "Is vanadium of human significance yet?" Journal of the American Dietetic Association, 1994, 94: 891-894.

Hoffman-LaRoche, Inc., "Diabetes and vitamin E., Diabetes, February 1995, 44 (2).

Jialal, I., and Fuller, C. J., "Vitamin E appears to reduce risk of heart disease in diabetics," press release from University of Texas Southwestern Medical Center, Dallas, April 29, 1995. Full article published in May 1995 issue of The American Journal of Clinical Nutrition.

Jialal, I., Fuller, C.J., & Huet, B., "Study determines lowest vitamin E dose for effect on LDL oxidation," press release from University of Texas Southwestern Medical Center, Dallas, February 10, 1995. Full article published in February 1995 issue of Arteriosclerosis, Thrombosis and Vascular Biology.

Bhatt, H.R, et cal, "Can faulty vitamin B12 (cobalamin) metabolism produce diabetic neuropathy?" Lancet (letter), 1983, 2: 572.

Petley, Ann, et al, "The pharmacokinetics of nicotinamide in humans and rodents," Diabetes, February 1995, 44: 152-155.

Ghannam, N., "The antidiabetic activity of aloes: Preliminary clinical and experimental observations," Hormone Research, 1986, 24:288-294.

Shanmugasundaram, E.R.B., et al, "Use of gymnema sylvestre leaf extract in the control of blood glucose in insulin-dependent diabetes mellitus," Journal of Ethnopharmacology, 1990, 30: 281-294.

Murphy, D.R., "Diagnosis and manipulative treatment in diabetic polyneuropathy and its relation to intertarsal joint dysfunction," Journal of Manipulative and Physiological Therapeutics, 1994, 17: 29-37.

Nelson, W.A., "Diabetes mellitus: two case reports," Chiropractic Technique, 1989, 1: 37-40.

Digestive and intestinal disorders

H. Spiro, "Clinical Gastroenterology," third edition, MacMillan, New York, 1983, 713-735.

Mayberry, J.F., et al, "Increased sugar consumption in Crohn's Disease," Digestion, 1980, 20: 323-326.

Jarnerot, J., et al, "Consumption of refined sugar by patients with Crohn's Disease, ulcerative colitis, or irritable bowel syndrome," Scandinavian Journal of Gastroenterology, 1983, 18: 999-1002.

Thornton, J.R., et al, "Diet and Crohn's Disease: Characteristics of the pre-illness diet," British Medical Journal, 1979, 279: 762-764.

Fedotin, M.S., "Helicobacter pylori and peptic ulcer disease: Re-examining the therapeutic approach," Postgraduate Medicine, 1993, 94 (3): 38-45.

Dew, M.J., et al, "Peppermint oil for the irritable bowel syndrome: A multicentre trial," British Journal of Clinical Practice, 1984, 38: 394-398.

Babineau, Timothy J., M.D., "Specific Nutrients For the Gastrointestinal Tract: Glutamine, Arginine, Nucleotides and Structured Lipids," Chapter 5 Enteral Nutrition, 1994;47-59.
Burkitt, Denis, and Trowell, H., " Western Diseases: Their Emergence and Prevention," Harvard University Press, Cambridge, MA, 1981.

Painter, N.S., "Bran and the irritable bowel," Lancet, 1976, 1: 540.
Shive, W., et al, "Glutamine in treatment of peptic ulcer," Texas State Journal of Medicine, 1957, 53:840-843.

Turpie, A.G., Runcie, J., and Thomson,T.J., "Clinical trial of deglycyrrhizinated licorice in gastric ulcer," Gut, 1969, 10: 299-303.

Winsor, H., "Sympathetic Segmental Disturbances; The Evidence of the Association in Dissected Cadavers of Visceral Disease with Vertebrae Deformities of the Same Sympathetic Segments," Medical Times, November 1921, 49: 1-7,

Ussher, N.T., "Spinal curvatures - visceral disturbances in relation thereto," California and Western Medicine, June 1933, 38 (16): 423-428.

Pikalov, A.A., Kharin, V.V., "Use of spinal manipulative therapy in the treatment of duodenal ulcer: a pilot study," Journal of Manipulative and Physiological Therapeutics, June 1994, 17 (5): 310-313.

Eriksen, Kirk, "Effects of upper cervical correction on chronic constipation," Chiropractic Research Journal, 1994, 3: 19-22.

Ippoliti, A.F., et al, "The effect of various forms of milk on gastric-acid secretion." Ann Intern Med 84: 286-289, 1976.

Patty, E., et al, "Controlled trial of vitamin A in gastric ulcer," Lancet, 1982, 2:876 (letter).

Crescenzo, V.M., Cayer, D., "Plasma vitamin C levels in patients with peptic ulcer. Response to oral load of ascorbic acid," Gastroenterology, 1947, 8:755-761.

McNulty, C.A.M., et al, "Susceptibility of clinical isolates of Campylobacter pyloridis to 11 antimicrobial agents," Antimicrobial Agents Chemother, 1985, 28: 837-838.

Reimann, H.J., Ewin, J., "Gastric mucosal reactions in patients with food allergy," American Journal of Gastroenterology, 1988, 83 (11): 1212-1219.

Husebye, E., "Gastrointestinal Motility Disorders and Bacterial Overgrowth," Journal of Internal Medicine, 1995, 237: 419-427.

"Sucrose permeability as a marker for nonsteroidal anti-inflammatory gastrointestinal injury: How sweet it is," Nutrition Reviews, 1995, 53:1.

Watanabe, Toshio, et al, "Zinc deficiency delays gastric ulcer healing in rats," Digestive Diseases and Sciences, June 1995, 40 (6):1340-1344.

Dizziness/vertigo

Mowrey, D. B., "Motion sickness, ginger and psychophysics," Lancet, 1982: 655-657.

Grontved, A., et al, "Ginger root against seasickness: A controlled trial on the open sea," Acta Otolaryngol, 1988, 105, 1-2:45-49.

Lewit, Karel, "Manipulative Therapy and Rehabilitation of the Locomotor System," Butterworths, London, 1985: 323-329.

Fitz-Ritson, D., "Neuroanatomy and neurophysiology of the upper cervical spine," in "Upper Cervical Syndrome," edited by H. Vernon, Williams and Wilkins, Baltimore, 1988, 48-85.

Fitz-Ritson, Don, "Assessment of Cervicogenic Vertigo," Journal of Manipulative and Physiological Therapies, 1991, 14 (3): 193-198.

Cote, Pierre, Mior, S.A., Fritz-Ritson, Don, "Cervicogenic vertigo: A report of three cases," Journal of the Canadian Chiropractic Association, 1991, 35: 89-94.

Ear infections

White, Linda, "Treatments for earaches: What every parent should know about children's ear infections," Vegetarian Times, March 1997, 34-39.

Townsend, E.H., and Radebaugh, J.F., "Prevention of complications of respiratory illness in pediatric practice: A double-blind study," New England Journal of Medicine, 1962, 266: 683.

Cantekin, E.I., McGuire, T.N., et al, "Antimicrobial therapy for otitis media with effusion," Journal of the American Medical Association, 1991, 266 (23): 3309-3317.

Tos, M., and Poulsen, G., "Secretory otitis media: Late effects of the treatment with grommets," Arch Otolaryngology, 1976, 102: 672.

Williams, R.L., et al, "Use of antibiotics in preventing recurrent otitis media and in treating otitis media with effusion," Journal of the American Medical Association, 1993, 270: 1344-1351.

Kempthorne, Jill, Giebink, G., "Pediatric approach to the diagnosis and management of otitis media," Otolaryngologic Clinics of North America, August 1991, 24 (4): 905-929.

English, G., "Choosing the right therapy for acute otitis media," The Journal of Respiratory Diseases, July 1985, 93-100.

Bluestone, C.D., "Otitis media in children: To treat or not to treat," New England Journal of Medicine, 1982, 306: 1399-1404.

Diamant, M. and B., "Abuse and timing of use of antibiotics in acute otitis media," Arch Otol, 1974, 100: 226-232.

Gravel, Judith S., et al. "Early otitis media and later educational risk," Acta Otolaryngol (Stockholm), 1995, 115: 279-281.

Milk allergy: Personal communication with Charles Attwood, M.D. For more information on the myth of milk drinking, see "Dr. Attwood's Low-Fat Prescription for Kids," Penguin Books, New York, 1995, 62.

Rapp, Doris, "Is This Your Child's World," Bantam Books, New York, 1996, 21.

Bellionin, P., et al, "Allergy: A leading role in otitis media with effusion," Allergol Immunol, 1987, 15: 205-208.

Duncan B, et al, "Exclusive breast-feeding for at least four months protects against otitis media," Pediatrics, 1993, 91: 867-872.

Guttman, G., "Blocked Atlanto Nerve Syndrome in Infants and Small Children," International Chiropractic Association Review, July 1990: 37-42.

Vanbreda, Wendy M., and Juan M., "A Comparative Study of the Health Status of Children Raised under the healthcare models of chiropractic and allopathic Medicine," Journal of Chiropractic Research, Summer 1989.

Fysh, Peter N., "Upper respiratory infections in children: A chiropractic approach to management," International Chiropractic Association Review, March/April, 1990.

Headaches and neck pain

Kennedy, Veronica (Newhouse News Service), "Bad news: Headache medication can cause headaches," The Oregonian, November 22, 1993.

Rubenstein, E., Federman, D.D., "Scientific American Medicine," Scientific American, New York, 1987, 11:XI: 1-3, CTM:II: 10.
Stewart, W., et al, "Prevalence of migraine headache in the United States," Journal of the American Medical Association, 1992, 267: 64-69.

Stang, P., Osterhaus, J., "Impact of migraine in the United States: Data from the National Health Interview Survey," Headache, 1993, 33: 29-35.

Sillanpää, M., Antilla, P.C., "Increasing prevalence of headache in 7 year old school children," Headache, 1996, 36: 466-470

Graff-Radford, S.B., et al, "Management of chronic head pain," Headache, 1987, 27: 186-190.

"How is your doctor treating you?" Consumer Reports, February 1995, 81-88.

Eisenberg, D.M., et al, "Unconventional medicine in the United States," New England Journal of Medicine, January 28, 1993, 238: 246-252.

Bogduk, N., Marsland, A., "On the concept of third occipital headache," Journal of Neurology, Neurosurgery, and Pschiatry, 1986, 15 (1): 67-70.

Chapman-Smith, David, "Primary headaches and cervical spine dysfunction," The Chiropractic Report, May 1995, 9 (3): 1-8. Including personal communication from Craig Nelson, D.C., of the Norwestern College of Chiropractic, Minneapolis, a leading researcher in the field of headaches.

Blau, J., et al, "Migraine and the neck," Headache, 1994, 34: 88-90.

Weingarten, S., et al, "The effectiveness of cerebral imaging in the diagnosis of chronic headaches," Archives of Internal Medicine, 1992, 152: 2457-2462.

Vernon, Howard, "Spinal manipulation and headaches of cervical origin: A review of the literature and presentation of cases," Journal of Manual Medicine, 1991, 6 (2): 73-79.

Baker, Barbara, "Manipulation beats acetaminophen for neck pain," Family Practice News, June 1, 1996: 14.

Boline, P.D., et al, "Spinal manipulation vs. Amitryptyline for the treatment of chronic tension-type headaches: A randomized clinical trial," Journal of Manipulation and Physiological Therapeutics, 1995, 18: 148-154. Also:

Boline, P.D., et al., "Abstract No. 90-30-1," Proceedings of the 1993 International Conference on Spinal Manipulation, Foundation for Chiropractic Education and Research, Arlington, VA. (paper submitted for publication).

Whittingham, W., Ellis, W.B., Molyneux, T.P., "The effect of manipulation (toggle recoil technique) for headaches with upper cervical joint dysfunction: A pilot study," Journal of Manipulation and Physiological Therapeutics, July/August, 1994, 17 (6): 369-375.

Parker, G.B., et al, "Why does migraine improve with a clinical trial? Further results from a trial of cervical manipulation for migraine," Australian Journal of Medicine, 1980, 10: 192-198.

Martelletti, P., LaTour, D., et al, "Spectrum of pathophysiological disorders in cervicogenic headache and its therapeutic indications," Journal of the Neuromusculoskeletal System, 1995, 3 (4): 182-187.

Lewit, Karel. "Manuelle Therapie," J.A. Barth, Leipzig, 1973, chapter 2.7, 50-54.

Coulter, I.D., et al, "The appropriateness of manipulation and mobilization of the cervical spine," RAND, 1996.

Dabbs, V., Lauretti, W.J., "A risk assessment of cervical manipulation vs. NSAIDs for the treatment of neck pain," Journal of Manipulation and Physiological Therapeutics, 1995, 18 (8): 530-536.

Braly, James, "Dr. Braly's Food Allergy & Nutrition Revolution," Keats Publishing, 1992, 380.

Egger, J., et al, "Is migraine food allergy?: A double-blind controlled trial of oligoantigenic diet treatment," Lancet, 1983, 2: 865-869.

Lipton, R., et al, "Aspartame as a dietary trigger of headache," Headache, 1989, 29: 90-92.

Murphy, J.J., et al, "Randomized double-blind placebo-controlled trial of feverfew in migraine prevention," Lancet,1988, ii:189-192.

Thys-Jacobs, Susan, "Vitamin D and calcium in menstrual migraine," Headache, October 1991, 34 (9): 544-546.

Gallai, Virgilio, et al, "Magnesium content of mononuclear blood cells in migraine patients," Headache, March, 1994, 34:160-165.

Heartburn, esophageal reflux and hiatal hernia

Maxton, D.G., et al, "Controlled trial of pyrogastrone and cimetidine in the treatment of reflex esophagitis," Gut, 1990, 31 (3): 351-354.

Hogan, W.J., et al, "Ethanol induced acute esophageal sphincter motor dysfunction," Journal of Applied Physiology, 1972, 32: 755-760.

Thomas, F.B., et al, "Inhibitory effect of coffee on lower esophageal sphincter pressure," Gastroenterology, 1980, 79 (6): 1262-1266.

Price, S.F., et al, "Food sensitivity in reflux esophagitis," Gastroenterology, 1978, 75 (2): 240-243.

Ippoliti, A.F., et al, "The effect of various forms of milk on gastric acid secretion," Annals of Internal Medicine, 1976, 84: 286-289.

Castell, D.O., "Diet and the lower esophageal sphincter," American Journal of Clinical Nutrition, 1975, 28: 1296-1298.

Burkitt, Denis P., James, P.A., "Low-residue diets and hiatus hernia," Lancet, 1973, 2:128.

High blood pressure

Whitaker, Julian, "Dr. Whitaker's Guide to Natural Healing," Prima Publishing, Rocklin CA, 1995: 271.

Helgeland, A., "Treatment of mild hypertension: A five-year controlled drug trial: The Oslo Study," American Journal of Medicine, 1980, 69: 725-32.

Fries, E.D., "Rationale against the drug treatment of marginal diastolic systemic hypertension," American

Journal of Cardiology, 1990, 66: 368-71.

Grossman, Ehud, Messerli, Franz H., "High Blood Pressure: A Side Effect of Drugs, Poisons, and Food," Archives of Internal Medicine, March 13, 1995, 155: 450-460.

Raeburn, Paul, "Blood pressure drugs may boost heart attack risk," Philadelphia Inquirer, March 11, 1995, 1.

Brody, Jane, "Heart Attacks:Turmoil beneath the calm," New York Times, June 21, 1983; III, 1.

Kaplan, N.M., "Non-drug treatment of hypertension," Annals of Internal Medicine, 1985, 102: 359-373.

Casdorph, Richard, Walker, Morton, "Toxic Metal Syndrome: How metal poisonings can affect your brain," Avery Books, Garden City Park, NY., 1995, 279-304.

Glauser, S.C., et al, "Blood cadmium levels in normotensive and untreated hypertensive humans," Lancet, 1976, 1: 717-718.

Harlan, W.R., et al, "Blood lead and blood pressure: Relationship in the adolescent and adult US population," Journal of the American Medical Association, 1985, 253 (4): 530-534.

Rouse, I.L., et al, "Vegetarian diet, blood pressure and cardiovascular risk," Austalian/ New Zealand Journal of Medicine, 1984, 14 (4): 439-443.

Appel, Lawrence, et al, "A clinical trial of the effects of dietary patterns on blood pressure," New England Journal of Medicine, April 17, 1997, 336 (16): 1117-1124.

Pietinen, Pirjo, "Dietary fat and blood pressure," Annals of Medicine, 1994, 26: 465-468.

Knapp, Howard R., "Fatty acids and hypertension," World Review of Nutrition and Diet, 1994, 76: 9-14.

Swain, Randall, and Kaplan, Barbara, "Vitamins as therapies in the 1990s," Journal of the American Board of Family Practice, May-June 1995, 8 (3): 206-216.

Tse, W. Y., et al, "Antioxidant status in controlled and uncontrolled hypertension and its relationship to endothelial damage," Journal of Human Hypertension, 1994;8:843-849.

Hamet, Pavel, et al, "The evaluation of the scientific evidence for a relationship between calcium and hypertension," The Journal of Nutrition, 1995,125: 311S-400S.

"Magnesium: The forgotten nutrient," The Nutrition Report, February 1995: 7.

Elin, R., "Magnesium: The 5th but forgotten electrolyte," American Journal of Clinical Pathology, 1994,102 (5): 616-622.

Wirell, M., et al, "Magnesium lowers blood pressure," The Nutrition Report, October 1994;77.

"Nutritional dose of magnesium in hypertensive patients on beta blockers lowers systolic blood pressure: A double-blind, cross-over study," Journal of Internal Medicine, August 1994, 236:189-195.

Whelton, Paul K., et al, "The effect of potassium supplementation in persons with a high normal blood pressure: Results from phase I of the trials of hypertension prevention (TOHP)," Annals of Epidemiology, 1995, 5: 85-95.

Rashid, A., Khan, A.A., "The mechanism of hypotensive effect of garlic extract," Journal of the Pakistan Medical Association, 1985, 35: 357.

Dubey, M.P., et al, "Pharmacological studies on coleonol, a hypotensive diterpene from Coleus forskohlii," Journal of Ethnopharmacology, 1981 (3): 1-13.

Yamagami, T., et al, "Bioenergetics in clinical medicine. Studies on coenzyme Q10 and essential hypertension," Res Commun Chem Pathol Pharmacol, 1975, 11: 273. Langsjoen, Peter, Molecular Aspects of Medicine, 1994, 15 (supplement).

Schneider, R.H., Staggers, F., et al., "A randomized controlled trial of stress reduction for hypertension in older African Americans," Hypertension, November 1995, 26: 820-827.

Saito, I., Ito, K., et al, "Hypothyroidism as a cause of hypertension," Hypertension, 1983, 5: 112.

Yates, R.G., et al. "Effects of chiropractic treatment on blood pressure and anxiety: A randomized, controlled trial," Journal of Manipulation and Physiological Therapeutics, December 1988, 11 (6): 484-488.

Plaugher, G., Bachman, T.R., "Chiropractic management of a hypertensive patient: A case study," Journal of Manipulation and Physiological Therapeutics, 1993.

Goodman, R., "Hypertension and the atlas subluxation complex," Chiropractic Research and Clinical Investigation, July 1992, 8 (2): 30-32.

McKnight, M.E., DeBoer, K.F., "Preliminary study of blood pressure changes in normotensive subjects undergoing chiropractic care," Journal of Manipulation and Physiological Therapeutics, 1988, 11: 261-266.

Mootz, R., "Conservative management of patients with mild hypertension," Topics in Clinical Chiropractic, March 1995, 2 (1): 37-44.

Hypoglycemia

Challem, Jack, "Paleolithic nutrition: Your future is in your dietary past," Nutrition Science News, April 1997: 186-187, quoting Eaton, S.B., Eaton III, S.B., et al, "An evolutionary perspective enhances understanding of human nutritional requirements," Journal of Nutrition, June 1996, 126: 1732-40.

Buehler, M.S, "Relative hypoglycemia: a clinical review of 350 cases," Lancet, July 1962: 289.

Zucker, Martin, "Food and mood — There's no mistaking the connection," Let's Live Magazine, December 1988, 12.

Schoenthaler, Stephen, "Diet and crime: An empirical examination of the value of nutrition in the control and treatment of incarcerated juvenile offenders," International Journal of Biosocial Research, 1983, 4: 25-39.

Hudspeth, W.J., Peterson, L.W., Soli, D.E., Trimbel, B.A., "Neurobiology of the hypoglycemia syndrome," Journal of Holistic Medicine, 1981, 3 (1): 60.

Anthony, D., et al, "Personality disorder and reactive hypoglycemia: a quantitative study," Diabetes, 1973, 22: 664.

Anderson, J.W., Gustafson, N.J., "Dietary fiber in disease prevention and treatment," Comparative Therapies, 1987, 13 (1): 43-53.

Shansky, A., "Vitamin B3 in the alleviation of hypoglycemia," Drug Cosmetic Industry, 1981, 129 (4): 68.

Breneman, J.C., "Basics of Food Allergy," Charles C. Thomas, Springfield, IL, 1978.

Hypothyroidism

Barnes, Broda O., Galton, Lawrence, "Hypothyroidism: The Unsuspected Illness," Harper and Row, New York, 1976.

Langer, Stephen E., "The reason behind weight gain, fatigue, muscle pain, depression, food allergies, infections..." Alternative Medicine Digest, January 1997, 16: 52-56.

Wiersinga, W.M., "Subclinical hypothyroidism and hyperthyroidism: Prevalence in clinical relevance," Netherlands Journal of Medicine, 1995, 46: 197-204.

Sawin, Clark T., "Subclinical hypothyroidism in older persons," Clinics in Geriatric Medicine, May 1995, 11 (2): 231-238.

Bastenie, P.A., et al, "Preclinical hypothyroidism: A risk factor for coronary heart disease," Lancet, 1971, 1: 203.

Schnert, Keith, Croft, Arthur, "Basal metabolic temperature vs. laboratory assessment in 'posttraumatic hypothyroidism," Journal of Manipulation and Physiological Therapeutics, 1996, 19 (1): 6-12.

Male sexual dysfunction

LeBan, M.M., et al, "Sexual impotence in men having low back syndrome," Archives Physical Medicine & Rehabilitation, November 1966; 715-723.

Shibata, S., et al, "Chemistry and pharmacology of Panax," Econ Med Plant Research, 1985, 1:217-284.

Sikora, R., et al, "Ginkgo biloba extract in the therapy of erectile dysfunction," Journal of Urology. 1989, 141:188A.

Reid, K., et al, "Double blind trial of yohimbine in treatment of psychogenic impotence," Lancet, 1987, ii: 421-423.

Susset, J.G., et al, "Effect of yohimbine hydrochloride on erectile impotence: A double-blind study," Journal of Urology, 1989, 141 (6):1360-1363.

NIH Consensus Conference Panel on Impotence. Journal of the American Medical Association, 1993, 270: 83-90.

Memory Problems — From Everyday mental malfunction to Alzheimer's Disease

Senility and pharmaceutical drugs, Mayo Clinic Proceedings, 1995, 69: 1137-1145.

Speck, Carl E., et al, "History of depression as a risk factor for Alzheimer's disease," Epidemiology, July 1995: 366-369.

Tedd Koren, "Spinal patterns as predictors of personality profiles: a pilot study," International Journal of Psychosomatics, 1992, 39: 10-17.

Thomas, M.D., Wood, J., "Upper cervical adjustments may improve mental function," Journal of Manual Medicine, 1992, 6: 215-216

Potthoff, S., Penwell, B., et al, "Panic attacks and the chiropractic adjustment: a case report," Journal of Chiropractic, December 1993, 30: 26-28.

Zhang, C., Wang, Y., et al, "Study on cervical visual disturbances and its manipulative treatment," Journal of Traditional Chinese Medicine, 1984: 205-210

Gorman, R.F., and Milne, E., "Chiropractic medicine for rejuvenation of the mind," Academy of Chiropractic Medicine, Darwin, 1983 (Privately published). Two medical doctors interested in chiropractic report on a wide range of physical and psychological conditions reponding to chiropractic care. They conclude that many people are functioning with diminished mental potential or are disabled by "mental illness which has a simple physical cause" — a restriction in blood flow to the brain due to vertebral misalignment that creates stress on the vertebral arteries. (Quoted in Tedd Koren's "Chiropractic and Spinal Research," spring 1995, Koren Publications).

Terrett, A.G.J., "Cerebral dysfunction: A theory to explain some effects of chiropractic manipulation," Journal of Chiropractic Technique, 1993, 5: 168-173. Also in letters section, same journal, August 1994.

Terrett, A.G.J., "The cerebral dysfunction theory," chapter in "Foundations of Chiropractic Subluxations.

Rasmusson, D.X., et al, "Head injury as a risk factor in Alzheimer's disease," Brain Injury, 1995, 9 (3):213-219.

Gurwitz, M.D., "Unconventional medicine in Alzheimer's disease," The Journal of American Geriatrics Society, 1995, 43: 829-830.

"Iron, B6 and Co-enzyme Q10 in Alzheimer's," The Nutrition Report, October 1994, 12 (10): 75.

"Vitamin B12 and Alzheimer's disease," The Nutrition Report, October 1994, 12 (10): 75.

Canty, David J., "Lecithin and choline in human health and disease," Nutrition Reviews, October 1994, 52 (10): 327-339.
Lietha, Roman, Zimmermann, Michael, "Neuropsychiatric disorders associated with folate deficiency in the presence of elevated serum and erythrocyte folate: A preliminary report," Journal of Nutritional Medicine, 1994, 4: 441-447.

Urakami, K., et al, "Cu, Zn, Superoxide Dismutase in patients with dementia of the Alzheimer type," Acta Neurol Scand, 1995, 91:165-168.

Frolich, L., Riederer, P., "Free radical mechanisms in dementia of the Alzheimer's type and the potential for antioxidative treatment," Drug Research, 1995, 45 (1) 3A: 443-446.

Sano, Mary, et al, "A controlled trial of Selegiline, alpha-tocopherol, or both as treatment for Alzheimer's disease," New England Journal of Medicine, April 24, 1997, 336 (17): 1216-1222)

Pettegrew, J.W., et al, "Clinical and neurochemical effects of Acetyl-l-carnitine in Alzheimer's disease," Neurobiology of Aging, 1995,16 (1): 1-4.

Zapatero, M.D., et al, "Serum aluminum levels in Alzheimer's disease and other senile dementias," Biological Trace Element Research, 1995, 47: 235-240.

Bleecker, Margit L., "Invited commentary: Solvent exposure as a risk factor for Alzheimer's disease: A multiple insult hypothesis," American Journal of Epidemiology, 1995,141 (11):1072-1074.

Menopause

Huppert, L.C., "Hormonal replacement therapy: benefits, risks, doses," Medical Clinics of North America, 1987, 71:23-39.

Zhy, D.P.Q., "Dong quai," Am Journal of Chinese Medicine, 1987, 15 (3-4):117-125.

Costello, C.H., Lynn, E.V., "Estrogenic substances from plants: I. Glycyrrhiza," Journal of American Pharm Soc, 1950, 39: 177-180.

Kumagai, A, et al, "Effect of glycyrrhizin on estrogen action," Endocrinol Japon, 1967, 14: 34-38.

Finkler, R.S., "The effect of vitamin E in the menopause," J Clin Endocrinol Metab, 1949, 9: 89-94.

Barnard, Neal, "Eat Right, Live Longer," Harmony Books, New York, 1995, 93-94.

Zhou, James, "Menopause relief from Chinese herbs," Health Supplement Retailer, March 1997: 42.)

Bullock, Carole, "Soybeans: An estrogen replacement alternative?" Family Practice News, April 6, 1995:11.

The Burke Study on soy reported in the Los Angeles Times, November 12, 1996.

Clarkson, Thomas B., et al, "Estrogenic soybean, isoflavones, and chronic disease risk and benefits," Trends in Endocrinology and Metabolism, 1995, 6:11-16.

Reitz, R. "Menopause: A Positive Approach." New York, Penguin Books, 1979.

Taylor, A., et al, "Zinc metabolism in post-menopausal women receiving hormone replacement therapy," Trace Elements and Electrolytes, 1995, 12 (1):47-51.

"Dehydroepiandrosterone (DHEA) and Aging," international conference of the New York Academy of Sciences, June 17-19, 1995, Annals of the New York Academy of Sciences, 1995, 774.

Multiple sclerosis (MS)

Sandyk, Reuven, "Chronic relapsing multiple sclerosis: A case of rapid recovery by application of weak electromagnetic fields," International Journal of Neuroscience, 1995, 82: 223-242.

Goldberg, P., et al, "Multiple sclerosis: Decrease relapse rate through dietary supplementation with calcium, magnesium and vitamin D," Medical Hypotheses, 1986, 21 (2):193-200.

Swank, R.L., Dugan, B.B., "Effect of low saturated fat diet in early and late cases of multiple sclerosis," Lancet, 1990, 336: 37-39.

Cendrowski, W., "Multiple sclerosis and Max EPA," British Journal of Clinical Practice, 1986, 40: 365-367.

Wolfgram, F., et al, "Serum linoleic acid in multiple sclerosis," Neurology, 1975, 25 (8): 786-788.

Agranoff, B., Goldberg, D., "Diet and the geographical distribution of multiple sclerosis," Lancet, 1974, 2:1061-1066.

Craelius, W., "Comparative epidemiology of multiple sclerosis and dental caries," Journal of Epidemiol Comm Health, 1972, 32:155-165.

Rio, J., et al. "Serum homocysteine levels and multiple sclerosis," Archives of Neurology, December 1994, 51:1181.

A discussion of neuromuscular conditions is contained in Tedd Koren's "Chiropractic and Spinal Research, Spring 1995 edition, 60.

Stude, D.E., et al., "Clinical presentation of the patient with multiple sclerosis and response to manual chiropractic adjustive therapies," Journal of Manipulative and Physiological Therapeutics, 1993, 16: 595-600.

Roberts, J.W., et al, "Multiple sclerosis and early diagnosis: A literature review," Journal of Chiropractic, June 1990, 27: 75-77.

Kirby, S.L., "A case study: the effects of chiropractic on multiple sclerosis," Chiropractic Research Journal, 1994; 3:7-12.

Weber, Marion, and Masarsky, Charles, editors of "Neurological Fitness," January 1995, 4 (2): 1.

Osteoporosis

Barnard, Neal, "Eat Right, Live Longer," Harmony Books, New York, 1995, p. 161.

"The Problem with Protein," Nutrition Action Healthletter, June 1993, p. 7.

Attwood, Charles, "Dr. Attwood's Low-Fat Prescription for Kids," Penguin Books, New York, 1995, 62-69.

Abelow, B. J., et al, "Cross-cultural association between dietary animal protein and hip fracture: a hypothesis," Calcified Tissue International, 1992, 50: 14-18.

Brattstrom LE, et al, "Folic acid responsive postmenopausal homocysteinemia," Metabol, 1985, 34:1073-1077.

Neilsen FH, et al, "Effect of dietary boron on mineral, estrogen, and testosterone metabolism in postmenopausal women," FASEB, 1987, 1: 394-397.

Hunt, I.F., et al, "Bone mineral content in postmenopausal women: Comparison of omnivores and vegetarians," American Journal of Clinical Nutrition, 1989, 50: 517-523.

Spencer, H., Kramer, L., "Osteoporosis: Calcium, fluoride, and aluminum interactions," Journal of the American College of Nutrition, 1985, 4 (1):121-128.

Recker, R.R., "Calcium absorption and achlorhydria," New England Journal of Medicine, 1985, 313 (2):70-73.

Chilibeck, Philip D., et al, "Exercise and bone mineral density," Sports Medicine, 1995, 19 (2):103-122.

Strause, L., et al, "Calcium, trace minerals minimize bone loss," The Nutrition Report, October 1994: 78. "Spinal bone loss in postmenopausal women supplemented with calcium and trace minerals," Journal of Nutrition, July 1994, 124: 1060-1064.

Kannus, Pekka, "Effect of starting age of physical activity on bone mass in the dominate arm of tennis and squash players," Annals of Internal Medicine, July 1, 1995, 123: 27-31.

Wimalawansa, Sunil J., et al, "Combined therapy with estrogen and etidronate has an additive effect on bone mineral density in the hip and vertebra: Four-year randomized study," The American Journal of Medicine, July 1995, 99: 36-42.

Nguyen, T.V., et al, "Lifestyle factors and bone density in the elderly: Implications for osteoporosis prevention," Journal of Bone and Mineral Research, 1994, 9 (9):1339-1345.

Binkley, N.C., Suttie, J.W., "Vitamin K nutrition and osteoporosis," Journal of Nutrition, 1995, 125: 1812-1821.

Bell, Norman, "Vitamin D metabolism, aging and bone loss," Journal of Clinical Endocrinology and Metabolism, 1995, 80 (4): 1051.

Garton, Mark, et al, "Bone mineral density in premenopausal women taking L-thyroxine replacement therapy," Clinical Endocrinology, 1994, 41: 747-755.

Premenstrual syndrome (PMS)

Goei, G.S., et al, "Dietary patterns of patients with premenstrual tension," Journal of Applied Nutrition, 1982, 34 (1): 4-11.

Mira, M., et al, "Vitamin and trace element status in premenstrual syndrome," American Journal of Clinical Nutrition, 1988, 47 (4): 636-641.

Wurtman, J.J., et al, "Effect of nutrient intake on premenstrual depression," American Journal of Obstetrics and Gynecology, 1989, 161 (5):1228-1234.

Chuong, C. James, Dawson, Earl B., "Magnesium levels in premenstrual syndrome," Nutrition Research, 1994,14 (11): 1623-1624.

Thys-Jacobs, Susan, "Vitamin D and calcium in menstrual migraine," Headache, October 1994, 34 (9); 544-546.

Brush, M.G., et al, "Abnormal essential fatty acid levels in plasma of women with premenstrual syndrome," American Journal of Obstetrics and Gynecology, 1984, 150 (4): 363-366.

London, R.S., et al, "The effect of alpha-tocopherol on premenstrual symptomatology: A double-blind study," Journal of the American College of Nutrition, 1983, 2 (2): 115-122.

Baker, Elizabeth R., et al, "Efficacy of progesterone vaginal suppositories in alleviation of nervous symptoms in patients with premenstrual syndrome," Journal of Assisted Reproduction and Genetics, 1995, 12 (3): 205-209.

Kokjohn, D., Schmid, D.M., et al, "The effect of spinal manipulation on pain and prostaglandin levels in women with primary dysmenorrhea," Journal of Manipulative and Physiological Therapeutics, June 1992, 15 (5): 279-285.

Whittier, M.A., "Chiropractic approach to premenstrual syndrome (PMS)," Journal of Chiropractic Research and Clinical Investigation, 1992, 8: 26-29.

Liebl, N.A., Butler, N.M., "A chiropractic approach to the treatment of dysmenorrhea," Journal of Manipulative and Physiological Therapeutics, 1990, 13: 101-106.

Thomason, P.R., Fisher, B.L., et al, "Effectiveness of spinal manipulative therapy in treatment of primary dysmenorrhea: A pilot study," Journal of Manipulative and Physiological Therapeutics, 1979, 2: 140-145.

Dvorak, N., "Theoretical considerations to the clinic and therapy of spinal disturbances in gynecology," Manuelle Medizin, 1973, vol. 1.

Prostate

Jaroff, Leon, "The Man's Cancer," Time Magazine, April 1, 1996, 58-65.

Hald, T., "Review of current treatment of benign prostatic hyperplasia," European Urology, 1994, 25 (supplement 1): 15-19.

Ball, A.J., Feneley, R.C., et al, "The natural history of untreated prostatism," British Journal of Urology, 1981, 53: 613-616.

Carani, C., et al, "Urological and sexual evaluation of treatment of benign prostatic disease using Pygeum africanum at high doses," Arch Ital Urol Nefrol Androl, 1991, 63 (3): 341-345.

"Commission E Monograph on saw palmetto," January 17, 1991, translated by the American Botanical Council (available on the ABC Internet website: www.herbalgram.org/

Braeckman, Johan, "The extract of Serenoa repens in the treatment of benign prostatic hyperplasia: A multicenter open study," Current Therapeutic Research, July 1994, 55 (7): 776-785.

Berges, R.R., et al, "Randomized, placebo-controlled, double-blind clinical trial of b-sitosterol in patients with benign prostatic hyperplasia," The Lancet, June 17, 1995, 345: 1529-1532.

Barnard, Neal, "Eat Right, Live Longer," (Harmony Books, New York, 1995), 120.

Gittleman, Ann Louise, "Super Nutrition For Men," (M. Evans and Company, New York, 1996), 59.

Irving M. Bush and associates, "Zinc and the prostate," Cook County Hospital, Chicago. Presented at the annual meeting of the American Medical Association, Chicago, 1974.

Dumrau, F., "Benign prostatic hyperplasia: Amino acid therapy for symptomatic relief," American Journal of Geriatrics, 1962, 10: 426-430.

Hart, J.P., Cooper, W.L., "Vitamin F in the treatment of prostatic hyperplasia." Report Number 1, Lee

Foundation for Nutritional Research, Milwaukee, WI., 1941.

Rheumatoid arthritis

Fries, J.F., Miller, S.R., et al, "Toward an epidemiology of gastropathy associated with nonsteroidal anti-inflammatory drug use," Gastroenterology, 1989, 96: 647-655.

Scott, D.L., Coulton, B.L., et al, "Long-term outcome of treating rheumatoid arthritis: Results after 20 years," Lancet, 1989: 1108-1111.

Bjarnason, I., et al, "Intestinal permeability and inflammation in rheumatoid arthritis: Effects of non-steroidal anti-inflammatory drugs," Lancet, 1984, 2:1171-1174.

Hartung, E.F., Steinbrocker, O., "Gastric acidity in chronic arthritis," Annals of Internal Medicine, 1935, 9:252-257.

Skoldstam L., "Fasting and vegan diet in rheumatoid arthritis," Scandinavian Journal of Rheumatology, 1987, 15 (2): 219-21.
Hazenberg, M.P., "Intestinal flora, bacteria and arthritis: Why the joint?" Scandinavian Journal of Rheumatology, 1995, 24 (supplement 101): 207-211.

Prudden, J.F., Balassa, L.L., "The biological activity of bovine cartilage preparations," Semin Arthritis Rheum, 1974, 3 (4): 287-321.

Bingham, Robert, et al, "Yucca plant saponin in the management of arthritis," Journal of Applied Nutrition, 1975, 27: 45-50.

Darlington, L.G., et al, "Clinical review of dietary therapy for rheumatoid arthritis," British Journal of Rheumatology, 1993, 32: 507-514.

Geusens, Piet, et al, "Long-term effect of omega-3 fatty acid supplementation in active rheumatoid arthritis: A 12-month, double-blind, controlled study," Arthritis and Rheumatism, June 1994, 37 (6): 824-829.

Kremer, J.M., et al, "Effects of high-dose fish oil on rheumatoid arthritis after stopping non-steroidal anti-inflammatory drugs. Clinical and immune correlates," Arthritis and Rheumatism, 1995, 38: 1107-1114.

Oldroyd, K.G., Dawes, P.T., "Clinically significant vitamin C deficiency in rheumatoid arthritis," British Journal of Rheumatology, 1985, 24: 362-363.

Barton-Wright, E.C., and Elliott, W.A., "The pantothenic acid metabolism of rheumatoid arthritis," Lancet, 1963, 2: 862-863.

Sinus infections

Dohlman, A.W., et al, "Subacute sinusitis: are antimicrobials necessary?" Journal of Allergic Clinical Immunology, 1993, 91: 1015-1023.

Rapp, Doris, "Is This Your Child's World: How You Can Fix the Schools and Homes that are Making Your Children Sick," Bantam Books, New York, 1996, 154.

Guttman, G., "The atlas fixation syndrome in the baby and infant," Manuelle Medizin, 1987,25: 5-10.

Vanbreda, Wendy M., and Juan M., "A Comparative Study of the Health Status of Children Raised under the healthcare models of chiropractic and allopathic Medicine," Journal of Chiropractic Research, Summer 1989.

Ryan, R.E., "A double-blind clinical evaluation of bromelains in the treatment of acute sinusitis," Headache, 1967, 7 (1):13-17.

Taub, S.J., "The use of bromelains in sinusitis: A double blind clinical evaluation," Eye Ear Nose Throat Mon, 1967, 46 (3): 361-362.

Pelikan, Z., "Nasal response to food ingestion challenge," Archives Otolaryngology Head Neck Surg, 1988,114 (5): 525-530.

Ogle, K.A., Bullock, J.D., "Children with allergic rhinitis and/or bronchial asthma treated with elimination diet: A five year follow up," Annals of Allergy, 1980, 44: 273-278.

Gillespie, B.R., Barnes, J.F., "Diagnosis and treatment of TMJ, head, neck and asthmatic symptoms in children," Journal of Craniomandibular Practice, October 1990, 8 (4).

Skin problems

Strosser, A.V., Nelson, L.S., "Synthetic vitamin A in the treatment of eczema in children," Annals of Allergy, 1952, 10:703-704.

Steinman, Haris A., et al, "The precipitation of symptoms by common foods in children with atopic dermatitis," Allergy Proceedings, July-August 1994, 15 (4): 203-210.

Morren, Marie-Anne, et al, "Atopic dermatitis: Triggering factors," Journal of the American Academy of Dermatology, September 1994, 31 (3, Part I): 467-473.

Stress and your adrenal glands

Ershoff, B.H., "Effects of vitamin A malnutriture on resistance to stress," Proceedings of Society Exp Biol Med, 1952,79: 580.

Wilmot, C.A., et al, "Ascorbic acid inhibits isolation-induced fighting in mice," Fed Proc, 1983, 42: 1160.

Van Rij, J.T., et al, "Zinc as an integral component of the metabolic response to trauma," Surg Gynecol Obstet, 1981,153: 677.

Baschetti, Riccardo, "Chronic fatigue syndrome and licorice," New Zealand Medical Journal, April 26, 1995; 157.

Tinnitus

Flynn, Rebecca, "Your Guide to Standardized Herbal Products," One World Press, Prescott, AZ, 1995, 30.

Yanick, Paul Jr., "Holistic applications to ear disorders," Journal of the International Academy of Preventive Medicine, 1983: 24-27.

Weille, F.R., "Hypoglycemia in Meniere's disease," Arch Otolaryngol, 1968, 87:129.

Lhole, E., "The influence of chronic vitamin A deficiency on human and animal ears," Arch Otolaryngol, 1982, 234: 167-173.

Lobel, M.J., "Is hearing loss due to nutritional deficiency?" Arch Otolaryngol, May, 1951: 515-526.

Brookes, G.B., "Vitamin D deficiency — A new cause of cochlear deafness," Journal of Laryngol Otol, 1983, 97 (5): 405-420.

Sun, A.H., et al, "Iron deficiency and hearing loss," ORL, 1987, 49: 118-122.

Debartolo, H.M. Jr., "Zinc and diet for tinnitus," American Journal of Otol, 1989, 10 (3): 256.

Shambaugh, G.E. Jr., "Zinc for tinnitus, imbalance and hearing loss in the elderly," American Journal of Otol , 1986, 7 (6): 476-477.

Duke, W.W., "Meniere's syndrome caused by allergy," Journal of the American Medical Association, 1923, 81: 2179.

Vision

Raymond, L.F., "Allergy and chronic simple glaucoma," Annals of Allergy, 1964, 22:146-150.

Asregadoo, E.R., "Blood levels of thiamine and ascorbic acid in chronic open angle glaucoma," Annals of Ophthalmology, 1979, 11 (7):1095-1100.

Evans, S.C., "Ophthalmic nutrition and prevention of eye disorder and blindness," Nutritional Metabolism, 1977, 21(supplement 1): 268-72.

Skalka H.W, Prchal, J.T., "Cataracts and riboflavin deficiency." American Journal of Clinical Nutrition, 1981, 34 (5): 861-863.
Jacques, P.T., Chylack, L.T. Jr., "Epidemiological evidence of a role for the antioxidant vitamins and caro-tenoids in cataract prevention," American Journal of Clinical Nutrition, 1991, 53:352S-355S.

Robertson, J..M., et al, "Vitamin E intake and risk of cataracts in humans," Annals of the New York Academy of Sciences, 1989, 570: 372-382.

Benninger, Jon, "Understanding bilberry," Health Supplement Retailer, March 1997, 54.

Zhang, C., Wang, Y., et al. "Study on cervical visual disturbances and its manipulative treatment," Journal of Traditional Chinese Medicine, 1984, 4: 205-210.

Briggs, L., Boone, W.R., "Effects of a chiropractic adjustment on changes in pupillary diameter: A model for evaluating somatovisceral response," Journal of Manipulative Physiological Therapies, 1988, 11 (3): 181-189.

Gilman, G., Bergstrand, J., "Visual recovery following chiropractic intervention," Journal of Behavioral Optometry, 1990, 1: 73-74.

Gorman, R. F., "An observer's view of the treatment of visual perception defect by spinal manipulation: A survey of 16 patients," Sydney, Australia, 1991 (Privately Published).

Stevens, D. and Gorman, R.F., "The prospective treatment of visual perception deficit by chiropractic spinal manipulation: A report on two juvenile patients," Chiropractic Journal of Australia, 1996, 26: 82-86.

Terrett, A. G. J., "Cerebral dysfunction: A theory to explain some effects of chiropractic manipulation," Chiropractic Technique, August 1994, 6 (3).

Yeast infections

Rippon, John W., "Medical Mycology," (second edition), W.B. Saunders, Philsadelphia, 1982.

Crook, William G., "The Yeast Connection: A Medical Breakthrough," Professional Books, 681 Skyline Drive, Jackson, TN 38301 (901-423-5400), 1988.

Brodsky, writing in foreword of "The Yeast Connection."

Crook, William G., "They say myth, I say fact," letter, Nutrition Insights (Let's Live Magazine), May 1997, 38.

Truss, C.O., "The role of candida albicans in human illness," Journal of Orthomolecular Psychiatry, 1981,10: 228-238.

Wolf, C., "Multiple chemical sensitivities: Is there a scientific basis?," International Archives of Occupational and Environmental Health, 1994, 66: 213-216.

Holti, G., "Candida allergy," in Winner and Hurley, editors, "Symposium on Candida Infections," Livingstone Publishers, Edinburgh, 1966.

Rippon, quoted in Crook, 73.

"Lactobacillus feeding alters human colonic bacterial enzyme activities," Nutrition Reviews, 1984, 42 (11): 374-376.

Bohler, K., et al, "Zinc levels of serum and cervicovaginal secretion in recurrent vulvovaginal candidiasis," Genitourin Medi, 1994, 70: 308-310.

Mikhail, Magdy S., et al, "Decreased beta carotene levels in exfoliated vaginal epithelial cells in women with vaginal candidiasis," American Journal of Reproductive Immunology, 1994, 32: 221-225.

Roesler, Joachim, et al, "Application of purified polysaccharides from cell cultures of the plant echinacea purpurea to mice; Mediates protection against systemic infections with Listeria Monocytogenes and Candida Albicans," International Journal of Immunopharmacology, 1991,13 (1): 27-37.

Stiles, J.C., "The inhibition of candida albicans by oregano," Journal of Applied Nutrition, 1995, 47 (4): 96-102.

Adetumbi, M.A., and Lau, B.H., "Allium sativum (garlic) — A natural antibiotic," Medical Hypotheses, 1983, 12: 227-237.

INDEX

ABOUT THE AUTHOR

Martin P. Gallagher, M.S., D.C., a chiropractic physician who specializes in clinical nutrition, has been in practice for more than 20 years. He received his undergraduate (B.A.) degree in psychology from Wheeling Jesuit College, his Masters degree (M.S.) in biology and nutrition from the University of Bridgeport, and his doctorate degree (D.C.) from Logan College of Chiropractic in St. Louis. Dr. Gallagher is a former faculty member in the Division of Clinical Services at Logan College, a current post-graduate faculty member at Logan College and the New York College of Chiropractic, a member of the American Chiropractic Association, the International Academy of Preventive Medicine, and the American Back Society. He has lectured internationally to chiropractors, medical doctors and osteopathic physicians. Dr. Gallagher and his wife, Charlotte Ciotti, D.C., are co-directors of Medical Wellness Associates, a multidisciplinary health facility staffed by 5 chiropractors, 2 medical doctors, 5 registered nurses, and 65 paraprofessionals. The Gallaghers reside near Pittsburgh with their son, Todd.